Imaging of Osteoarthritis

Guest Editor

ALI GUERMAZI, MD

RADIOLOGIC CLINICS
OF NORTH AMERICA

www.radiologic.theclinics.com

July 2009 • Volume 47 • Number 4

SAUNDERS an imprint of ELSEVIER, Inc.

W.B. SAUNDERS COMPANY
A Division of Elsevier Inc.

1600 John F. Kennedy Boulevard ● Suite 1800 ● Philadelphia, Pennsylvania 19103-2899

http://www.theclinics.com

RADIOLOGIC CLINICS OF NORTH AMERICA Volume 47, Number 4
July 2009 ISSN 0033-8389, ISBN 13: 978-1-4377-1403-6, ISBN 10: 1-4377-1403-X

Editor: Barton Dudlick
Developmental Editor: Theresa Collier

Radiologic Clinics of North America (ISSN 0033-8389) is published bimonthly in January, March, May, July, September, and November by Elsevier Inc., 360 Park Avenue South, New York, NY 10010-1710. Business and Editorial Offices: 1600 John F. Kennedy Boulevard., Suite 1800, Philadelphia, PA 19103-2899. Customer Service Office: 11830 Westline Industrial Drive, St. Louis, MO 63146. Periodicals postage paid at New York, NY and additional mailing offices. Subscription prices are USD 328 per year for US individuals, USD 487 per year for US institutions, USD 160 per year for US students and residents, USD 383 per year for Canadian individuals, USD 611 per year for Canadian institutions, USD 473 per year for international individuals, USD 611 per year for international institutions, and USD 230 per year for Canadian and foreign students/residents. To receive student and resident rate, orders must be accompanied by name of affiliated institution, date of term and the signature of program/residency coordinatior on institution letterhead. Orders will be billed at individual rate until proof of status is received. Foreign air speed delivery is included in all *Clinics* subscription prices. All prices are subject to change without notice. **POSTMASTER:** Send address changes to *Radiologic Clinics of North America*, Elsevier Journals Customer Service, 11830 Westline Industrial Drive, St. Louis, MO 63146. **Customer Service: 1-800-654-2452 (US and Canada). From outside of the United States and Canada, call 1-314-453-7041. Fax: 1-314-453-5170. E-mail: JournalsCustomerService-usa@elsevier.com (for print support) and JournalsOnlineSupport-usa@elsevier. com (for online support).**

Reprints. For copies of 100 or more of articles in this publication, please contact the Commercial Reprints Department, Elsevier Inc., 360 Park Avenue South, New York, New York 10010-1710. Tel.: (+1) 212-633-3812; Fax: (+1) 212-462-1935; E-mail: reprints@elsevier.com.

Radiologic Clinics of North America also published in Greek Paschalidis Medical Publications, Athens, Greece.

Radiologic Clinics of North America is covered in *MEDLINE/PubMed (Index Medicus), EMBASE/Excerpta Medica, Current Contents/Life Sciences, Current Contents/Clinical Medicine, RSNA Index to Imaging Literature, BIOSIS, Science Citation Index,* and *ISI/BIOMED.*

Contributors

GUEST EDITOR

ALI GUERMAZI, MD
Associate Professor of Radiology; Section Chief,
Musculoskeletal Imaging; and Director,
Quantitative Imaging Center (QIC), Department
of Radiology, Boston University School
of Medicine, Boston, Massachusetts

AUTHORS

BERND BITTERSOHL, MD
Department of Orthopedic Surgery, University
of Bern, Freiburgstrasse, Switzerland; and
Department of Orthopedic Surgery, University
of Düsseldorf, Duseldorf, Germany

ALAN BRETT, PhD
Optasia Medical, Manchester, United Kingdom

DEBORAH BURSTEIN, PhD
Associate Professor of Radiology and Health
Sciences and Technology, Department of
Radiology, Beth Israel Deaconess Medical Center,
Harvard Medical School, Boston, Massachusetts

**PHILIP G. CONAGHAN, MBBS, PhD, FRACP,
FRCP**
Professor, Section of Musculoskeletal Disease,
Leeds Institute of Molecular Medicine, University
of Leeds, Chapel Allerton Hospital, Chapeltown
Road, Leeds, United Kingdom

MICHEL D. CREMA, MD
Fellow in Musculoskeletal Radiology, Quantitative
Imaging Center, Department of Radiology, Boston
University School of Medicine, Boston,
Massachusetts

BERNARD DARDZINSKI, PhD
Senior Director of Imaging, Bone, Respiratory,
Immunology, and Endocrinology, Merck, Inc.,
West Point, Pennsylvania

JEAN-LUC DRAPÉ, MD, PhD
Professor and Chairman, Department of Radiology
B, Cochin Hospital, Paris Descartes University,
Paris, France

JEFF DURYEA, PhD
Brigham and Women's Hospital, Harvard Medical
School, Boston, Massachusetts

FELIX ECKSTEIN, MD
Institute of Anatomy and Musculoskeletal
Research, Paracelsus Medical University,
Salzburg, Austria; and Chondrometrics GmbH,
Ainring, Germany

MARTIN ENGLUND, MD, PhD
Musculoskeletal Sciences, Department of
Orthopedics, Clinical Sciences Lund, Lund
University Hospital, Lund, Sweden; and Clinical
Epidemiology Research and Training Unit, Boston
University School of Medicine, Boston,
Massachusetts

ANTOINE FEYDY, MD, PhD
Associate Professor, Department of Radiology B,
Cochin Hospital, Paris Descartes University, Paris,
France

MARTHA GRAY, PhD
J.W. Kieckhefer Professor of Medical and
Electrical Engineering, Massachusetts Institute of
Technology, Cambridge, Massachusetts

HENRI GUERINI, MD
Clinical Assistant Professor, Department of
Radiology B, Cochin Hospital, Paris Descartes
University, Paris, France

ALI GUERMAZI, MD
Associate Professor of Radiology; Section Chief,
Musculoskeletal Imaging; and Director,
Quantitative Imaging Center (QIC), Department of
Radiology, Boston University School of Medicine,
Boston, Massachusetts

DAVID J. HUNTER, MBBS, FRACP, PhD
Chief of Research, Division of Research, New
England Baptist Hospital, Boston, Massachusetts

HELEN I. KEEN, MBBS, FRACP
School of Medicine and Pharmacology, University
of Western Australia, Perth, Australia

YOUNG-JO KIM, MD, PhD
Department of Orthopedic Surgery, Children's
Hospital, Harvard Medical School, Boston,
Massachusetts

FRÉDÉRIC LECOUVET, MD, PhD
Department of Radiology, Cliniques Universitaires
Saint-Luc, Université Catholique de Louvain,
Brussels, Belgium

**MARIE-PIERRE HELLIO LE GRAVERAND, MD,
DSc, PhD**
Senior Director, Clinical Development and Medical
Affairs, Inflammation, Specialty Care Business
Unit, Pfizer Inc., New London, Connecticut

THOMAS M. LINK, MD
Professor of Radiology, Department of Radiology
and Biomedical Imaging, University of California at
San Francisco, San Francisco, California

STEFAN L. LOHMANDER, MD, PhD
Musculoskeletal Sciences, Department of
Orthopedics, Clinical Sciences Lund, Lund
University Hospital, Lund, Sweden

TALLAL C. MAMISCH, MD
Department of Orthopedic Surgery, University of
Bern, Freiburgstrasse, Switzerland; and
Department of Radiology, Sonnenhof Clinics,
Bern, Switzerland

MONICA D. MARRA, MD
Fellow in Musculoskeletal Radiology, Quantitative
Imaging Center, Department of Radiology, Boston
University School of Medicine, Boston,
Massachusetts

STEVE MAZZUCA, PhD
Indiana University School of Medicine,
Indianapolis, Indiana

GUSTAVO A. MERCIER, MD, PhD
Department of Radiology, Nuclear Medicine and
Molecular Imaging, Boston University Center,
Boston, Massachusetts

TIM MOSHER, MD
Professor of Radiology and Orthopaedics; Vice
Chair for Radiology Research; and Chief of
Musculoskeletal Imaging and MRI, Pennsylvania
State College of Medicine, The Milton S. Hershey
Medical Center, Hershey, Pennsylvania

PATRICK OMOUMI, MD
Department of Radiology, Cliniques Universitaires
Saint-Luc, Université Catholique de Louvain,
Brussels, Belgium; and Department of Radiology,
Centre Hospitalo-Universitaire de Tours, Tours,
France

ETIENNE PLUOT, MD
Fellow of Radiology, Department of Radiology B,
Cochin Hospital, Paris Descartes University,
Paris, France

FRANK W. ROEMER, MD
Associate Professor of Radiology; Co-Director,
Quantitative Imaging Center (QIC), Department of
Radiology, Boston University School of Medicine,
Boston, Massachusetts; Attending Radiologist
and Section Chief, MRI, Department of Radiology,
Klinikum Augsburg, Augsburg, Germany; and
Director of Research and Vice President
Musculoskeletal Radiology, Boston Imaging Core
Laboratory, LLC, Boston, Massachusetts

MARK SCHWEITZER, MD
Professor and Chair of Radiology, Department of
Diagnostic Imaging, The Ottawa Hospital, General
Campus, University of Ottawa, Ottawa, Canada

ADNAN SHEIKH, MD
Assistant Professor in Musculoskeletal Radiology,
Department of Diagnostic Imaging, The Ottawa
Hospital, General Campus, University of Ottawa,
Ottawa, Canada

KLAUS A. SIEBENROCK, MD, PhD
Department of Orthopedic Surgery, University
of Bern, Freiburgstrasse, Switzerland

PAOLO SIMONI, MD
Department of Radiology, Cliniques Universitaires
Saint-Luc, Université Catholique de Louvain,
Brussels, Belgium

BRUNO C. VANDE BERG, MD, PhD
Department of Radiology, Cliniques Universitaires
Saint-Luc, Université Catholique de Louvain,
Brussels, Belgium

STEFAN WERLEN, MD
Department of Radiology, Sonnenhof Clinics,
Bern, Switzerland

DAVID R. WILSON, DPhil
Associate Professor, Department of
Orthopaedics, University of British Columbia
and Vancouver Coastal Health Research
Institute, Vancouver, British Columbia,
Canada

CHRISTOPH ZILKENS, MD
Department of Orthopedic Surgery, University
of Düsseldorf, Duseldorf, Germany; and
Department of Orthopedic Surgery, Children's
Hospital, Harvard Medical School, Boston,
Massachusetts

Contents

This article highlights recent studies, particularly those with an emphasis on MR imaging, that are providing unique insights into the relation between structures identified on imaging and symptoms and disease genesis. It is becoming increasingly apparent that the subchondral bone, periosteum, periarticular ligaments, periarticular muscle spasm, synovium, and joint capsule are all richly innervated and are the likely source of nociception in osteoarthritis. It is also apparent that local tissue alterations in the bone and meniscus and alignment of the lower extremity are important in terms of disease genesis. This article represents the literature in that much of the focus and understanding is knee centric with less focus on the hip and hand.

Osteoarthritis is widely believed to result from local mechanical factors acting within the context of systemic susceptibility. This article delineates current understanding of the etiopathogenesis of osteoarthritis and more specifically examines the critical role of biomechanics in disease pathogenesis. There are several ways that mechanical forces across the joint can be measured, including many that rely heavily on imaging methods. These are described and methods to advance the field are proposed.

Accurate and highly reproducible measurements of the rate of progression of osteoarthritis is crucial to assessing structural change, and requires adherence to exacting standards of positioning, which include specifications for flexion and rotation of the joint, and angulation of the x-ray beam. The progression of osteoarthritis traditionally has been measured using radiographic joint space width (JSW). Over the past two decades, numerous knee radiographic protocols have been developed with various levels of complexity and performance as they relate to detecting JSW loss (ie, joint space narrowing). Semiautomated software has been developed to improve the accuracy of JSW measurement over manual methods. JSW measurements include minimum JSW, mean JSW or joint space area and JSW at fixed locations.

This article outlines the benefits of imaging osteoarthritis with ultrasonography and some of the limitations. Pathologic structures able to be identified in osteoarthritis with ultrasonography are reviewed, with a focus on the validity of the technique. Common ultrasonographic abnormalities seen in osteoarthritis in specific joint regions are discussed. Finally, future research agendas are considered. With improving technology, accessibility of ultrasonography, increasing evidence regarding the validity, and use of ultrasonography in osteoarthritis mean that ultrasonography is likely increasingly used in the clinical trial setting and routine clinical practice to aid the diagnosis and management of osteoarthritis.

CT arthrography and MR arthrography are accurate methods for the study of surface cartilage lesions and cartilage loss. They also provide information on subchondral bone and marrow changes, and ligaments and meniscal lesions that can be associated with osteoarthritis. Nuclear medicine also offers new insights in the assessment of the disease. This article discusses the strengths and limitations of CT arthrography and MR arthrography. It also highlights nuclear medicine methods that may be relevant to the study of osteoarthritis in research and clinical practice.

Whole-organ assessment of a joint with osteoarthritis (OA) requires tailored MR imaging hardware and imaging protocols to diagnose and monitor degenerative disease of the cartilage, menisci, bone marrow, ligaments, and tendons. Image quality benefits from increased field strength, and 3.0-T MR imaging is used increasingly for assessing joints with OA. Dedicated surface coils are required for best visualization of joints affected by OA, and the use of multichannel phased-array coils with parallel imaging improves image quality and/or shortens acquisition times. Sequences that best show morphologic abnormalities of the whole joint include intermediate-weighted fast-spin echo sequences. Also quantitative sequences have been developed to assess cartilage volume and thickness and to analyze cartilage biochemical composition.

Whole-organ semiquantitative (SQ) assessment by expert readers has become a powerful research tool in understanding the natural history of osteoarthritis (OA). SQ morphologic scoring has been applied to observational large cross-sectional and longitudinal epidemiologic studies in addition to interventional clinical trials. In comparison to quantitative and biochemical assessment of cartilage, SQ whole-organ scoring also analyzes additional joint structures that are potentially relevant as surrogate outcome measures for interventional approaches. Resources needed for SQ scoring rely on the MR imaging protocol, image quality, experience of the expert readers, method of documentation, and individual scoring system that is applied. This article discusses the different available OA whole-organ scoring systems, focusing on MR imaging of the knee, and also reviews alternative approaches.

Whereas the strength of scoring systems in osteoarthritis (OA) lies in detecting local changes, involving small parts of the structures of interest (ie, cartilage lesions), quantitative measures are powerful where minute changes occur homogeneously throughout large structures. Cartilage measurements at 1.5 or 3 Tesla are technically accurate, reproducible, and sensitive to change. The rate of change in knee OA was found to be 1% to 2% annually. Risk factors of cartilage loss include a high BMI, meniscal pathology, malalignment, advanced radiographic OA, bone marrow alterations, and focal cartilage lesions. MRI of articular tissues represents a potent tool in experimental, epidemiological and pharmacological intervention studies; however, it is only with the availability of disease modifying drugs that it will play a relevant role in clinical practice.

Osteoarthritis involves ongoing degradative and healing processes that occur at the molecular level in multiple tissues in the joint in response to a number of biochemical and mechanical factors. Understanding these dynamic processes before they affect the structural aspects of the joint motivates the need for metrics to better visualize the compositional and structural molecular aspects of the tissues in vivo. As reviewed here, most of the work to date in this regard has been focused on magnetic resonance imaging approaches for interrogating molecular features of cartilage, including T2 mapping, T1rho mapping, delayed gadolinium-enhanced magnetic resonance imaging of cartilage (dGEMRIC), and sodium imaging. Specific examples illustrate new opportunities and insights emerging from these methods.

Osteoarthritis of the knee has to be considered a disease of the whole joint. Magnetic resonance imaging allows superior assessment of all joint tissues that may be involved in the disease process, such as the subchondral bone, synovium, ligaments, and periarticular soft tissues. Reliable MR imaging-based scoring systems are available to assess and quantify these structures and associated pathology. Cross-sectional and longitudinal evaluation has enabled us to understand their relevance in explaining pain and structural progression.

The menisci play a critical protective role for the knee joint through shock absorption and load distribution. Asymptomatic meniscal tears are common and are frequent incidental findings on knee MR imaging of the middle-aged or older patient. A meniscal tear can lead to knee osteoarthritis (OA), but knee OA can also lead to a spontaneous meniscal tear through breakdown and weakening of meniscal structure. A degenerative meniscal lesion in the middle-aged or older patient could suggest early stage knee OA and should be treated accordingly. Surgical resection of non-obstructive degenerate lesions may only remove evidence of the disorder while the OA and associated symptoms proceeds.

Osteoarthritis of the hip joint is caused by a combination of intrinsic factors and extrinsic factors. Different surgical techniques are being performed to delay or halt osteoarthritis. Success of salvage procedures of the hip depends on the existing cartilage and joint damage before surgery; the likelihood of therapy failure rises with advanced osteoarthritis. For imaging of intra-articular hip pathology, MR imaging represents the best technique because of its ability to directly visualize cartilage, superior soft tissue contrast, and the prospect of multidimensional imaging. This article gives an overview on the standard MR imaging techniques used for diagnosis of hip osteoarthritis and their implications for surgery.

Although osteoarthritis (OA) of the wrist and fingers is routinely diagnosed using plain film, a thorough assessment of cartilage injuries using CT-arthrography, MR imaging, or MR-arthrography remains necessary before any surgical procedure. MR imaging is ideally suited for delineating the presence, extent, and complications of degenerative spinal disease, including OA of the spine involving the disc space, vertebral endplates, facet joints, or supportive and surrounding soft tissues. Other imaging modalities such as CT, dynamic radiography, myelography, and discography may provide complimentary information in selected cases. This article focuses on imaging of OA of the wrist and hand and the lumbar spine, with an emphasis on current MR imaging grading systems available for the assessment of discovertebral lesions.

Within the recent years, advances in imaging technology have increased its applicability to diagnose musculoskeletal disease. The modification of imaging techniques and improved image quality has led to increased use of computed tomography and magnetic resonance imaging in the assessment of postoperative complications related to orthopedic procedures. This article discusses the indications, pre- and post-operative imaging findings and post-operative complications of knee and hip arthoplasty, articular cartilage repair and high tibial osteotomy.

GOAL STATEMENT

The goal of the *Radiologic Clinics of North America* is to keep practicing radiologists and radiology residents up to date with current clinical practice in radiology by providing timely articles reviewing the state of the art in patient care.

ACCREDITATION

The *Radiologic Clinics of North America* is planned and implemented in accordance with the Essential Areas and Policies of the Accreditation Council for Continuing Medical Education (ACCME) through the joint sponsorship of the University of Virginia School of Medicine and Elsevier. The University of Virginia School of Medicine is accredited by the ACCME to provide continuing medical education for physicians.

The University of Virginia School of Medicine designates this educational activity for a maximum of 15 *AMA PRA Category 1 Credits*™ for each issue, 90 credits per year. Physicians should only claim credit commensurate with the extent of their participation in the activity.

The American Medical Association has determined that physicians not licensed in the US who participate in this CME activity are eligible for a maximum of *15 AMA PRA Category 1 Credits*™ for each issue, 90 credits per year.

Credit can be earned by reading the text material, taking the CME examination online at http://www.theclinics.com/home/cme, and completing the evaluation. After taking the test, you will be required to review any and all incorrect answers. Following completion of the test and evaluation, your credit will be awarded and you may print your certificate.

FACULTY DISCLOSURE/CONFLICT OF INTEREST

The University of Virginia School of Medicine, as an ACCME accredited provider, endorses and strives to comply with the Accreditation Council for Continuing Medical Education (ACCME) Standards of Commercial Support, Commonwealth of Virginia statutes, University of Virginia policies and procedures, and associated federal and private regulations and guidelines on the need for disclosure and monitoring of proprietary and financial interests that may affect the scientific integrity and balance of content delivered in continuing medical education activities under our auspices.

The University of Virginia School of Medicine requires that all CME activities accredited through this institution be developed independently and be scientifically rigorous, balanced and objective in the presentation/discussion of its content, theories and practices.

All authors/editors participating in an accredited CME activity are expected to disclose to the readers relevant financial relationships with commercial entities occurring within the past 12 months (such as grants or research support, employee, consultant, stock holder, member of speakers bureau, etc.). The University of Virginia School of Medicine will employ appropriate mechanisms to resolve potential conflicts of interest to maintain the standards of fair and balanced education to the reader. Questions about specific strategies can be directed to the Office of Continuing Medical Education, University of Virginia School of Medicine, Charlottesville, Virginia.

The faculty and staff of the University of Virginia Office of Continuing Medical Education have no financial affiliations to disclose.

The authors/editors listed below have identified no financial or professional relationships for themselves or their spouse/partner:
Bernd Bittersohl, MD; Philip G. Conaghan, MBBS, PhD, FRACP, FRCP; Jean-Luc Drapé, MD, PhD; Barton Dudlick (Acquisitions Editor); Jeffrey Duryea, PhD; Martin Englund, MD, PhD; Antoine Feydy, MD, PhD; Martha Gray, PhD; Henri Guerini, MD; Theodore E. Keats, MD (Test Author); Frederic Lecouvet, MD, PhD; Thomas M. Link, MD; Steven Mazzuca, PhD; Gustavo A. Mercier, MD, PhD; Timothy J. Mosher, MD; Patrick Omoumi, MD; Etienne Pluot, MD; Mark E. Schweitzer, MD; Adnan Sheikh, MD; Klaus A. Siebenrock, MD, PhD; Paolo Simoni, MD; Bruno C. Vande Berg, MD, PhD; Stefan Werlen, MD; and, Christoph Zilkens, MD.

The authors/editors listed below have identified the following financial or professional relationships for themselves or their spouse/partner:
Alan Brett, PhD is employed by Optasia Medical Ltd.
Deborah Burstein, PhD is a consultant for Sanofi and is an industry funded research/investigator for Pfizer, Stryker, and Geleta.
Michel D. Crema, MD is a shareholder with Boston Imaging Core Lab, LLC.
Bernard J. Dardzinski, PhD is employed by and his spouse is employed by Merck Research Laboratories.
Felix Eckstein, MD is employed by and is a shareholder (CEO) with Chondrometrics GmbH, and is a consultant for Merck Serono, Novartis, and Pfizer.
Ali Guermazi, MD (Guest Editor) is the president and founder of Boston Imaging Core Lab, LLC, owns stock in Synarc, Inc., has received a grant from General Electrics, and is a consultant for Merck Serono.
David J. Hunter, MBBS, FRACP, PhD is an industry funded research/investigator for Pfizer, Wyeth, and Astra Zeneca and owns a patent with DonJoy.
Helen I. Keen, MBBS, FRACP serves on the Speakers Bureau for Abbott, Roche, and Sanofi Aventis, and is an industry funded research/investigator for CBIO.
Young-Jo Kim, MD, PhD is an industry funded research/investigator and serves on the Advisory Committee for Siemens Health Care.
Marie-Pierre Hellio Le Graverand, MD, DSc, PhD is employed by Pfizer.
Stefan L. Lohmander, MD, PhD is an industry funded research/investigator for Pfizer and AstraZeneca, serves on the Speakers Bureau for AstraZeneca, and serves on the Advisory Board for Tigenix and Wyeth.
Tallal C. Mamisch, MD is a consultant for Siemens Healthcare AG.
Monica D. Marra, MD is a shareholder with Boston Imaging Core Lab, LLC.
Frank W. Roemer, MD is the vice president and shareholder of Boston Imagine Core Lab, LLC.
David R. Wilson, DPhil is an industry funded research/investigator for Benvenue Medical.

Disclosure of Discussion of Non-FDA Approved Uses for Pharmaceutical Products and/or Medical Devices.
The University of Virginia School of Medicine, as an ACCME provider, requires that all faculty presenters identify and disclose any off-label uses for pharmaceutical and medical device products. The University of Virginia School of Medicine recommends that each physician fully review all the available data on new products or procedures prior to clinical use.

TO ENROLL

To enroll in the Radiologic Clinics of North America Continuing Medical Education program, call customer service at 1-800-654-2452 or sign up online at http://www.theclinics.com/home/cme. The CME program is available to subscribers for an additional annual fee USD 205.

Radiologic Clinics of North America

THE CLINICS ARE NOW AVAILABLE ONLINE!

Access your subscription at:
www.theclinics.com

Preface

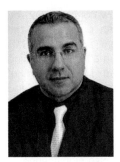

Ali Guermazi, MD
Guest Editor

Osteoarthritis (OA) remains an enigmatic disease. A simplified definition based on clinical and radiographic findings has been used for decades but seems to represent only the advanced stages of the disease. So far, only symptomatic therapy is available, and it is accepted dogma that OA is a chronic and nontreatable disease of almost every elderly person. OA affects an estimated 30 million Americans,[1,2] and recent estimates suggest that symptomatic knee OA occurs in 6% of adults aged over 30 years[3] and 13% of persons aged 60 and over.[1,4] Prevalence is expected to increase even further with the obesity epidemic and the aging of the baby-boomer generation.[5]

And yet, despite 2 decades of research, there is still no effective treatment of OA. An air of gloom has descended on the world of OA research. Effective prevention seems unreachable, clinical trials consume time and resources and result in outcomes that are unclear, and a true understanding of the pathophysiology of OA is elusive. Many pharmaceutical companies and clinical and basic researchers are abandoning OA research. Despite the sense of frustration, work continues and, though progress is slow and incremental, we continue to learn more about this sometimes frustrating, often mysterious disease.

In this issue of *Radiologic Clinics of North America*, David Hunter presents new insights from imaging in epidemiology and pathophysiology of OA. David Hunter and David Wilson then write extensively on alignment and biomechanics in OA and implications for imaging.

Marie-Pierre Hellio Le Graverand and colleagues describe the role of radiographs in grading and measuring joint space width in OA. Both the US

Food and Drug Administration and the European Agency for the Evaluation of Medicinal Products currently recommend joint space narrowing (JSN) measurement as the imaging end point for clinical trials of disease-modifying OA drugs. Even though radiographs represent a proven methodology and are widely used in clinical trials, their drawbacks make their use an unlikely focus of research in the near future. Radiographs lack sensitivity to change and do not visualize key features of OA (eg, bone marrow lesions [BMLs], the menisci, synovitis). Furthermore, reproducibility of radiograph positioning in large multicenter trials is still problematic.[6] Radiograph assessment remains relevant as a way to define the progression of radiographic JSN, the current gold standard for measuring clinical efficacy in therapy.[7] A shift in paradigm is necessary and research needs to focus on an acceptable definition of OA and the natural history of the disease. Radiographs still play an important role in inclusion and as a means of stratification in clinical trials.

Ultrasound in OA, as presented by Helen Keen and colleagues, will likely play an important role in the assessment of structural changes in OA, especially concerning evaluation of synovitis. Nevertheless, ultrasound, too, has its drawbacks: user-dependency, poor visualization of bone anatomy and deep intra-articular structures, as well as its difficult documentation, which relies on subjective screenshots. These make its use in clinical trials difficult and unrealistic.

Patrick Omoumi and colleagues, in their article, describe some of the advantages of CT- and MR-arthrography over MR imaging for visualizing cartilage focal defects. However, the price of these advantages is articular contrast injection, another

Radiol Clin N Am 47 (2009) xiii–xvii
doi:10.1016/j.rcl.2009.06.007

hurdle in clinical trials. Fludeoxyglucose positron emission tomography (FDG-PET) and scintigraphy also may help us understand the inflammatory nature of OA with regards to better visualization of synovitis, but these techniques remain nonspecific.

It is now accepted that MR imaging has the most promise for understanding the natural history of OA, and it has been shown to be a sensitive biomarker of the disease at diagnosis, progression, and after therapy. On the other hand, and unlike radiographs, MR imaging is a complex modality that heavily depends on the hardware and sequences used. These facts are well covered in the article by Thomas Link.

Cartilage is one component of the puzzle of OA, but MR imaging can visualize the whole joint. Validated, semiquantitative scoring systems for whole-joint assessment of the knee are in use today, and Frank Roemer and Ali Guermazi describe these scoring systems, with insights on possible application to other joints. Semiquantitative assessment has taught us some counterintuitive lessons (eg, that focal cartilage defects are better visualized on conventional water-sensitive MR imaging sequences than on cartilage-dedicated MR imaging sequences [Fig. 1]).

Quantitative assessment of cartilage still plays an important role in assessing OA progression, and is especially sensitive in Kellgren-Lawrence grades 3 and 4. Felix Eckstein and colleagues describe quantitative methods for analyzing cartilage and other features of knee OA and also possible application to other joints.

Several researchers are now concentrating on early and preclinical OA, with cartilage as the main focus of interest. There are several MR image–based compositional methods, including delayed gadolinium-enhanced MR imaging of cartilage (dGEMRIC), T2 mapping, sodium, and T1 rho. Deborah Burstein and colleagues report on special software and hardware needed to acquire these types of images. The authors discuss current and possible future applications. Although rich with possibilities, the precise significance of these methods is still being investigated, and trials will be needed to determine their clinical utility.

Cartilage pathology alone cannot explain OA. Indeed, cartilage is an aneural structure and is not useful in helping us understand pain, which is part of the very definition of OA. Michel Crema and colleagues have studied noncartilage OA features, including BMLs, synovitis, effusion, and periarticular cysts and bursa. They share their insights on imaging of these features and their relevance to OA research. Subchondral BMLs have especially become a focus of research as they are potentially reversible and are strongly associated with pain. BMLs also play a role in predicting and influencing structural outcome.[8,9] The authors emphasize the importance of technology and protocol selection when quantifying and assessing BMLs. In this context, it is crucial to know that only water-sensitive fat-suppressed

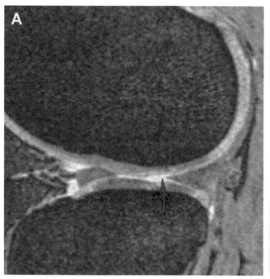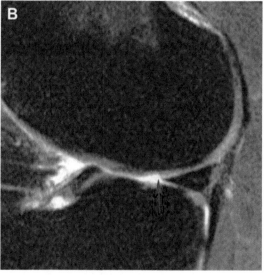

Fig. 1. Superficial cartilage focal defect. (A) Sagittal dual-echo in the steady-state MR image only barely depicts the central lateral femur defect (arrow). (B) Superior delineation concerning size and conspicuity of focal cartilage defect (arrow) on sagittal fat-suppressed intermediate-weighted MR image.

MR imaging sequences should be applied[10] (Fig. 2). The importance of intravenous gadolinium administration for the assessment of synovitis has only recently been recognized. In large epidemiological OA studies, synovitis—defined as inflammation of the synovial membrane—is commonly assessed on non–contrast-enhanced MR images using a surrogate of nonspecific hyperintensity on proton density-, intermediate-, and T2-weighted images of Hoffa's fat pad[11] (Fig. 3).

Several recent publications have turned to meniscal damage to understand the natural history of OA. One recent article showed that 38% of the elderly in the United States have asymptomatic meniscal tears.[12] Meniscal damage is strongly associated with development of frequent knee pain.[13] Meniscal damage and malposition are associated with increased risk of cartilage loss[14] and incidental OA.[15] In their article, Martin Englund and colleagues describe different meniscal lesions and their appearance in different MR imaging sequences. They describe the pathophysiology of meniscal anomalies and how those anomalies affect the knee joint. They also suggest some future research on meniscal pathology as a means of understanding the natural history of OA.

Most imaging in OA research has concentrated on the knee because its anatomy is easy to image and it has the thickest cartilage of all the diarthrodial joints. Charles Mamisch and colleagues,

however, have explored OA in the hip. They describe the anatomical variants that are known risk factors for hip OA, as well as some of the imaging features of early and late OA in the hip. They also provide insights and perspective on the role of imaging in surgical planning for hip OA. The next article, by Antoine Feydy and colleagues, covers imaging of OA in the hand, wrist, and spine.

In the final article, Adnan Sheikh and Mark Schweitzer describe imaging problems and procedures of total and partial joint replacements and high tibial osteotomy as therapies for OA. They also describe the postoperative appearance and complications of joint replacements.

For several decades, clinical researchers and pharmaceutical companies have relied on radiographic JSN as the accepted surrogate outcome biomarker. However, radiographs are not very responsive to change and at most correlate only moderately with clinical end points. Therapeutic development has essentially stalled for lack of a better biomarker, and the lack of progress has been so discouraging that some of the major participants are leaving the field. Collaborative interdisciplinary work, concentrating above all on imaging and especially on MR imaging, is needed to define a valid and sensitive biomarker of OA. Large ongoing research endeavors, such as the Osteoarthritis Initiative, will foster such collaboration and

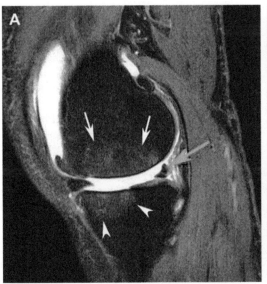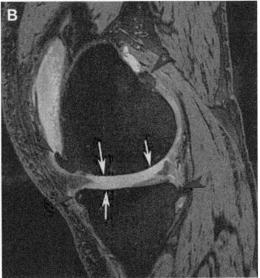

Fig. 2. Bone marrow lesion. (*A*) Sagittal fat-suppressed intermediate-weighted MR image shows hyperintense bone marrow lesions at the central medial femur (*white arrows*) and at the central and anterior medial tibia (*white arrowheads*). These bone marrow lesions are not seen on (*B*) sagittal dual-echo in the steady-state MR image. There is an extensive cartilage loss of the medial femur and tibia (*yellow arrows*), osteophytosis (*red arrowheads*), maceration of the posterior horn of the medial meniscus (*green arrow*), and mild joint effusion.

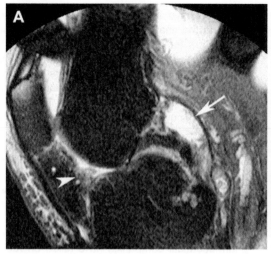 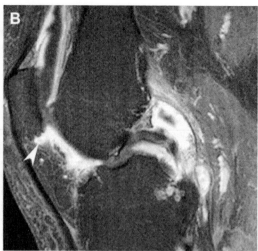

Fig. 3. Synovitis. (*A*) Sagittal fat-suppressed proton density-weighted extremity MR image shows an effusion posterior to the posterior cruciate ligament (*arrow*), which turns out to be the thick synovitis on (*B*) sagittal contrast-enhanced T1-weighted MR image. There is a small intercondylar synovitis (*arrowhead*) and no infrapatellar synovitis on the sagittal extremity MR image (*A*). The intercondylar synovitis is obviously more important with infrapatellar synovitis (*arrowhead*) on the sagittal contrast-enhanced T1-weighted MR image (*B*). (*Courtesy of* the Multicenter Osteoarthritis [MOST] study.)

accelerate understanding of the natural history of the disease. Presumably, the fruits of such work will motivate researchers and pharmaceutical companies to reinvest in this exciting field and we will have several effective therapies that will flourish in the market.

We hope the readers of *Radiologic Clinics of North America* will find this issue a valuable source of information on state-of-the-art imaging of OA. The latest results from clinical research and clinical trials should also be of interest.

Ali Guermazi, MD
Musculoskeletal Imaging
Quantitative Imaging Center
Department of Radiology
Boston University School of Medicine
820 Harrison Avenue
FGH Building, Third Floor
Boston, MA 02118, USA

E-mail address:
ali.guermazi@bmc.org (A. Guermazi)

REFERENCES

1. Centers for Disease Control and Prevention (CDC). Prevalence and impact of chronic joint symptoms—seven states, 1996. MMWR Morb Mortal Wkly Rep 1998;47:345–51.

2. Lawrence RC, Helmick CG, Arnett FC, et al. Estimates of the prevalence of arthritis and selected musculoskeletal disorders in the United States. Arthritis Rheum 1998;41:778–99.

3. Felson DT, Lawrence RC, Dieppe PA, et al. Osteoarthritis: new insights. Part 1: the disease and its risk factors. Ann Intern Med 2000;133:635–46.

4. Dunlop DD, Manheim LM, Song J, et al. Arthritis prevalence and activity limitations in older adults. Arthritis Rheum 2001;44:212–21.

5. Centers for Disease Control and Prevention (CDC). Arthritis prevalence and activity limitations—United States, 1990. MMWR Morb Mortal Wkly Rep 1994; 43:433–8.

6. Guermazi A, Hunter DJ, Roemer FW. Plain radiography and magnetic resonance imaging diagnostics in osteoarthritis: validated staging and scoring. J Bone Joint Surg Am 2009;91(Suppl 1):54–62.

7. Food and Drug Administration. Guidance for Industry. Clinical development programs for drugs, devices, and biological products intended for the treatment of osteoarthritis (OA). http://www.fda.gov/Cber/gdlns/osteo.htm.

8. Roemer FW, Guermazi A, Javaid MK, et al. Change in MRI–detected subchondral bone marrow lesions is associated with cartilage loss—the MOST study. A longitudinal multicenter study of knee osteoarthritis. Ann Rheum Dis 2008 Oct 1 [Epub ahead of print].

9. Felson DT, Niu J, Guermazi A, et al. Correlation of the development of knee pain with enlarging bone

marrow lesions on magnetic resonance imaging. Arthritis Rheum 2007;56:2986–92.

10. Roemer FW, Hunter DJ, Guermazi A. MRI-based semiquantitative assessment of subchondral bone marrow lesions in osteoarthritis research. Osteoarthritis Cartilage 2009;17:414–5.

11. Roemer FW, Guermazi A, Zhang Y, et al. Hoffa's fat pad: evaluation on unenhanced MR images as a measure of patellofemoral synovitis in osteoarthritis. Am J Roentgenol AJR 2009;192:1696–700.

12. Englund M, Guermazi A, Gale D, et al. Incidental meniscal findings on knee MRI in middle-aged and elderly persons. N Engl J Med 2008;359:1108–15.

13. Englund M, Niu J, Guermazi A, et al. Effect of meniscal damage on the development of frequent knee pain, aching, or stiffness. Arthritis Rheum 2007;56: 4048–54.

14. Hunter DJ, Zhang YQ, Niu JB, et al. The association of meniscal pathologic changes with cartilage loss in symptomatic knee osteoarthritis. Arthritis Rheum 2006;54:795–801.

15. Englund M, Guermazi A, Roemer FW, et al. Meniscal tear in knee without surgery and the development of radiographic osteoarthritits among middle-aged and elderly persons: The Multicenter Osteoarthritis Study. Arthritis Rheum 2009;60:831–9.

Insights from Imaging on the Epidemiology and Pathophysiology of Osteoarthritis

David J. Hunter, MBBS, FRACP, PhD

KEYWORDS

• Epidemiology • Pathophysiology • Osteoarthritis
• Knee • Imaging

Osteoarthritis (OA) is the most common form of arthritis in the United States, affecting approximately 15% of the population overall, 50% of those aged 65 years and older, and 85% of those 75 years and older. Symptomatic OA causes substantial physical and psychosocial disability.[1] In the early 1990s, over 7 million Americans were limited in their ability to participate in their main daily activities, such as going to school or work or maintaining their independence, simply because of their arthritis.[2] Interestingly, the risk for disability (defined as needing help walking or climbing stairs) attributable to knee OA is as great as that attributable to cardiovascular disease and greater than that caused by any other medical condition in elderly persons.[1] Knee OA is already the leading cause of functional disability, and its prevalence is projected to double by the year 2020, caused in part by increases in obesity and longevity. Like arthritis prevalence, the prevalence of arthritis-related disability is also expected to rise by the year 2020, when an estimated 11.6 million people will be affected.[2]

The synovial joint is an organ, and OA represents failure of that organ and can be initiated by abnormalities arising in any of its constituent tissues.[3] This highly prevalent disease occurs when the dynamic equilibrium between the breakdown and repair of the synovial joint tissues is overwhelmed.[4] In OA, inflammatory changes are secondary and are caused by particulate and soluble breakdown products of cartilage and bone. OA should not be considered to be a "degenerative joint disease" insofar as the cells of the cartilage and bone are normal and, if the inciting breakdown mechanism is reduced, can restore the damaged tissue to normal.

This article briefly describes the epidemiology and pathophysiology of OA. It also delineates what knowledge imaging has brought to these scientific areas in recent years. The predominant symptom in most patients presenting with OA is pain. Over recent years a number of imaging-based studies have narrowed the discord between knowledge about structural findings on imaging and symptoms. In addition, a number of new risk factors seen with imaging methods that portend to more rapid structural progression have been identified. Much of the research and understanding of OA is centered on the knee and most of the content of this article similarly is less focused on the hand and hip.

EPIDEMIOLOGY

In epidemiologic investigation, OA is typically defined using conventional radiographs, and less frequently self report. The reported prevalence of OA varies according to the evaluation method used. The characteristic features of OA scored on radiographs are osteophytes (osteocartilaginous growths); subchondral sclerosis; and joint space narrowing (**Fig. 1**).

Orthopedic Department, Division of Research, New England Baptist Hospital, 125 Parker Hill Avenue, Boston, MA 02120, USA
E-mail address: djhunter@caregroup.harvard.edu

Radiol Clin N Am 47 (2009) 539–551
doi:10.1016/j.rcl.2009.03.004
0033-8389/09/$ – see front matter © 2009 Elsevier Inc. All rights reserved.

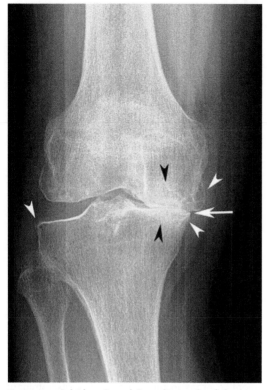

Fig. 1. A weight-bearing plain radiograph of the knee depicting the characteristic features seen in OA: medial tibiofemoral joint space narrowing (*arrow*), marginal femoral and tibial osteophytosis (*white arrowheads*), and medial tibial and femoral subchondral sclerosis (*black arrowheads*).

Kellgren and Lawrence grade progression as a measure of disease progression should best be avoided.

Understanding the radiographic method of disease definition becomes important when one considers that osteophytes, typically the first feature identified on radiographs, are not necessarily a deleterious finding and may represent an effort on the part of the joint to promote stability. They are important, however, if they represent a source of symptoms, and yet most of the epidemiologic research in OA is based on the presence of self-reported OA or radiographic osteophytes and not on symptomatic OA, defined as the concomitant presence of pain and radiographic features. It is the presence of symptomatic OA that is important clinically, not simply the radiographic identification of osteophyte formation or self-reported OA (where misclassification is even more problematic than the commonly used radiographic OA definition). In addition, marked osteoarthritic damage must be present to detect characteristic changes with conventional radiographs, and they are not sensitive diagnostic tests.[6–11]

During a 1-year period, 25% of people over 55 years have a persistent episode of knee pain, of whom about one in six consult their general practitioner.[12] In this British sample, symptomatic knee OA defined as pain on most days and radiographic features consistent with OA occurred in approximately 12% of those aged over 55.[12] From United States estimates about 6% of adults aged greater than 30 years[13] and 13% of persons aged 60 and over[14] have symptomatic knee OA.

Although OA is common in the knee, it is even more prevalent in the hands, especially the distal and proximal interphalangeal joints and the base of the thumb (carpometacarpal). When symptomatic, especially so for the base of thumb joint, hand OA is associated with functional impairment.[15,16] OA of the thumb carpometacarpal joint is a common condition that can lead to substantial

The presence and severity of OA is typically classified using the Kellgren and Lawrence grading system,[5] a system that is heavily dependent on the osteophytes for classification of disease (Table 1). This system suffers from limitations based on invalid assumptions by mixing distinct constructs (osteophytes, joint space narrowing, subchondral sclerosis, subchondral bone shape changes, cysts, and so forth) into one scale. Further, the scale is not linear and the use of

Table 1	
The Kellgren and Lawrence grading system	
Grade 0	Normal
Grade 1	Doubtful narrowing of joint space and possible osteophytic lipping
Grade 2	Definite osteophytes and possible narrowing of joint space
Grade 3	Moderate multiple osteophytes, definite narrowing of joint space and some sclerosis, and possible deformity of bone ends
Grade 4	Large osteophytes, marked narrowing of joint space, severe sclerosis, and definite deformity of bone ends

From Kellgren JH, Lawrence JS. Atlas of standard radiographs. Oxford: Blackwell Scientific; 1963; with permission.

pain, instability, deformity, and loss of motion.[17] Over the age of 70 years, approximately 5% of women and 3% of men have symptomatic OA affecting this joint with impairment of hand function.[15]

The prevalence of hip OA is about 9% in white populations.[18] In contrast, studies in Asian, black, and East Indian populations indicate a very low prevalence of hip OA.[19] The prevalence of symptomatic hip OA is approximately 4%.[14] It has been suggested that the lower rates detected among certain ethnic groups may be caused by lower rates of congenital or developmental abnormalities and, in some cultures, the common use of squatting postures, which force the hip through extreme ranges of motion.[20]

The prevalence of OA is expected to increase as the population ages and the prevalence of obesity rises (this being an important risk factor, as discussed next). By 2020, it is expected that the number of people with OA may have doubled.[2,21]

Risk Factors for Osteoarthritis

OA is perhaps best understood as resulting from excessive mechanical stress applied in the context of systemic susceptibility (Fig. 2). Susceptibility to OA may be increased in part by genetic inheritance (a positive family history increases risk); age, ethnicity; diet; and female gender.[22]

In persons vulnerable to the development of knee OA, local mechanical factors, such as abnormal joint congruity, malalignment (varus or valgus deformity), muscle weakness, or alterations in the structural integrity of the joint environment,

such as meniscal damage, bone marrow lesions, or ligament rupture, can facilitate the progression of OA. Loading can also be affected by obesity and joint injury (either acutely as in a sporting injury or after repetitive overuse, such as occupational exposure), both of which can increase the likelihood of development or progression of OA.

Insights from Imaging on Epidemiology

Bearing in mind that radiographs are notoriously insensitive to the earliest pathologic features of OA, the absence of positive radiographic findings should not be interpreted as confirming the complete absence of symptomatic disease. Conversely, the presence of positive radiographic findings does not guarantee that an osteoarthritic joint is also the active source of the patient's current knee or hip symptoms where other sources of pain including periarticular sources, such as pes anserine bursitis at the knee and trochanteric bursitis at the hip, often contribute.[23] According to the American College of Rheumatology criteria for classification of hand OA (unlike the hip and knee where radiographs enhance the sensitivity and specificity), radiographs are less sensitive and specific than physical examination in the diagnosis of symptomatic hand OA.[24] The usefulness of radiographs relates more importantly to the exclusion of other diagnostic possibilities rather than confirmation of osteoarthritic disease.[25] In clinical practice the diagnosis of OA should be made on the basis of history and physical examination and the role of radiography is to confirm this clinical suspicion and rule out other conditions.

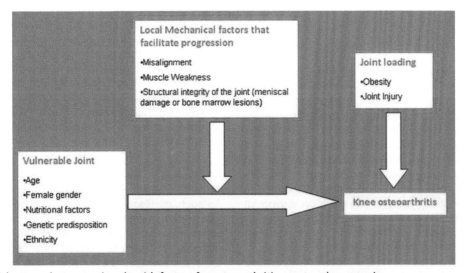

Fig. 2. Schemata demonstrating the risk factors for osteoarthritis onset and progression.

Recent imaging studies have provided new insights into disease genesis. This section focuses on these as they pertain to the hip and hand, with the remainder of the article providing a larger focus on the knee.

Hip OA is a major cause of disability in the United States,[26] and the major reason for the approximately 200,000 hip replacements performed annually.[27] Recent evidence highlights the importance of local mechanical factors including acetabular dysplasia, which may account for up to 40% of hip OA.[28,29] In dysplasia, the shallow acetabulum leads to increased abnormal loading of the articular cartilage, leading to its damage and degradation.

OA of the thumb carpometacarpal joint is a common condition that can lead to substantial pain, instability, deformity, and loss of motion.[17] The agility of the thumb is afforded mainly by the mobility of the trapeziometacarpal joint or so-called "base of thumb" joint.[30–32] Eaton and Littler[30] proposed that instability of the trapeziometacarpal joint combined with strenuous use could potentially lead to OA. The author recently confirmed this suspicion and demonstrated that radial subluxation predisposes to subsequent OA of the trapeziometacarpal joint in men.[33]

A recent study using high-resolution MR imaging and surface coils adapted for clinical scanners, with an in-plane resolution of 80 to 100 mm, identified early phenotypic features of hand OA where enthesophytic changes were prominent.[34] The most striking abnormalities were in the collateral ligaments (abnormalities ranging from thickening to frank disruption) and capsules of the distal and proximal interphalangeal joints, rather than in the articular cartilage or subchondral bone.

PATHOPHYSIOLOGY OF OSTEOARTHRITIS

Early investigators tended to regard OA as an isolated disease of articular cartilage. Although cartilage loss is a prominent feature of OA, contemporary models recognize that the entire synovial joint organ is affected by OA. OA can be viewed as the clinical and pathologic outcome of a range of disorders that results in structural and functional failure of the synovial joint organ with loss and erosion of articular cartilage; subchondral bone alteration; meniscal degeneration; a synovial inflammatory response; and bone and cartilage overgrowth (osteophytes).[35] This highly prevalent disease occurs when the dynamic equilibrium between the breakdown and repair of joint tissues is overwhelmed.[4] The resulting progressive joint failure may cause pain, physical disability, and psychologic distress,[1] although many persons with structural changes consistent with OA are asymptomatic.[23] The reasons why there is this disconnect between disease severity and the level of reported pain and disability is largely unknown, although recent imaging studies are beginning to shed light.

INSIGHTS FROM IMAGING ON SYMPTOM GENESIS

The structural determinants of pain and mechanical dysfunction in OA are not well understood, but are believed to involve multiple interactive pathways that are best framed in a biopsychosocial framework (posits that biologic, psychologic, and social factors all play a significant role in pain in OA).[36,37] Local to the joint there are a number of tissues that contain nociceptive fibers and these are the likely sources of pain in OA. The subchondral bone, periosteum, periarticular ligaments, periarticular muscle, synovium, and joint capsule are all richly innervated and are the likely source of nociception in OA.

In population studies there is a significant discordance between radiographically diagnosed OA and knee pain.[23] Although radiographic evidence of joint damage predisposes to joint pain, it is clear that the severity of joint damage on radiographs bears little relation to the severity of the pain experienced. Using other imaging modalities, however, such as MR imaging, significant structural associations, such as subchondral bone marrow lesions,[38,39] subarticular bone attrition,[40] synovitis, and effusion,[41,42] have been related to knee pain. It remains unclear which of these local tissue factors predominate because until recently these analyses did not account for the fact that much of the structural change is collinear (a person who has more severe disease has worse structural change in multiple tissues including the bone, synovium, and so forth) and were not adjusting for other tissue changes. A recent analysis confirmed most beliefs that it is likely that changes in the subchondral bone and synovial activation-effusion predominate.[43] The different tissues within the joint and their respective contribution to symptoms are discussed next.

Hyaline Articular Cartilage

Articular cartilage is both aneural and avascular. As such, cartilage is incapable of directly generating pain, inflammation, stiffness, or any of the symptoms that patients with OA typically describe.[44] Given its relative unimportance to OA's symptomatic presentation, it is ironic that articular cartilage has received so much attention, whereas other common symptom sources in the joint are ignored. Some studies have suggested a relation between cartilage morphometry and lesions and the symptoms of OA.[45] It is important to note that this disease of the whole joint concurrently affects other tissues that do contain nociceptors. The studies that have demonstrated a relation of cartilage damage to pain have traditionally investigated the role of cartilage in predisposing to symptoms in isolation from other tissues and as such are fundamentally flawed. A recent study suggested that areas of denuded cartilage are related to symptoms.[46] Again, the likely mechanism for symptom genesis is through secondary mechanisms, such as (1) exposing the underlying subchondral bone and the inherent symptom genesis from this structural alteration, (2) vascular congestion of subchondral bone leading to increased intraosseous pressure, and (3) synovitis secondary to articular cartilage damage with activation of synovial membrane nociceptors.

Subchondral Bone

Periarticular bone changes associated with OA can be segregated into distinct patterns based on the anatomic location and pathogenic mechanisms. These alterations include progressive increase in subchondral plate thickness; alterations in the architecture of subchondral trabecular bone; formation of new bone at the joint margins (osteophytes); development of subchondral bone cysts; and advancement of the tidemark associated with vascular invasion of the calcified cartilage.

Of these lesions that which has the most supportive evidence for a role in symptom genesis is the bone marrow lesion (Fig. 3). Lesions in the bone marrow play an integral if not pivotal role in the symptoms that emanate from knee OA and its structural progression.[38] Bone marrow lesions were found in 272 (77.5%) of 351 persons with painful knees compared with 15 (30%) of 50 persons with no knee pain ($P <.001$). Large lesions were present almost exclusively in persons with knee pain (35.9% versus 2%; $P <.001$). After adjustment for severity of radiographic disease, effusion, age, and gender, all lesions and in particular large lesions remained associated with the occurrence of knee pain. More recently their relation to pain severity[39] and incident pain[47] was also demonstrated. There are conflicting data albeit from smaller studies with different methods suggesting no relation of bone marrow lesions to pain[48,49]; however, the balance of data supports a strong relation of bone marrow lesions to pain.

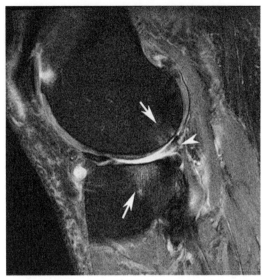

Fig. 3. Sagittal fat-suppressed intermediate-weighted MR image depicts diffuse ill-defined hyperintensities (*arrows*) abutting the subchondral plate in the weight-bearing lateral tibia and femur characteristic of bone marrow lesions. There is also an extensive osteophytosis and cartilage defect of the lateral tibial plateau and femoral condyle and bone attrition of the tibial plateau. There is an oblique tear of the partially macerated posterior horn of the lateral meniscus (*arrowhead*).

Other bone-related causes of pain include periostitis associated with osteophyte formation,[50] subchondral microfractures,[51] bone attrition,[40] and bone angina caused by decreased blood flow and elevated intraosseous pressure.[52] The particular bone pathology most responsible for pain remains elusive; however, identifying this would be a major advance in delineating appropriate therapeutic targets. One likely source that remains underexplored is that of intraosseous hypertension. The pathophysiology remains unclear, although phlebographic studies in OA indicate impaired vascular clearance from bone and raised intraosseous pressure in the bone marrow near the painful joint.[52–55] What may subsequently cause pain is as yet unknown. Increased trabecular bone pressure, ischemia, and inflammation are all possible stimuli.

Synovitis and Effusion

The synovial reaction in OA includes synovial hyperplasia; fibrosis; thickening of synovial capsule; activated synoviocytes; and in some cases lymphocytic infiltrate (B and T cells and plasma cells).[56] The site of infiltration of the synovium is of obvious relevance because one of the most densely innervated structures of the joint is the white adipose tissue of the fat pad, which also shows evidence of inflammation and can act as a rich source of inflammatory adipokines.[57] Synovial causes of pain include irritation of sensory nerve endings within the synovium from osteophytes and synovial inflammation that is caused, at least in part, by the release of prostaglandins, leukotrienes, proteinases, neuropeptides, and cytokines.[37,58]

Synovitis and effusion are frequently present in OA and correlate with pain and other clinical outcomes (**Fig. 4**).[41] Synovial thickening around the infrapatellar fat pad using noncontrast MR imaging has been shown on biopsy to represent mild chronic synovitis.[59] A semiquantitative measure of synovitis from the infrapatellar fat pad is associated with pain severity and similarly change in synovitis is associated with change in pain severity.[42] This study assessed 270 subjects (158 men, 112 women) with at least one follow-up MR image. Mean age was 66.8 (9.2) years; body mass index was 31.5 (5.7); and visual analogue scale pain score was 44.7 (25.2) mm. Mean synovitis score at baseline was 3.3 (1.9) with an average change of 0.15 (1.5). There was a correlation of baseline synovitis with baseline pain score (Pearson correlation coefficient

$r = 0.20, P = 0.0005$). Changes in summary synovitis score were associated with changes in pain over time ($P = 0.005$). An increase of one unit in summary synovitis score resulted in a 3.11-mm increase in visual analogue scale pain score (0–100 scale). Of the three locations for synovitis, changes in the infrapatellar fat pad were most strongly related to pain change (4.2-mm increase in pain per unit increase in synovitis).

In an important caveat to this analysis a recent study compared nonenhanced fat-suppressed proton density weighted MR imaging with fat-suppressed contrast-enhanced T1-weighted MR imaging for semiquantitative assessment of peripatellar synovitis in OA.[60] These data suggested that signal alterations in Hoffa's fat pad on nonenhanced MR imaging do not always represent synovitis as seen on contrast-enhanced T1-weighted MR imaging but are a rather nonspecific albeit sensitive finding. This study concluded that semiquantitative scoring of peripatellar synovitis in OA ideally should be performed using contrast-enhanced T1-weighted MR imaging and should include scoring of synovial thickness.

Meniscus

The meniscus has many functions in the knee, including load bearing, shock absorption, stability enhancement, and lubrication.[61,62] The menisci transmit anywhere from 45% to 60% of the compressive loads in the knee.[61] If the meniscus does not cover the articular surface that it is designed to protect because of change in position, or if a tear leaves it unable to resist axial loading, it does not perform this role. The absence of a functioning meniscus increases peak and average contact stresses in the medial compartment of the knee in a range of 40% to 700%.[63–65]

Knee OA after meniscectomy-meniscal repair is traditionally considered a result of the joint injury that leads to the meniscectomy in the first instance and the increased cartilage contact stress caused by the loss of meniscal tissue.[66–68] Meniscectomy is often accompanied by the onset of OA because of the high focal stresses imposed on articular cartilage and subchondral bone subsequent to excision of the meniscus. The studies that have explored the relationship between the meniscus and risk of disease progression in OA provide a clear indication of the risk inherent with damage to this vital tissue.[69–71] Each aspect of meniscal abnormality (whether change in position or damage) (**Fig. 5**) had a major effect on risk of cartilage loss in OA.

The intact and functional meniscus is clearly important to the preservation of joint integrity and

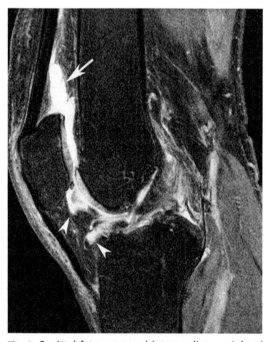

Fig. 4. Sagittal fat-suppressed intermediate-weighted MR image shows knee joint effusion (*arrow*) and infrapatellar synovitis (*arrowhead*). On this noncontrast MR image the magnitude of synovitis is difficult to determine.

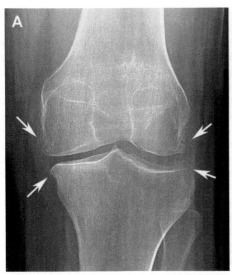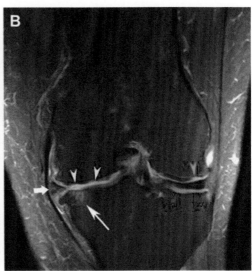

Fig. 5. (A) Anteroposterior left knee radiograph shows diffuse marginal osteophytosis of the tibia and femur (*arrows*). There is a mild to moderate medial tibiofemoral joint space narrowing. (B) Coronal fat-suppressed proton density weighted MR image performed the same day shows subchondral bone marrow lesion (*thin arrow*) at the medial tibial plateau just subjacent to a focal full-thickness cartilage defect. There are multiple partial-thickness defects of the medial femoral condyle cartilage (*yellow arrowheads*). Surprisingly, there are more extensive focal full-thickness cartilage defects (*green arrowhead*) at the lateral femoral condyle and almost complete denudation (*red arrowheads*) subchondral bone at the lateral tibia, as opposed to a radiographically normal-appearing lateral tibiofemoral joint space width. Indeed, most of the joint space narrowing of the medial tibiofemoral joint is secondary to a partially macerated and extruded medial meniscus (*thick arrow*). There is attrition of the medial and lateral tibial plateaus and marginal osteophytosis.

prevention of further joint damage. In contrast, the meniscus plays a much smaller role in symptom genesis. An unfortunate consequence of the frequent use of MR imaging in clinical practice is the frequent detection of meniscal tears.[72] Degenerative lesions, described as horizontal cleavages, flap (oblique), or complex tears or meniscal maceration or destruction, are associated with older age and are almost universal in persons with OA.[72] In asymptomatic subjects with a mean age of 65 years, a tear was found in 67% using MR imaging, whereas in patients with symptomatic knee OA, a meniscal tear was found in 91%.[73] In the interests of preserving menisci an important cautionary note: meniscal tears are nearly universal in persons with knee OA and are unlikely to be a cause of increased symptoms.[73,74] The penchant to remove menisci is to be avoided, unless there are symptoms of locking or extension blockade, at which point surgical treatment often becomes necessary.[75]

The Role of Other Tissues

Periarticular muscles influence joint loading, and impairments in muscle function have been observed in people with OA.[76] Various studies have investigated the role of muscle strength on joint integrity and some have explored the impact on physical functioning. Sharma and colleagues[77] conducted a 3-year longitudinal cohort study investigating factors contributing to poor physical functioning in 257 patients with knee OA. They found that in addition to such factors as age, reduced absolute quadriceps and hamstrings strength, and poor proprioceptive acuity increased the likelihood of poor physical functioning as measured by the time to perform five repetitions of rising and sitting in a chair. In addition to their exploration in observational studies there is ample evidence from clinical trials demonstrating that muscle-strengthening exercises result in improvements in pain, physical function, and quality of life in people with knee OA.[78,79]

Obesity is the single most important risk factor for development of severe OA of the knee and more so than other potentially damaging factors including heredity.[80] Even if it is usually accepted that mechanical loading contributes to joint destruction in overweight patients, recent advances in the physiology of adipose tissue add further insights in understanding the relationship between obesity and OA. Indeed, the positive association between overweight or obesity and OA is observed not only for knee joints but also for non–weight bearing joints, such as hands.[81,82]

Furthermore, if weight loss may prevent the onset of OA, the loss of body fat is more closely related to symptomatic benefit than is the loss of body weight.[83] Local fat depots may play an important role in disease and symptoms genesis. Among these tissues, the synovium and infrapatellar fat pad seem to produce large amounts of adipokines.[84] Until recently, the fat pad, which is an extrasynovial but an intra-articular tissue, had been neglected. This adipose tissue, however, is able to release growth factors, cytokines, and adipokines.[57] Because obese individuals have higher concentrations of inflammatory markers, inflammation may contribute to functional limitation and disease progression in those with OA.[85] Besides direct effects on the joint, inflammatory mediators can affect muscle function and lower the pain threshold.

Another source of joint pain in OA may be from the nerves themselves. Following joint injury in which there is ligamentous rupture, the nerves that reinnervate the healing soft tissues contain an overabundance of algesic chemicals, such as substance P and calcitonin gene-related peptide. An interesting observation of these new nerves was that their overall morphology was abnormal with fibers appearing punctate and disorganized.[86,87] Because these phenomena are consistent with the innervation profiles described in nerve injury models, injured joints may develop neuropathic pain posttrauma. Indeed, treatment of inflamed joints with the neuropathic pain analgesic gabapentin can also relieve arthritis pain.[88]

INSIGHTS FROM IMAGING ON DISEASE PATHOGENESIS

Traditionally, measurement of OA structural change has been performed using radiographs. Standardized techniques for measuring joint space width in the medial tibiofemoral compartment, using standardized radiographic protocols, have become accepted for quantifying changes in knee OA.[89] Because of inherent limitations in conventional radiograph technology, further research and development has investigated other techniques that may improve the assessment of disease, its early development, and its progression. Foremost among these is MR imaging, a noninvasive three-dimensional method for assessing joint morphology that may supplant the widespread use of conventional radiographs in clinical trials.[90] Although MR imaging has enormous potential, recent studies provide a note of caution for its immediate ability to supersede the weight-bearing radiograph. The responsiveness of different measures of cartilage morphometry may not be as great as early data suggested.[7,91,92]

Because of limitations in the responsiveness of both radiographic and MR imaging measures of progression, efforts are being made to stratify those with the highest risk of progression. Several studies have suggested that baseline clinical, biomarker, and imaging features are predictive of progression of cartilage loss in the medial compartment of the knee and could be used to provide greater study power by selecting a population at greater risk for more rapid progression. These include increased body mass index,[93] an increased level of type II collagen C-terminal degradation products detected in the urine,[94] the presence of varus malalignment at the tibiofemoral joint,[95,96] the presence on MR imaging of subchondral bone marrow lesions,[97] or meniscal abnormalities.[71] A discussion of constructs identified on imaging studies that provide insights into factors that predispose to disease progression follows.

Alignment

Mechanical factors are the dominant risk factor for structural progression. Varus and valgus malalignment have been shown to increase the risk of subsequent medial and lateral knee OA radiographic progression, respectively.[95] Varus malalignment has been shown to lead to a fourfold amplification of focal medial knee OA progression, whereas valgus malalignment has been shown to predispose to a twofold to fivefold increase in lateral OA progression.[95,98] In an MR imaging–based study, varus malalignment predicted medial tibial cartilage volume and thickness loss, and tibial and femoral denuded bone increase, after adjusting for other local factors (meniscal damage and extrusion, laxity).[96] Understanding the role alignment plays in OA progression is important because it modulates the effect of standard risk factors for knee OA progression including obesity,[99] quadriceps strength,[100] laxity,[100] and stage of disease.[95,98]

Meniscal Damage

The absence of a functioning meniscus increases peak and average contact stresses in the medial compartment in a range of 40% to 700%.[63–65] Biswal and colleagues[69] studied 43 subjects and demonstrated that the 26 subjects who had sustained meniscal tears had a higher average rate of progression of cartilage loss (22%) than that seen in those who had intact menisci (14.9%; $P \leq .018$). Berthiaume and colleagues[70] investigated the relation between knee meniscus structural damage and cartilage degradation in 32 subjects and found similar effects. The author demonstrated a strong association of meniscal position and meniscal damage and cartilage loss[71] with the highest quartile of medial meniscal damage having an odds of medial progression of 6.3 (3.1–12.6). Each aspect of meniscal abnormality (whether change in position or damage) had a major effect on risk of cartilage loss.

Bone Marrow Lesions

Bone marrow lesions have also been found to be associated with compartment-specific OA cartilage progression measured semiquantitatively.[97,101] Medial tibiofemoral compartment bone marrow lesions occurred mostly in those with varus malalignment, and lateral tibiofemoral lesions in those with valgus limbs. Of 75 knees with medial lesions, 25 (36%) showed medial progression versus only 12 (8.1%) of 148 knees without lesions (odds ratio for progression = 6.5; 95% confidence interval, 3–14). A total of 69% of knees destined to progress medially had medial lesions. Lateral lesions conferred a similar marked risk of lateral progression. These increased risks were attenuated by 30% to 50% after adjusting for limb alignment. This demonstrates that bone marrow lesions are a potent risk factor for predicting progression in knee OA, and its relation to progression is explained, in part, by its association with limb alignment.

Stage of Disease

A recent longitudinal analysis demonstrated that by selecting persons with Kellgren and Lawrence grading system grade 3 at baseline this group demonstrated the greatest change in joint space width over 12 months.[102] A recent MR imaging study demonstrates that by selecting participants and regions with the presence of a full-thickness cartilage defect (denuded area) the ability to demonstrate change in cartilage loss in that plate was markedly improved. Before stratification the highest standardized response mean for any region was 0.35[91] and after stratification and selection of those with a denuded area this improved to 0.62.

Other Risk Factors or Profiling Indices

Synovitis is frequently present in OA and may correlate with pain and other clinical outcomes.[41,42] Although synovitis may play a role in mediating symptoms its role in predisposing to further structural progression seems limited,[42] so using this as a method for identifying those at high risk of progression is not optimal.

Among those with established knee OA, an estimated 20% to 35% have an incidental anterior cruciate ligament tear identified by MR imaging.[103] The effect of an incidental complete anterior cruciate ligament tear on the risk for cartilage loss seems to be mediated by concurrent meniscal pathology,[104] so using this as a method for identifying those at high risk of progression is not optimal.

SUMMARY

Recent studies, particularly those with an emphasis on MR imaging, are providing unique insights into the relation between structure identified on imaging and symptom and disease genesis. The traditional predominant focus of imaging studies and preclinical investigation is on hyaline cartilage. The subchondral bone, periosteum, periarticular ligaments, periarticular muscles, synovium, and joint capsule are all richly innervated, however, and are the likely source of nociception in OA. In addition, local tissue alterations in the bone, meniscus, and alignment of the lower extremity are important in terms of disease genesis.

Although imaging studies have provided many insights much remains unknown and uncertain. Imaging developments in OA are an important rate-limiting step to further therapeutic development. If and when structure-modifying agents are available their efficacy will need to be determined using appropriate structure constructs. Some of these fundamental questions include (1) What structural changes on MR imaging are consistent with the diagnosis of OA? (2) How does one define early disease on MR imaging? (3) What metrics of structural change (on either conventional radiograph or MR imaging) are most useful at different stages of disease and for clinical trial application? (4) What are the optimal platforms and sequences for specific structural features? It is hoped that over the years to come clinicians will develop answers to these questions and the field will move forward with these advances.

REFERENCES

1. Guccione AA, Felson DT, Anderson JJ, et al. The effects of specific medical conditions on the functional limitations of elders in the Framingham Study. Am J Public Health 1994;84:351–8.
2. Centers for Disease Control and Prevention (CDC). Arthritis prevalence and activity limitations—United States, 1990. MMWR Morb Mortal Wkly Rep 1994; 43:433–8.

3. Brandt KD, Dieppe P, Radin EL. Etiopathogenesis of osteoarthritis. Rheum Dis Clin North Am 2008; 34:531–59 [review].

4. Eyre DR. Collagens and cartilage matrix homeostasis. Clin Orthop Relat Res 2004;(Suppl 427):S118–22 [review].

5. Kellgren JH, Lawrence JS. Atlas of standard radiographs. Oxford: Blackwell Scientific; 1963.

6. Pessis E, Drape JL, Ravaud P, et al. Assessment of progression in knee osteoarthritis: results of a 1 year study comparing arthroscopy and MRI. Osteoarthritis Cartilage 2003;11:361–9.

7. Eckstein F, Burstein D, Link TM. Quantitative MRI of cartilage and bone: degenerative changes in osteoarthritis. NMR Biomed 2006;19:822–54 [review].

8. Karachalios T, Zibis A, Papanagiotou P, et al. MR imaging findings in early osteoarthritis of the knee. Eur J Radiol 2004;50:225–30.

9. Hunter DJ, Patil V, Niu JB, et al. The etiology of knee pain in the community. Arthritis Rheum 2004;50:1885.

10. Reichenbach S, Guermazi A, Niu J, et al. Prevalence of bone attrition on knee radiographs and MRI in a community-based cohort. Osteoarthr Cartil 2008;16:1005–10.

11. Amin S, LaValley MP, Guermazi A, et al. The relationship between cartilage loss on magnetic resonance imaging and radiographic progression in men and women with knee osteoarthritis. Arthritis Rheum 2005;52:3152–9.

12. Peat G, McCarney R, Croft P. Knee pain and osteoarthritis in older adults: a review of community burden and current use of primary health care. Ann Rheum Dis 2001;60:91–7.

13. Hunter D, Felson D. Osteoarthritis. BMJ 2006;332: 639–42 [review].

14. Lawrence RC, Helmick CG, Arnett FC, et al. Estimates of the prevalence of arthritis and selected musculoskeletal disorders in the United States. Arthritis Rheum 1998;41:778–99 [see comments].

15. Zhang Y, Niu J, Kelly-Hayes M, et al. Prevalence of symptomatic hand osteoarthritis and its impact on functional status among the elderly: The Framingham Study. Am J Epidemiol 2002;156:1021–7.

16. Cunningham LS, Kelsey JL. Epidemiology of musculoskeletal impairments and associated disability. Am J Public Health 1984;74:574–9.

17. Armstrong AL, Hunter JB, Davis TR. The prevalence of degenerative arthritis of the base of the thumb in post-menopausal women. J Hand Surg [Br] 1994;19:340–1.

18. Felson DT, Zhang Y. An update on the epidemiology of knee and hip osteoarthritis with a view to prevention. Arthritis Rheum 1998;41:1343–55 [review].

19. Nevitt MC, Xu L, Zhang Y, et al. Very low prevalence of hip osteoarthritis among Chinese elderly in Beijing, China, compared with whites in the United States: the Beijing Osteoarthritis Study. Arthritis Rheum 2002;46:1773–9.

20. Zhang Y, Hunter DJ, Nevitt MC, et al. Association of squatting with increased prevalence of radiographic tibiofemoral knee osteoarthritis: the Beijing Osteoarthritis Study. Arthritis Rheum 2004;50: 1187–92.

21. Badley E, DesMeules M. Arthritis in Canada: an ongoing challenge 2003. Ottawa (ON): Scientific Publication and Multimedia Services, Population and Public Health Branch, Health Canada. Report.

22. Felson DT. An update on the pathogenesis and epidemiology of osteoarthritis. Radiol Clin North Am 2004;42:1–9 [review].

23. Hannan MT, Felson DT, Pincus T. Analysis of the discordance between radiographic changes and knee pain in osteoarthritis of the knee. J Rheumatol 2000;27:1513–7.

24. Altman RD. Classification of disease: osteoarthritis. Semin Arthritis Rheum 1991;20:40–7 [review].

25. Cibere J. Do we need radiographs to diagnose osteoarthritis? Best Pract Res Clin Rheumatol 2006;20:27–38 [review].

26. Centers for Disease Control and Prevention (CDC). Prevalence of self-reported arthritis or chronic joint symptoms among adults—United States, 2001. MMWR Morb Mortal Wkly Rep 2002;51:948–50.

27. Fortin PR, Clarke AE, Joseph L, et al. Outcomes of total hip and knee replacement: preoperative functional status predicts outcomes at six months after surgery. Arthritis Rheum 1999;42:1722–8.

28. Harris WH. Etiology of osteoarthritis of the hip. Clin Orthop Relat Res 1986;20–33.

29. Solomon L. Patterns of osteoarthritis of the hip. J Bone Joint Surg Br 1976;58:176–83.

30. Eaton RG, Littler JW. Ligament reconstruction for the painful thumb carpometacarpal joint. J Bone Joint Surg Am 1973;55:1655–66.

31. Cooke KS, Singson RD, Glickel SZ, et al. Degenerative changes of the trapeziometacarpal joint: radiologic assessment. Skeletal Radiol 1995; 24(7):523–7.

32. Glickel SZ. Clinical assessment of the thumb trapeziometacarpal joint. Hand Clin 2001;17(2):185–95 [review].

33. Hunter DJ, Zhang Y, Sokolove J, et al. Trapeziometacarpal subluxation predisposes to incident trapeziometacarpal osteoarthritis (OA): the Framingham Study. Osteoarthritis Cartilage 2005;13:953–7.

34. Tan AL, Grainger AJ, Tanner SF, et al. High-resolution magnetic resonance imaging for the assessment of hand osteoarthritis. Arthritis Rheum 2005; 52:2355–65.

35. Nuki G. Osteoarthritis: a problem of joint failure. Z Rheumatol 1999;58:142–7 [review].

36. Dieppe PA, Lohmander LS. Pathogenesis and management of pain in osteoarthritis. Lancet 2005;365:965–73 [Review].

37. Hunter DJ, McDougall JJ, Keefe FJ. The symptoms of osteoarthritis and the genesis of pain. Rheum Dis Clin North Am 2008;34:623–43.

38. Felson DT, Chaisson CE, Hill CL, et al. The association of bone marrow lesions with pain in knee osteoarthritis. Ann Intern Med 2001;134:541–9.

39. Hunter D, Gale D, Grainger G, et al. The reliability of a new scoring system for knee osteoarthritis MRI and the validity of bone marrow lesion assessment: BLOKS (Boston Leeds Osteoarthritis Knee Score). Ann Rheum Dis 2008;67:206–11.

40. Torres L, Dunlop DD, Peterfy C, et al. The relationship between specific tissue lesions and pain severity in persons with knee osteoarthritis. Osteoarthritis Cartilage 2006;14:1033–40.

41. Hill CL, Gale DG, Chaisson CE, et al. Knee effusions, popliteal cysts, and synovial thickening: association with knee pain in osteoarthritis. J Rheumatol 2001;28:1330–7.

42. Hill CL, Hunter DJ, Niu J, et al. Synovitis detected on magnetic resonance imaging and its relation to pain and cartilage loss in knee osteoarthritis. Ann Rheum Dis 2007;66:1599–603.

43. Lo G, McAlindon T, Niu J, et al. Strong association of bone marrow lesions and effusion with pain in osteoarthritis. Arthritis Rheum 2008;56(9):S790 [abstract].

44. Felson D. The sources of pain in knee osteoarthritis. Curr Opin Rheumatol 2005;17:624–8 [review].

45. Hunter DJ, March L, Sambrook PN. The association of cartilage volume with knee pain. Osteoarthritis Cartilage 2003;11:725–9.

46. Moisio K, Eckstein F, Song J, et al. The relationship of denuded subchondral bone area to knee pain severity and incident frequent knee pain. Arthritis Rheum 2008;58(9):S237–8 [abstract].

47. Felson DT, Niu J, Guermazi A, et al. Correlation of the development of knee pain with enlarging bone marrow lesions on magnetic resonance imaging. Arthritis Rheum 2007;56:2986–92.

48. Link TM, Steinbach LS, Ghosh S, et al. Osteoarthritis: MR imaging findings in different stages of disease and correlation with clinical findings. Radiology 2003;226:373–81.

49. Kornaat PR, Bloem JL, Ceulemans RY, et al. Osteoarthritis of the knee: association between clinical features and MR imaging findings. Radiology 2006;239:811–7.

50. Cicuttini FM, Baker J, Hart DJ, et al. Association of pain with radiological changes in different compartments and views of the knee joint. Osteoarthritis Cartilage 1996;4:143–7.

51. Burr DB. The importance of subchondral bone in the progression of osteoarthritis. J Rheumatol Suppl 2004;70:77–80 [review].

52. Simkin P. Bone pain and pressure in osteoarthritic joints. Novartis Found Symp 2004;260:179–86 [review].

53. Arnoldi CC, Lemperg K, Linderholm H. Intraosseous hypertension and pain in the knee. J Bone Joint Surg Br 1975;57:360–3.

54. Arnoldi CC, Djurhuus JC, Heerfordt J, et al. Intraosseous phlebography, intraosseous pressure measurements and 99mTC-polyphosphate scintigraphy in patients with various painful conditions in the hip and knee. Acta Orthop Scand 1980;51:19–28.

55. Arnoldi CC. Vascular aspects of degenerative joint disorders: a synthesis. Acta Orthop Scand Suppl 1994;261:1–82 [review].

56. Roach HI, Aigner T, Soder S, et al. Pathobiology of osteoarthritis: pathomechanisms and potential therapeutic targets. Curr Drug Targets 2007;8:271–82 [Review].

57. Ushiyama T, Chano T, Inoue K, et al. Cytokine production in the infrapatellar fat pad: another source of cytokines in knee synovial fluids. Ann Rheum Dis 2003;62:108–12.

58. McDougall J. Arthritis and pain: neurogenic origin of joint pain. Arthritis Res Ther 2006;8:220 [review].

59. Fernandez-Madrid F, Karvonen RL, Teitge RA, et al. Synovial thickening detected by MR imaging in osteoarthritis of the knee confirmed by biopsy as synovitis. Magn Reson Imaging 1995;13:177–83.

60. Roemer F, Hunter D, Guermazi A, et al. Semiquantitative assessment of peripatellar synovitis in osteoarthritis: a comparative study of non-enhanced vs. contrast-enhanced MRI. Ann Rheum Dis, in press.

61. Seedhom BB, Dowson D, Wright V. Proceedings: functions of the menisci. A preliminary study. Ann Rheum Dis 1974;33:111.

62. Verstraete KL, Verdonk R, Lootens T, et al. Current status and imaging of allograft meniscal transplantation. Eur J Radiol 1997;26:16–22 [review].

63. Baratz ME, Fu FH, Mengato R. Meniscal tears: the effect of meniscectomy and of repair on intraarticular contact areas and stress in the human knee: a preliminary report. Am J Sports Med 1986;14(4):270–5.

64. Fukubayashi T, Kurosawa H. The contact area and pressure distribution pattern of the knee: a study of normal and osteoarthrotic knee joints. Acta Orthop Scand 1980;51(6):871–9.

65. Kurosawa H, Fukubayashi T, Nakajima H. Load-bearing mode of the knee joint: physical behavior of the knee joint with or without menisci. Clin Orthop Relat Res 1980;(149):283–90.

66. Tapper EM, Hoover NW. Late results after meniscectomy. J Bone Joint Surg Am 1969;51:517–26.

67. Johnson RJ, Kettelkamp DB, Clark W, et al. Factors effecting late results after meniscectomy. J Bone Joint Surg Am 1974;56:719–29.

68. Englund M, Roos EM, Lohmander LS. Impact of type of meniscal tear on radiographic and

symptomatic knee osteoarthritis: a sixteen-year followup of meniscectomy with matched controls. Arthritis Rheum 2003;48:2178–87.

69. Biswal S, Hastie T, Andriacchi TP, et al. Risk factors for progressive cartilage loss in the knee: a longitudinal magnetic resonance imaging study in forty-three patients. Arthritis Rheum 2002;46:2884–92.

70. Berthiaume MJ, Raynauld JP, Martel-Pelletier J, et al. Meniscal tear and extrusion are strongly associated with progression of symptomatic knee osteoarthritis as assessed by quantitative magnetic resonance imaging. Ann Rheum Dis 2005;64:556–63.

71. Hunter DJ, Zhang YQ, Niu JB, et al. The association of meniscal pathologic changes with cartilage loss in symptomatic knee osteoarthritis. Arthritis Rheum 2006;54:795–801.

72. Englund M, Guermazi A, Gale D, et al. Incidental meniscal findings on knee MRI in middle-aged and elderly persons. N Engl J Med 2008;359:1108–15.

73. Bhattacharyya T, Gale D, Dewire P, et al. The clinical importance of meniscal tears demonstrated by magnetic resonance imaging in osteoarthritis of the knee. J Bone Joint Surg Am 2003;85-A:4–9 [comment].

74. Englund M, Niu J, Guermazi A, et al. Effect of meniscal damage on the development of frequent knee pain, aching, or stiffness. Arthritis Rheum 2007;56:4048–54.

75. Englund M, Lohmander LS. Risk factors for symptomatic knee osteoarthritis fifteen to twenty-two years after meniscectomy. Arthritis Rheum 2004; 50:2811–9.

76. Hurley MV. The role of muscle weakness in the pathogenesis of osteoarthritis. Rheum Dis Clin North Am 1999;25:283–98 [review].

77. Sharma L, Cahue S, Song J, et al. Physical functioning over three years in knee osteoarthritis: role of psychosocial, local mechanical, and neuromuscular factors. Arthritis Rheum 2003;48:3359–70.

78. Roddy E, Zhang W, Doherty M, et al. Aerobic walking or strengthening exercise for osteoarthritis of the knee? A systematic review. Ann Rheum Dis 2005;64:544–8 [see comment] [review].

79. Roddy E, Zhang W, Doherty M, et al. Evidence-based recommendations for the role of exercise in the management of osteoarthritis of the hip or knee: the MOVE consensus. Rheumatology 2005; 44:67–73 [see comment] [review].

80. Coggon D, Reading I, Croft P, et al. Knee osteoarthritis and obesity. Int J Obes Relat Metab Disord 2001;25:622–7.

81. Cicuttini FM, Baker JR, Spector TD. The association of obesity with osteoarthritis of the hand and knee in women: a twin study. J Rheumatol 1996; 23:1221–6.

82. Sayer AA, Poole J, Cox V, et al. Weight from birth to 53 years: a longitudinal study of the influence on

clinical hand osteoarthritis. Arthritis Rheum 2003; 48:1030–3.

83. Toda Y, Toda T, Takemura S, et al. Change in body fat, but not body weight or metabolic correlates of obesity, is related to symptomatic relief of obese patients with knee osteoarthritis after a weight control program. J Rheumatol 1998;25:2181–6.

84. Presle N, Pottie P, Dumond H, et al. Differential distribution of adipokines between serum and synovial fluid in patients with osteoarthritis: contribution of joint tissues to their articular production. Osteoarthritis Cartilage 2006;14:690–5.

85. Spector TD, Hart DJ, Nandra D, et al. Low-level increases in serum C-reactive protein are present in early osteoarthritis of the knee and predict progressive disease. Arthritis Rheum 1997;40: 723–7.

86. McDougall JJ, Bray RC, Sharkey KA. Morphological and immunohistochemical examination of nerves in normal and injured collateral ligaments of rat, rabbit, and human knee joints. Anat Rec 1997;248:29–39.

87. McDougall JJ, Yeung G, Leonard CA, et al. A role for calcitonin gene-related peptide in rabbit knee joint ligament healing. Can J Physiol Pharmacol 2000;78:535–40.

88. Hanesch U, Pawlak M, McDougall JJ, et al. Gabapentin reduces the mechanosensitivity of fine afferent nerve fibres in normal and inflamed rat knee joints. Pain 2003;104:363–6.

89. Guermazi A, Burstein D, Conaghan P, et al. Imaging in osteoarthritis. Rheum Dis Clin North Am 2008;34:645–87 [review].

90. Eckstein F, Mosher T, Hunter D. Imaging of knee osteoarthritis: data beyond the beauty. Current opinion in rheumatology 2007;19:435–43 [review].

91. Hunter DJ, Niu J, Zhang Y, et al. Change in cartilage morphometry: a sample of the progression cohort of the Osteoarthritis Initiative. Ann Rheum Dis 2009;68(3):349–56.

92. Hunter D, Conaghan P, Peterfy C, et al. Responsiveness, effect size, and smallest detectable difference of magnetic resonance imaging in knee osteoarthritis. Osteoarthritis Cartilage 2006; 1(Suppl 14):112–5.

93. Felson DT. Obesity and osteoarthritis of the knee. Bull Rheum Dis 1992;41:6–7 [review].

94. Garnero P, Ayral X, Rousseau JC, et al. Uncoupling of type II collagen synthesis and degradation predicts progression of joint damage in patients with knee osteoarthritis. Arthritis Rheum 2002;46: 2613–24 [comment].

95. Sharma L, Song J, Felson DT, et al. The role of knee alignment in disease progression and functional decline in knee osteoarthritis. [erratum appears in JAMA 2001 Aug 15;286(7):792]. JAMA 2001;286: 188–95.

96. Sharma L, Eckstein F, Song J, et al. Relationship of meniscal damage, meniscal extrusion, malalignment, and joint laxity to subsequent cartilage loss in osteoarthritic knees. Arthritis Rheum 2008;58: 1716–26.

97. Felson DT, McLaughlin S, Goggins J, et al. Bone marrow edema and its relation to progression of knee osteoarthritis. Ann Intern Med 2003;139:330–6.

98. Cerejo R, Dunlop DD, Cahue S, et al. The influence of alignment on risk of knee osteoarthritis progression according to baseline stage of disease. Arthritis Rheum 2002;46:2632–6.

99. Sharma L, Lou C, Cahue S, et al. The mechanism of the effect of obesity in knee osteoarthritis: the mediating role of malalignment. Arthritis Rheum 2000; 43:568–75.

100. Sharma L, Dunlop DD, Cahue S, et al. Quadriceps strength and osteoarthritis progression in maligned and lax knees. Ann Intern Med 2003;138: 613–9 [see comment] [summary for patients in Ann Intern Med 2003 Apr 15;138(8):I1; PMID: 12693914].

101. Hunter D, Zhang Y, Niu J, et al. Increase in bone marrow lesions is associated with cartilage loss: a longitudinal MRI study in knee osteoarthritis. Arthritis Rheum 2006;54:1529–35.

102. Hellio Le Graverand MP, Vignon E, Brandt KD, et al. Head-to-head comparison of the Lyon-Schuss and fixed flexion radiographic techniques: long-term reproducibility in normal knees and sensitivity to change in osteoarthritic knees. Ann Rheum Dis 2008;67:1562–6.

103. Hill CL, Seo GS, Gale D, et al. Cruciate ligament integrity in osteoarthritis of the knee. Arthritis Rheum 2005;52:794–9.

104. Amin S, Guermazi A, LaValley M, et al. Complete anterior cruciate ligament tear and the risk for cartilage loss and progression of symptoms in men and women with knee osteoarthritis. Osteoarthritis Cartilage 2008;16:897–902.

Role of Alignment and Biomechanics in Osteoarthritis and Implications for Imaging

David J. Hunter, MBBS, FRACP, PhD[a],*, David R. Wilson, DPhil[b]

KEYWORDS

- Alignment • Biomechanics • Osteoarthritis
- Imaging • Knee

Osteoarthritis (OA) affects an estimated 21 million Americans,[1,2] and recent estimates suggest that symptomatic knee OA occurs in 13% of persons aged 60 and over.[1,3] The prevalence of hip OA is approximately 9% in white populations.[4] The risk for mobility disability (defined as needing help walking or climbing stairs) attributable to knee OA alone is greater than that due to any other medical condition in people aged 65 and over.[5,6] Although this prevalence is high, it is expected to increase even further with the increasing prevalence of obesity and the aging of the community.[7] Despite its frequency, OA is a condition that is poorly understood and, heretofore, a condition for which few safe and effective therapeutic options have been available.

OA is widely believed the result of local mechanical factors acting within the context of systemic susceptibility. Several studies have highlighted mechanical factors in the etiopathogenesis of this disease.[8–13] Knee alignment and the stance-phase adduction moment[14] are key determinants of the disproportionate medial transmission of load.[15]

This review focuses on the influence of biomechanics on the etiology of OA and on the imaging methods that may be used to quantify these forces. Although it is recognized that joint mechanics are critical in disease pathogenesis, and there are some tools that enable modeling joint mechanics, there is a need for further imaging method advances to allow critically evaluating the forces within the joint under more physiologic loading conditions and evaluating the impact of targeted therapeutics on them. This review focuses on measurements and steps that may facilitate movement toward the goal of improved understanding of joint mechanics.

ETIOPATHOGENESIS OF OSTEOARTHRITIS

OA is a significant public health challenge, ranked as the leading cause of disability in elders.[5] Recent estimates suggest that symptomatic knee OA occurs in 6% of adults 30 years of age or older[16] and 13% of persons 60 years of age and over.[3] The prevalence of OA is expected to increase as the United States population ages and the prevalence of obesity rises. By 2020, the number of people who have OA may double.[7,17]

OA occurs in joints when the dynamic equilibrium between the breakdown and repair of joint tissues becomes unbalanced.[18] This progressive joint failure may cause pain and disability,[6] although many persons who have structural changes consistent with OA are asymptomatic.[19]

[a] Division of Research, New England Baptist Hospital, 125 Parker Hill Avenue, Boston, MA 02120, USA
[b] Department of Orthopaedics, University of British Columbia and Vancouver Coastal Health Research Institute, Vancouver, BC V5Z 1L8, Canada
* Corresponding author. Division of Research, New England Baptist Hospital, 125 Parker Hill Avenue, Boston, MA 02120.
E-mail address: djhunter@caregroup.harvard.edu (D.J. Hunter).

Radiol Clin N Am 47 (2009) 553–566
doi:10.1016/j.rcl.2009.04.006
0033-8389/09/$ – see front matter © 2009 Elsevier Inc. All rights reserved.

OA can occur in any synovial joint in the body but is most common in the knees, hips, and hands.

THE ROLE OF MECHANICS IN THE ETIOLOGY OF KNEE OSTEOARTHRITIS

OA is perhaps best understood as resulting from excessive mechanical stress applied in the context of systemic susceptibility. Susceptibility to OA may be increased in part by genetic inheritance (a positive family history increases risk), age, ethnicity, nutritional factors, and female gender.[20]

The susceptibility to OA also can, in theory, be influenced by the mechanical environment. For example, the predilection for OA being more prevalent in women than men may be explained partly on the basis of the female knee being more mechanically vulnerable to OA. Quadriceps strength in men is greater than in women and this difference may play a role in reducing postural sway and improving joint stability.[21] The higher fat mass and lower muscle mass in women may explain some of the gender difference in OA susceptibility although this is conjectural and needs to be formally tested.[22] Other gender differences that have an impact on joint loading include pelvic dimensions, knee morphology, Q angle, and neuromuscular strength.[23] For instance, disproportionate loading of the lateral compartment in women likely arises from differences in knee stability/stiffness that is reduced in women as a result of decreased neuromuscular strength and increased ligamentous laxity.[23–25]

Local mechanical factors, such as the adduction moment, malalignment, and quadriceps strength, potentially make the knee joint vulnerable to the development and progression of OA.[26] Local mechanical factors also mediate the impact of more systemic factors, such as obesity on the knee.[27]

The human knee is a complex joint with considerable forces on the articular surfaces during weight bearing. The knee has three joint compartments: the patellofemoral (PF) and the medial and lateral tibiofemoral joints. The medial compartment is subjected to more stress than the lateral compartment, which may account, in part, for why OA affects the medial tibiofemoral compartment more often than the lateral compartment in men and women (75% of knee OA affects the medial compartment as opposed to 25% affecting the lateral compartment).[28]

In theory, any shift from a neutral or collinear alignment of the hip, knee, and ankle affects load distribution at the knee.[29] The load-bearing mechanical axis is traditionally represented on radiographs by a line drawn from the center of the femoral head to the center of the ankle talus.

In neutrally aligned limbs, this line passes through a midpoint between the tibial spines. The medial compartment bears a resultant 60% to 70% of the force across the neutrally aligned knee during weight bearing[14] and, because it is subjected to more load than the lateral compartment, this may play a role in the predisposition to medial tibiofemoral compartment progression in OA.[28] In a varus knee, this axis passes medial to the knee and a moment arm is created, which further increases force across the medial compartment. In contrast, in a valgus knee, the load-bearing axis passes lateral to the knee, and the resulting moment arm increases force across the lateral compartment.[29] The neutral full-limb (mechanical) alignment in those who do not have OA is approximately 1° varus and, as a result, by convention neutral is typically categorized as 0° to 2° varus.[30]

The acquisition and measurement of the mechanical axis of the knee is technically difficult and requires a full-limb radiograph, which is considered the gold-standard method for assessing knee alignment (Fig. 1). More recently, some studies have assessed anatomic alignment on short-film

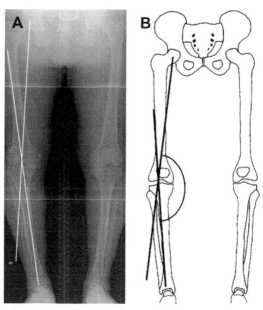

Fig. 1. Long limb film (A) and schematic (B) of varus malaligned right knee. Hip-knee-ankle alignment contributes to the load distribution across the knee articular surface by proportionally dividing load between the medial and lateral compartments. The load-bearing mechanical axis is traditionally represented on radiographs by a line drawn from the center of the femoral head to the center of the ankle talus. In a varus knee, this axis passes medial to the knee and a moment arm is created, which further increases force across the medial compartment.

radiographs centered at the knee (Fig. 2).[31] These measures on the short film do not capture proximal and distal anatomy but do avoid unwanted pelvic radiation, high cost, and specialized equipment. A study by Kraus and colleagues[31] demonstrated strong correlation between data obtained from full-limb measures of the mechanical axis and short-film measures of the anatomic axis. In this study, the anatomic axis was offset by a mean 4.21° valgus from the mechanical axis (3.5° in women, 6.4° in men). The high correlation in this study suggests that the more easily obtainable, standard knee films can be substituted for the more cumbersome full-length radiographs during the radiographic assessment of knee alignment.[32] Although these measures may correlate strongly there are differences, however, and optimal exploration of the relationship between knee alignment (mechanical axis) and OA should be pursued using measures of mechanical axis, which may afford greater precision.

EFFECT OF TIBIOFEMORAL MALALIGNMENT ON DISEASE PROGRESSION

Varus and valgus malalignment have been shown to increase the risk for, respectively, subsequent medial and lateral knee OA radiographic progression.[33] That is, in the presence of existing knee OA, abnormal alignment is associated with accelerated structural deterioration in the compartment subjected to abnormally increased compressive stress. Varus malalignment has been shown to lead to a fourfold amplification of focal medial knee OA progression, whereas valgus malalignment has been shown to predispose to a two- to fivefold increase in lateral OA progression.[33,34] In an MR imaging–based study, varus malalignment predicted medial tibial cartilage volume and thickness loss, and tibial and femoral denuded bone increase, after adjusting for other local factors (meniscal damage and extrusion and laxity).[35]

Malalignment has consequences beyond the direct effects on cartilage, including alteration in other knee-related tissues, such as bone marrow lesions, which further propagate OA disease.[36,37] These changes in the cartilage and other local tissues about the knee lead to further malalignment, and it is this vicious cycle that is the major determinant of the rate of structural progression in knee OA. Understanding the role alignment plays in OA etiopathogenesis is important because it modulates the effect of standard risk factors for knee OA progression, including obesity,[38] quadriceps strength,[39] laxity,[39] and stage of disease.[33,34]

IMPACT OF DYNAMIC MOMENTS ON DISEASE PROGRESSION

Malalignment provides only a static impression of the mechanical forces being imparted on the joint in one plane. To appropriately determine these forces in more than one plane requires 3-D analysis. During the stance phase of gait, the force acting at the foot during gait passes medial to the center of the knee joint in a normally aligned leg. The perpendicular distance from the line of action of this force and the center of the knee joint is the lever arm of this force about the joint center. This force combined with this lever arm produces a moment that tends to adduct the knee joint.[14] This moment can be substantial and provide a major contribution to the total loading across the knee joint, which usually is labeled the adduction (or external varus) moment at the knee.

The mean maximum magnitude of the adduction moment during normal gait is approximately 3.3% body weight times height[15] and is greater than either of the moments tending to flex or extend the knee. Studies of patients who have medial knee OA show that they have, on average, a higher adduction moment (4.2% body weight × height) than those who do not have OA.[15,40] This translates to a higher maximum reaction force on the medial compartment by 25% over normal values in those who have medial knee OA.[41,42]

Progressive varus alignment of the lower limb by medial joint space narrowing increases the perpendicular distance of the ground reaction force from

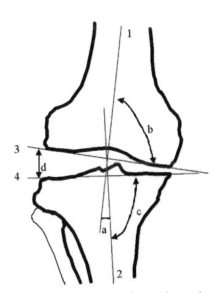

Fig. 2. Measures of alignment depicted on a short film of a typical varus knee. 1, femoral anatomic axis line; 2, tibial anatomic axis line; 3, condylar line; 4, tibial plateau line; a, anatomic axis angle; b, condylar angle; c, tibial plateau angle; d, condylar plateau angle.

the center of the knee joint and, as a result, is associated with an increase in the magnitude of the peak knee adduction moment.[41,42] Only 50% of knee adduction moment variability in subjects who have medial tibiofemoral OA is accounted for by the mechanical axis of the lower limb, however, emphasizing the need for dynamic evaluation of the knee joint loading environment.[42] The adduction moment also might be affected by habitual postures during locomotion or by more distal malalignments, such as tibial or calcaneal varum.

Higher maximum adduction moments at the knee are related to OA disease severity and to a higher rate of progression of knee OA.[41,43] Of the risk factors known to be associated with disease progression, the adduction moment is potentially the most potent that has been identified.[41] In addition to the effects this has on joint space it also seems strongly associated with remodeling in the subchondral bone as measured by bone mineral density.[40]

THE RELATIONSHIP BETWEEN MECHANICS AND KNEE SYMPTOMS

A full understanding of the risk factors for pain and other symptoms in knee OA requires consideration of a range of biopsychosocial factors.[44] The symptoms of knee OA typically are described as mechanical (ie, they occur with physical activity). Subjects who have the same degree of structural damage experience widely different levels of pain, however, a phenomenon that is poorly understood. Differences in joint forces and joint stress during functional activities may assist in explaining the dissociation between radiographic structural findings and pain. Malalignment previously has been shown to be a predictor for functional decline in knee OA and may play a role in the "mechanical" nature of OA-related pain.[33]

Knee OA may lead to adaptive strategies in gait to reduce the loading in an otherwise vulnerable joint.[42,45] These strategies include adopting a toe-out gait or slower walking speed. They can be reinforced or learned by appropriate rehabilitation and offer a potential for another conservative approach to knee OA therapy.

In addition to strategies adopted by patients, prescribed medication may alter knee loading. Commensurate with reductions in pain, nonsteroidal anti-inflammatory drugs (NSAIDs) also offer improvements in a person's walking speed.[46] Some of the increase in joint loading may be a direct consequence of faster walking speeds after the use of the NSAIDs, but previous analyses have also demonstrated increase in the adduction moment and quadriceps moment in persons who experienced pain relief with piroxicam.[47] Of particular concern is that anti-inflammatory or analgesic therapy may be associated with an increase in joint forces. Whether or not this is the mechanism that explains the potential for increased structural damage associated with NSAID use remains unclear.[48]

RELATION OF JOINT MECHANICS TO PATELLOFEMORAL OSTEOARTHRITIS

The PF joint transmits relatively high forces through relatively small contact areas. The PF joint reaction force (JRF) increases with increasing knee flexion. The JRF during walking (10°–15° of flexion) is approximately 50% of body weight. Walking up stairs (60°), the JRF is 3.3 times body weight. During squats (130°), the JRF is 7.8 times body weight.[49] It is, therefore, not surprising that the patella is involved in more than half of cases of symptomatic knee OA, with combined tibiofemoral and PF OA found in 41% of subjects and isolated PF disease found in 11% of subjects.[50]

Contemporary surgical and conservative treatment of PF OA is based, to a large extent, on Ficat's hypothesis that pain and cartilage degeneration occur when abnormal kinematics (lateral patellar tilt) produces excessive pressure on the lateral patellar facet.[51,52] Several studies have demonstrated that the relation of the patella with reference to the femur plays a critical role in determining the rate of disease progression and predisposing to symptoms in persons who have PF OA.[53–56] The patellar alignment measures are associated with markers of PF OA,[54] medial displacement and tilt of the patella are associated with medial PF compartment OA progression, and lateral displacement is associated with lateral PF compartment OA progression. The few studies that have explored PF OA show that the lateral PF compartment is affected more frequently than the medial.[57–59] Less directly, a radiographic study found that OA in the lateral PF compartment was associated with valgus malalignment, whereas medial OA was associated with varus malalignment.[57] The results were not entirely consistent, however. Approximately 25% of patients who had medial PF OA had valgus malalignment. These results suggest that anatomic variability between patients may influence PF load.

RELATION OF JOINT MECHANICS TO HIP OSTEOARTHRITIS

There is strong evidence that mechanical and structural changes around the hip are major etiologic factors in the development of OA.[60,61]

Childhood diseases, such as Legg-Perthes disease and slipped capital femoral epiphysis, predispose the hip to OA at a young age.[62–65] Acetabular dysplasia is well known as a major precursor of OA.[60,66] In patients who have acetabular dysplasia, overload of the acetabular rim is the pathomechanism that ultimately leads to OA.[67] These structural deformities can be corrected with a range of operative strategies, including pelvic and femoral osteotomies, in an effort to improve patient symptoms and delay OA progression.[68] It was originally assumed that 50% of hip OA was idiopathic (not associated with any obvious deformity).[69] More recent studies have found that 90% or more of hip OA cases can be attributed to anatomic abnormalities (discussed later).[60,61,70]

One of the most provocative new hypotheses in orthopedics is that femoroacetabular impingement (FAI) accounts for most cases of idiopathic hip OA.[71] This hypothesis has gained prominence over the past 5 years because of its many implications for prevention and treatment of OA. FAI describes repetitive abutment between the proximal femur and the acetabular rim due to abnormal hip morphology or excessive hip motion in patients who have no childhood history of hip pathology.[72,73] Patients, typically young (20s and 30s[74]), active adults, generally present with groin pain.[72] FAI is estimated to affect 10% to 15% of the general population,[75] suggesting that not all cases lead to OA.

The diagnosis of FAI currently is based on a history of groin pain, decreased range of motion on clinical examination, "impingement test" (pain elicited by combined flexion to 90°, adduction, and internal rotation), and radiographic evidence.[72] Several recent reviews have described the clinical examination process for FAI in detail with considerations of other potential overlapping diagnoses.[72,76,77] Recommendations include supplementing the standard impingement test with a complete examination of the affected limb and spine to rule out other sources of hip pain and performing a thorough examination of the lower abdominal musculature to rule out the possibility of a hernia.[77] A detailed systematic examination can identify the origin of pain in the hip and groin area.[78] Conventional radiographs often are used to assess the lack of femoral offset that characterizes FAI, but they may miss important abnormalities.[79] MR imaging can quantify the femoral neck "bump" in FAI.[80] A study using CT showed the value of 3-D reconstruction of the hip in understanding the morphologic deformities in cases of FAI.[81]

Recent evidence has demonstrated links between cartilage degeneration and the clinical symptoms and morphologic characteristics of FAI, but many questions about the association between FAI and cartilage degeneration remain. Two mechanisms by which the cartilage and labrum are affected by FAI have been described.[71,80,82,83] Cam impingement is a result of a nonspherical femoral head abutting against the acetabular rim in flexion and internal rotation (Fig. 3A). The abutment creates shear forces resulting in damage to the anterosuperior acetabular cartilage. Pincer impingement occurs as a result of

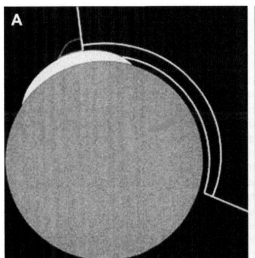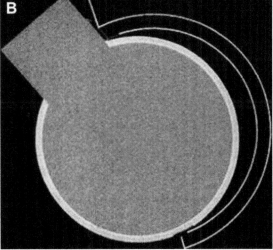

Fig. 3. Schematic illustrations of cam impingement (*A*) and pincer impingement (*B*). (*From* Ganz R, Parvizi J, Beck M, et al. Femoroacetabular impingement: a cause for osteoarthritis of the hip. Clin Orthop 2003;112–20; with permission.)

linear contact between the femoral head-neck junction and the acetabular rim (see **Fig. 3**B). Repeated abutment leads to degeneration of the labrum and circumferential cartilage damage. In a study of 149 hips with mild or no radiographic OA, patients who had radiologic features of cam impingement (26 hips) had damage to the antero-superior acetabular cartilage, whereas patients who had radiologic features of pincer impinge-ment (16 hips) had a narrow strip of circumferential cartilage damage.[84] Most patients had features of both mechanisms and showed a combination of these patterns of damage. Similar patterns of damage were confirmed in a recent arthrographic study of 50 patients who had cam or pincer impingement.[85] In 25 patients diagnosed with FAI (including cam and pincer mechanisms), histologic examination showed degeneration of the acetab-ular labrum and radiographic examination showed that most had mild to moderate OA.[86] A histologic study of cartilage taken from the femoral heads of 22 young patients diagnosed with FAI showed degenerative changes similar to those seen in OA.[87] A retrospective review of 117 patients who had FAI showed a high prevalence of juxta-artic-ular fibrocystic changes in the region close to the impingement site.[88] Positive impingement tests (hip pain produced by combined flexion, internal rotation and adduction) correlated with labral tears on magnetic resonance arthrograms, which corre-sponded to the location of impingement.[63] Major limitations of current understanding are that most of these studies have assessed only patients who have required surgery and that these assess-ments were made at a single time point (at surgery). It is not clear how many patients who have symptoms of FAI have cartilage changes, at what stage osteoarthritic changes begin in FAI, how they progress, and whether or not they can be prevented or reversed.

ROLE OF IMAGING IN ASSESSMENT OF JOINT BIOMECHANICS
What We Would Like to Measure and Why it Cannot be Done

There are several hypotheses about the links between mechanics and OA, and these hypoth-eses define the mechanical quantities of primary interest to researchers. Unfortunately, the most interesting quantities are among the most difficult to measure. Force on the joint surfaces is a key quantity in many hypotheses, but it can only be measured directly by implanting a measurement device into the joint, which is too interventional (in the case of the natural joint) for most in vivo studies of humans. Force distribution on the

cartilage surface is also widely believed important—a moderate force transmitted through a small contact area may produce local stresses that cause cartilage damage, whereas the same force transmitted through a large contact area would produce no cartilage injury. Although there are sensors available to measure force distribu-tion,[89] they also must be implanted, which carries the same limitations in vivo as direct measure-ments of force. Loading rate has been postulated to play a role in OA.[90] Assessing loading rate requires rapid measurements of force (typically every hundredth of a second or faster), which is considerably more challenging than static force measurements. There also is substantial interest in how force is transmitted through joint structures, such as cartilage and bone (stress). Measuring stress in simple machines and structures is a chal-lenge, and stress has not been measured in joints in vivo. Some approaches are emerging for measuring strain or deformation of the joint tissues in response to stress,[91] but the relationship between stress and strain is more complex in joint tissues than in, for example, steel, which makes it difficult to use strain measurements to predict stress. Kinematics (joint movement) is easier to measure and several methods for accurately quantifying joint kinematics in vivo have been developed in recent years. Kinematics describes how the bones that make up the joint move relative to each other, which can reflect where load is transmitted through the surfaces and the lines of action of structures that transmit forces. Kine-matics may have a more direct influence on oste-oarthritis, and relative velocity in the joint has been implicated in OA progression.[92]

Ex Vivo Studies and Joint Models

Current understanding of joint mechanics is founded on ex vivo studies, which are inappro-priate for linking mechanics with clinical symp-toms. In ex vivo studies, kinematics and contact mechanics have been measured in cadaver spec-imens loaded in mechanical rigs.[93–100] Although studies of this type have helped understanding of the biomechanics of healthy joints, their central limitation for studying OA is that morphologic adaptations due to the disease process or the healing process and mechanical links to clinical symptoms, such as pain, and ongoing processes, such as cartilage degeneration, cannot be studied in cadavers. An alternative, which avoids some of the limitations of mechanical measurements that can be made in vivo, is to predict joint mechanics using mathematical models. Models are limited primarily by the assumptions that must be made to formulate them. Models incorporating sophisticated descriptions of joint structures have been developed and validated[101–106] and used to answer specific clinically motivated questions.[107–110] Two primary limitations of mathematical models are that (1) many simplifying assumptions must be made about the properties of the joint, which limits their validity and applicability, and (2) like ex vivo studies, they are inappropriate for studying links with ongoing in vivo symptoms and processes, unless these changes are measured and incorporated into the model.

Radiographic Measures of Alignment

Most of the measures used clinically to quantify joint mechanics assess joint alignment. For example, tibiofemoral alignment often is quantified with the femorotibial angle or hip-knee-ankle angle.[111] A range of measures has emerged for quantifying PF alignment, with particular emphasis on medial-lateral position and patellar tilt. A central limitation of this approach is that the measures describe the joint (whose primary function is to move) at only one static position. In addition, although it is intuitive that these alignment measures are related to how load is transmitted in the joint, it is unclear how any given change in alignment measure would change force distribution in the joint. A further limitation is that the accuracy and repeatability of these measures is affected by their 2-D nature. 2-D radiographic measurements are prone to errors due to magnification and subject positioning. MR imaging and CT collect 3-D information about joint anatomy, which has been used in such applications as quantifying femoral neck deformities believed associated with hip OA.[80] In many cases, however, the 3-D data still are reduced to a 2-D measurement, which does not describe 3-D deformities adequately. This limitation is true for many measures, including patellar tilt, Q angle, anatomic alignment of the tibiofemoral joint, and the hip center-edge angle.

Gait Analysis

Gait analysis (often referred to more generally as motion analysis) is an important modality for estimating joint mechanics in activity. In motion analysis, movement of the joint segments is tracked with an optical, magnetic, or optoelectronic system and loads applied to the body (such as ground reaction forces) are measured. Mechanical analysis then can be used to assess the resultant forces and moments at the joints. The resultant forces and moments at the joints, which are output by the majority of commercial motion analysis systems, are entirely different from the contact forces in the joint. Determining contact forces requires the resultant forces and moments determined from motion analysis and further analysis using joint models.[112] The advantage of gait analysis is that movement is relatively unconstrained by the measurement system and, therefore, a large range of activities can be analyzed. One key limitation of gait analysis is that joint movement typically is measured with markers fixed to the skin, which move substantially relative to the bones and, therefore, can introduce substantial error. Large groups of skin-mounted markers has reduced the error due to skin movement.[113] A second key limitation is that the models and analysis required for determination of joint contact loads require many simplifications and assumptions, limiting the accuracy with which these can be measured. Typically, only general, rather than subject-specific, models are used, limiting the usefulness of these methods when pathologic joints are involved.

In Vivo Radiographic Measurement of Kinematics

Some of the limitations of motion analysis have been addressed with radiographic-based methods of measuring motion, including biplanar radiography and fluoroscopy. 3-D knee kinematics has been measured during activity in vivo using fluoroscopy and subsequent image processing. This has been done in joints after arthroplasty[114] and in normal joints.[115] A limitation of this approach is that measurement errors out of the imaging plane are large. The most accurate measurements of kinematics are made with biplanar radiography, which has been used to study kinematics in several joints.[116,117] Although many biplanar radiography studies are done with a series of static positions, recent work using high-speed biplanar radiography has made accurate measurements of kinematics during dynamic activity possible.[118] Because these measurements are so accurate, combining kinematics with known joint geometry yields predictions of joint contact interactions.[119] One key limitation of these approaches is that markers (typically small tantalum spheres) need to be implanted into the bones, an invasive procedure. A second key limitation is that these approaches expose patients to ionizing radiation, which always carries some risk and limits the number of repeat assessments that can be made.

MR Imaging Measurements of Kinematics

Several different approaches have been described using MR imaging to assess joint kinematics. They are distinguished from each other by whether or not they measure 2-D or 3-D movement, whether or not kinematics is measured when the joint is actively loaded, and whether or not the movement is measured continuously. Some 2-D measurements of patellar tracking have been made in loaded flexion, but these do not describe the movement of the patella completely because they are planar.[120,121] 2-D studies of the PF joint have shown that patterns of patellar tracking are different in loaded flexion as opposed to unloaded flexion,but found that patterns measured in very slow flexion are not different from those measured in rapid flexion.[121] The primary limitation of 2-D studies is that they neglect at least half of the movement— completely describing any joint's movement requires six quantities of movement (typically three rotations and three translations). Planar studies can measure a maximum of three quantities. One 3-D kinematic approach includes cine phase-contrast MR imaging[122–127] and fast phase-contrast MR imaging,[128] in which velocity information is extracted from MR imaging and used to measure 3-D tracking of the joint. Applications have focused on the knee. Although promising, these techniques have some limitations; most notably, subjects must flex their knees through many cycles, limiting the magnitude of load that can be applied and the applicability of the technique in symptomatic subjects. Subject interexamination variability ranges from 0.8° to 2.4° for fast phase-contrast MR imaging and 1.3° to 6.1° for cine phase-contrast MR imaging.[128] Another approach involves imaging the joint statically at several positions of loaded flexion. Although some variations of this method[129,130] have not quantified its accuracy in real knees, the accuracy and repeatability of other variations have been measured.[131–133] A limitation of this approach is that movement is not measured during continuous flexion. One of the limitations of all of these MR imaging–based approaches is that kinematics is measured when participants are supine in the confined cylindric bore of an MR imaging scanner. Some recent work has explored using open-configuration MR imaging scanners with a vertical gap, in which participants can stand and load their weight-bearing joints while being scanned.[134] Although this configuration provides a superior simulation of active weight bearing to that simulated in closed-bore scanners, open scanners have lower field strengths than standard closed-bore scanners, which limits the image quality that can be obtained.

MR Imaging Measurements of Contact Area

Several methods for assessing cartilage contact area from MR imaging in vivo have been described, although most methods have not yet been validated extensively. Contact area can be used to infer force distribution and some measurement approaches describe where contact occurs in the joint, which also may be relevant in OA. Although MR imaging has been used to measure contact area in animals, the applicability of measurements in cats[135] and dogs[136] to humans is difficult because of differences in geometry. In one study in humans, knees of healthy volunteers were imaged in a 1.5-T MR imaging scanner at several angles of flexion while they pressed against a weighted foot pedal to simulate standing load.[130] Area was assessed by constructing B-spline curves along the contact boundary of the PF joint in each slice and integrating across all of the slices to calculate area. A simplified version of this technique[137] defined cartilage contact with straight-line segments along the PF joint and then multiplied this contact length by the slice thickness, which was summed across all slices to determine total contact area. An in vitro validation study of this method using Fujifilm in cadavers[138] found an average measurement difference of 10.9% between the methods and no consistent directional difference between the MR imaging and pressure-sensitive film techniques. The same group has used the technique in other studies,[139,140] and a second group applied the method to standing volunteers in a 0.5-T open MR imaging scanner.[141,142] They validated their measurements using a phantom model with known contact areas and reported a coefficient of variation of 3%. In a study using a 0.2-T open MR imaging scanner to examine the knees of healthy volunteers at 30° and 90° of flexion while an external torque was applied distal to the knee joint, the coefficient of variation was less than 9% for contact areas in repeated scans.[143] Most approaches have focused on the PF joint; although contact areas in the elbow have been studied,[144] there is little work on the hip, shoulder, wrist, or the tibiofemoral joint (due in part to the presence of the meniscus). Most contact area measurement techniques have not been validated adequately with assessments of accuracy, which limits their usefulness.

THE WAY FORWARD

The OA community has been taking tools available in imaging tools and using them to try to image the joint. The most obvious impact has been on reliance on plain radiography to delineate the presence and severity of disease for OA.This also is true for much of the effort thus far in MR imaging, however, where the attention has been on applying MR imaging metrics used for other disease areas to OA. These are characteristically static images obtained in what often are not physiologically functional positions.

In addition, many of the tissues of the joint are unlike those of other organ systems in several inherent and important ways. For example, many MR imaging contrast mechanisms are dependent on the cellular/interstitial volume ratios; articular cartilage is almost acellular and, therefore, these contrast mechanisms may not be applicable to the study of cartilage. Furthermore, in most other systems, the function of the organ is that of cellular function (ie, cellular contraction, filtering, and electrical transmission); however, in the joint, the function of the tissues is biomechanical and generally provided by the characteristics of the extracellular matrix itself (although the cells are responsible for producing that matrix). As a result, many of the indices and contrast mechanisms that have been used for other body systems may not provide the information/contrast needed to study OA.

Although it is clear that malalignment is critical in determining disease progression, less is known of factors that contribute to alignment. Certain local factors within the joint, such as the tibiofemoral congruence (through bone and cartilage disease), anterior cruciate ligament integrity, and meniscal degeneration and position, seem to play a role in determining alignment. These same factors govern load distribution across the articular cartilage of a given joint.[145] Further elucidation of the factors that influence alignment may contribute to knowledge about OA pathophysiology and provide insight into therapeutic options.

Clinicians managing knee OA should make an effort, where possible, to influence modifiable risk factors. At present, there are several therapeutic options that can modify joint forces, including braces, wedges, and osteotomies for the knee and surgical correction of hip deformity associated with FAI syndrome. Through altering joint mechanics, the rate of disease progression may be altered. More importantly, there is substantial opportunity for further therapeutic development in this area, which, at present, needs imaging methods to quantify the impact these therapeutic advances have on joint mechanics.

Clearly biomechanics (by whatever measure or construct is used for quantifying) plays a critical role in the etiopathogenesis of OA. Unfortunately, the most interesting quantities are among the most difficult to measure. Although force, force distribution, and loading rate figure most prominently in mechanical hypotheses about OA, the methods to measure them in vivo are limited.

In order to improve the understanding of the relationship between biomechanics and OA and, more importantly, to develop, test, and disseminate therapies aimed at modifying biomechanics, the methods of acquisition currently available need to be improved, requiring a much-needed discourse between imaging manufacturers, imaging scientists, biomechanists, and OA clinical researchers to a new path.

SUMMARY

The pathogenesis of OA seems to be the result of a complex interplay between mechanical, cellular, and biochemical forces. Of these factors, mechanical forces are paramount. Extensive investigation of femorotibial alignment has demonstrated its pivotal role in knee OA progression. Understanding of the pivotal role of mechanical loading under physiologic and functional loading conditions is more limited, in part because of limitations in measurement technology. Greater attention to the role of mechanical factors in OA etiopathogenesis is required in order to find ways of reducing the public health impact of this condition. Therapies directed at unloading or reducing the forces in the knee are not used as frequently as they should be; there is substantial opportunity for further therapeutic development in this area and limitations in imaging methods to measure the impact of these interventions, need to be explored.

REFERENCES

1. Prevalence and impact of chronic joint symptoms—seven states, 1996. MMWR Morb Mortal Wkly Rep 1998;47:345–51.

2. Lawrence RC, Helmick CG, Arnett FC, et al. Estimates of the prevalence of arthritis and selected musculoskeletal disorders in the United States. Arthritis Rheum 1998;41:778–99.

3. Dunlop DD, Manheim LM, Song J, et al. Arthritis prevalence and activity limitations in older adults. Arthritis Rheum 2001;44:212–21.

4. Felson DT, Zhang Y. An update on the epidemiology of knee and hip osteoarthritis with a view to prevention. Arthritis Rheum 1998;41:1343–55.

5. Prevalence of disabilities and associated health conditions among adults—United States, 1999. MMWR Morb Mortal Wkly Rep 2001;50:120–5 [erratum appears in MMWR Morb Mortal Wkly Rep 2001 Mar 2;50(8):149].

6. Guccione AA, Felson DT, Anderson JJ, et al. The effects of specific medical conditions on the functional limitations of elders in the Framingham Study. Am J Public Health 1994;84:351–8.

7. Arthritis prevalence and activity limitations—United States, 1990. MMWR Morb Mortal Wkly Rep 1994; 43:433–8.

8. Kerin A, Patwari P, Kuettner K, et al. Molecular basis of osteoarthritis: biomechanical aspects. Cell Mol Life Sci 2002;59:27–35.

9. Jackson BD, Wluka AE, Teichtahl AJ, et al. Reviewing knee osteoarthritis—a biomechanical perspective. J Sci Med Sport 2004;7:347–57.

10. Teichtahl A, Wluka A, Cicuttini FM. Abnormal biomechanics: a precursor or result of knee osteoarthritis? Br J Sports Med 2003;37:289–90.

11. Carter DR, Beaupre GS, Wong M, et al. The mechanobiology of articular cartilage development and degeneration. Clin Orthop Relat Res 2004;(Suppl 427):S69–77.

12. Shakoor N, Moisio K. A biomechanical approach to musculoskeletal disease. Best Pract Res Clin Rheumatol 2004;18:173–86.

13. Andriacchi TP, Mundermann A, Smith RL, et al. A framework for the in vivo pathomechanics of osteoarthritis at the knee. Ann Biomed Eng 2004;32: 447–57.

14. Andriacchi TP. Dynamics of knee malalignment. Orthop Clin North Am 1994;25:395–403 [review] [28 refs].

15. Schipplein OD, Andriacchi TP. Interaction between active and passive knee stabilizers during level walking. J Orthop Res 1991;9:113–9.

16. Felson DT, Lawrence RC, Dieppe PA, et al. Osteoarthritis: new insights. Part 1: the disease and its risk factors. Ann Intern Med 2000;133:635–46.

17. Badley E, DesMeules M. Arthritis in Canada: an ongoing challenge. Ottawa, Canada: Scientific Publication and Multimedia Services, Population and Public Health Branch, Health Canada; 2003.

18. Eyre DR. Collagens and cartilage matrix homeostasis. Clin Orthop Relat Res 2004;(Suppl 427): S118–22.

19. Hannan MT, Felson DT, Pincus T. Analysis of the discordance between radiographic changes and knee pain in osteoarthritis of the knee. J Rheumatol 2000;27:1513–7.

20. Felson DT. An update on the pathogenesis and epidemiology of osteoarthritis. Radiol Clin North Am 2004;42:1–9.

21. Hassan BS, Doherty SA, Mockett S, et al. Effect of pain reduction on postural sway, proprioception, and quadriceps strength in subjects with knee osteoarthritis. Ann Rheum Dis 2002;61:422–8.

22. Madsen OR, Brot C, Petersen MM, et al. Body composition and muscle strength in women scheduled for a knee or hip replacement. A comparative study of two groups of osteoarthritic women. Clin Rheumatol 1997;16:39–44 [erratum appears in Clin Rheumatol 1997 Nov;16(6):640].

23. Huston LJ, Greenfield ML, Wojtys EM. Anterior cruciate ligament injuries in the female athlete. Potential risk factors. Clin Orthop Relat Res 2000; 372:50–63.

24. Hewett TE. Neuromuscular and hormonal factors associated with knee injuries in female athletes. Strategies for intervention. Sports Med 2000;29: 313–27.

25. Shelbourne KD, Davis TJ, Klootwyk TE. The relationship between intercondylar notch width of the femur and the incidence of anterior cruciate ligament tears. A prospective study. Am J Sports Med 1998;26:402–8.

26. Felson DT. Risk factors for osteoarthritis: understanding joint vulnerability. Clin Orthop Relat Res 2004;(Suppl 427):S16–21.

27. Felson DT, Goggins J, Niu J, et al. The effect of body weight on progression of knee osteoarthritis is dependent on alignment. Arthritis Rheum 2004;50:3904–9.

28. Ledingham J, Regan M, Jones A, et al. Radiographic patterns and associations of the knee in patients referred to hospital. Ann Rheum Dis 1993;52:520–6.

29. Tetsworth K, Paley D. Malalignment and degenerative arthropathy. Orthop Clin North Am 1994;25: 367–77.

30. Cooke TD, Sled EA, Scudamore RA. Frontal plane knee alignment: a call for standardized measurement. J Rheumatol 2007;34:1796–801.

31. Kraus VB, Vail TP, Worrell T, et al. A comparative assessment of alignment angle of the knee by radiographic and physical examination methods. Arthritis Rheum 2005;52:1730–5.

32. Hinman RS, May RL, Crossley KM, et al. Is there an alternative to the full-leg radiograph for determining knee joint alignment in osteoarthritis? Arthritis Rheum 2006;55:306–13.

33. Sharma L, Song J, Felson DT, et al. The role of knee alignment in disease progression and functional decline in knee osteoarthritis. JAMA 2001;286: 188–95 [erratum appears in JAMA 2001 Aug 15;286(7):792].

34. Cerejo R, Dunlop DD, Cahue S, et al. The influence of alignment on risk of knee osteoarthritis progression according to baseline stage of disease. Arthritis Rheum 2002;46:2632–6.

35. Sharma L, Eckstein F, Song J, et al. Relationship of meniscal damage, meniscal extrusion, malalignment, and joint laxity to subsequent cartilage loss in osteoarthritic knees. Arthritis Rheum 2008;58: 1716–26.

36. Felson DT, McLaughlin S, Goggins J, et al. Bone marrow edema and its relation to progression of knee osteoarthritis. Ann Intern Med 2003;139: 330–6.

37. Hunter D, Zhang Y, Niu J, et al. Increase in bone marrow lesions is associated with cartilage loss: a longitudinal MRI study in knee osteoarthritis. Arthritis Rheum 2006;54:1529–35.

38. Sharma L, Lou C, Cahue S, et al. The mechanism of the effect of obesity in knee osteoarthritis: the mediating role of malalignment. Arthritis Rheum 2000; 43:568–75.

39. Sharma L, Dunlop DD, Cahue S, et al. Quadriceps strength and osteoarthritis progression in maligned and lax knees. Ann Intern Med 2003;138: 613–9 [summary for patients in Ann Intern Med. 2003 Apr 15;138(8):I1; PMID: 12693914].

40. Wada M, Maezawa Y, Baba H, et al. Relationships among bone mineral densities, static alignment and dynamic load in patients with medial compartment knee osteoarthritis. Rheumatology 2001;40: 499–505.

41. Miyazaki T, Wada M, Kawahara H, et al. Dynamic load at baseline can predict radiographic disease progression in medial compartment knee osteoarthritis. Ann Rheum Dis 2002;61:617–22.

42. Hurwitz DE, Ryals AB, Case JP, et al. The knee adduction moment during gait in subjects with knee osteoarthritis is more closely correlated with static alignment than radiographic disease severity, toe out angle and pain. J Orthop Res 2002;20:101–7.

43. Sharma L, Hurwitz DE, Thonar EJ, et al. Knee adduction moment, serum hyaluronan level, and disease severity in medial tibiofemoral osteoarthritis. Arthritis Rheum 1998;41:1233–40.

44. Dieppe PA, Lohmander LS. Pathogenesis and management of pain in osteoarthritis. Lancet 2005;365:965–73.

45. Mundermann A, Dyrby CO, Hurwitz DE, et al. Potential strategies to reduce medial compartment loading in patients with knee osteoarthritis of varying severity: reduced walking speed. Arthritis Rheum 2004;50:1172–8 [erratum appears in Arthritis Rheum. 2004 Dec;50(12):4073].

46. Blin O, Pailhous J, Lafforgue P, et al. Quantitative analysis of walking in patients with knee osteoarthritis: a method of assessing the effectiveness of non-steroidal anti-inflammatory treatment. Ann Rheum Dis 1990;49:990–3.

47. Schnitzer TJ, Popovich JM, Andersson GB, et al. Effect of piroxicam on gait in patients with osteoarthritis of the knee. Arthritis Rheum 1993;36:1207–13.

48. Huskisson EC, Berry H, Gishen P, et al. Effects of antiinflammatory drugs on the progression of osteoarthritis of the knee. LINK Study Group. Longitudinal investigation of nonsteroidal antiinflammatory drugs in knee osteoarthritis. J Rheumatol 1995;22:1941–6.

49. Grelsamer RP, Weinstein CH. Applied biomechanics of the patella. Clin Orthop Relat Res 2001;389:9–14.

50. McAlindon T, Zhang Y, Hannan M, et al. Are risk factors for patellofemoral and tibiofemoral knee osteoarthritis different? J Rheumatol 1996;23:332–7.

51. Ficat RP, Hungerford DS. Disorders of the patellofemoral joint. Baltimore (MD): The Williams and Wilkins Co.; 1977.

52. Ficat P. [The syndrome of lateral hyperpressure of the patella]. Acta Orthop Belg 1978;44:65–76 [in French].

53. Kalichman L, Zhu Y, Zhang Y, et al. The association between patella alignment and knee pain and function: an MRI study in persons with symptomatic knee osteoarthritis. Osteoarthritis Cartilage 2007; 15:1235–40.

54. Kalichman L, Zhang YQ, Niu JB, et al. The association between patellar alignment on magnetic resonance imaging and radiographic manifestations of knee osteoarthritis. Arthritis Res Ther 2007;9(2):R26.

55. Hunter DJ, Zhang YQ, Niu JB, et al. Patella malalignment, pain and patellofemoral progression: the Health ABC Study. Osteoarthritis Cartilage 2007;15:1120–7.

56. Niu J, Zhang YQ, Nevitt M, et al. Patellar malalignment and knee pain among subjects with no radiographic knee osteoarthritis: The Beijing Osteoarthritis Study [abstract]. Arthritis Rheum 2005;52:S455–1191.

57. Elahi S, Cahue S, Felson DT, et al. The association between varus-valgus alignment and patellofemoral osteoarthritis. Arthritis Rheum 2000;43: 1874–80.

58. Harrison MM, Cooke TD, Fisher SB, et al. Patterns of knee arthrosis and patellar subluxation. Clin Orthop Relat Res 1994;309:56–63.

59. Iwano T, Kurosawa H, Tokuyama H, et al. Roentgenographic and clinical findings of patellofemoral osteoarthrosis. With special reference to its relationship to femorotibial osteoarthrosis and etiologic factors. Clin Orthop Relat Res 1990;252:190–7.

60. Harris WH. Etiology of osteoarthritis of the hip. Clin Orthop Relat Res 1986;213:20–33.

61. Tanzer M, Noiseux N. Osseous abnormalities and early osteoarthritis: the role of hip impingement. Clin Orthop Relat Res 2004;429:170–7.

62. Goodman DA, Feighan JE, Smith AD, et al. Subclinical slipped capital femoral epiphysis. Relationship to osteoarthrosis of the hip. J Bone Joint Surg Am 1997;79:1489–97 [erratum appears in J Bone Joint Surg Am 1999 Apr;81(4):592].

63. Leunig M, Werlen S, Ungersbock A, et al. Evaluation of the acetabular labrum by MR arthrography. J Bone Joint Surg Br 1997;79:230–4 [erratum appears in J Bone Joint Surg Br 1997 Jul;79(4): 693].

64. Rab GT. The geometry of slipped capital femoral epiphysis: implications for movement, impingement, and corrective osteotomy. J Pediatr Orthop 1999;19:419–24.

65. Snow SW, Keret D, Scarangella S, et al. Anterior impingement of the femoral head: a late

phenomenon of Legg-Calve-Perthes' disease. J Pediatr Orthop 1993;13:286–9.

66. Cooperman DR, Wallensten R, Stulberg SD. Acetabular dysplasia in the adult. Clin Orthop Relat Res 1983;175:79–85.

67. Klaue K, Durnin CW, Ganz R. The acetabular rim syndrome. A clinical presentation of dysplasia of the hip. J Bone Joint Surg Br 1991;73:423–9.

68. Millis MB, Kim YJ. Rationale of osteotomy and related procedures for hip preservation: a review. Clin Orthop Relat Res 2002;405:108–21.

69. Lloyd-Roberts GC. Osteoarthritis. J Bone Joint Surg Br 1955;37:8–47.

70. Solomon L. Patterns of osteoarthritis of the hip. J Bone Joint Surg Br 1976;58:176–83.

71. Ganz R, Parvizi J, Beck M, et al. Femoroacetabular impingement: a cause for osteoarthritis of the hip. Clin Orthop Relat Res 2003;417:112–20.

72. Crawford JR, Villar RN. Current concepts in the management of femoroacetabular impingement. J Bone Joint Surg Br 2005;87:1459–62.

73. Lavigne M, Parvizi J, Beck M, et al. Anterior femoroacetabular impingement: part I. Techniques of joint preserving surgery. Clin Orthop Relat Res 2004;418:61–6.

74. Sampson TG. Arthroscopic treatment of femoroacetabular impingement: a proposed technique with clinical experience. Instr Course Lect 2006; 55:337–46.

75. Leunig M, Beck M, Dora C, et al. [Femoroacetabular impingement: trigger for the development of coxarthrosis]. Orthopade 2006;35:77–84.

76. Beall DP, Sweet CF, Martin HD, et al. Imaging findings of femoroacetabular impingement syndrome. Skeletal Radiol 2005;34:691–701.

77. Guanche CA, Bare AA. Arthroscopic treatment of femoroacetabular impingement. Arthroscopy 2006;22:95–106.

78. Holmich P, Dienst M. [Differential diagnosis of hip and groin pain. Symptoms and technique for physical examination]. Orthopade 2006;35:8, 10–5 [in German].

79. Meyer DC, Beck M, Ellis T, et al. Comparison of six radiographic projections to assess femoral head/neck asphericity. Clin Orthop Relat Res 2006;445: 181–5.

80. Ito K, Minka MA, Leunig M, et al. Femoroacetabular impingement and the cam-effect. A MRI-based quantitative anatomical study of the femoral head-neck offset. J Bone Joint Surg Br 2001;83: 171–6.

81. Beaule PE, Zaragoza E, Motamedi K, et al. Three-dimensional computed tomography of the hip in the assessment of femoroacetabular impingement. J Orthop Res 2005;23:1286–92.

82. Leunig M, Casillas MM, Hamlet M, et al. Slipped capital femoral epiphysis: early mechanical damage to the acetabular cartilage by a prominent femoral metaphysis. Acta Orthop Scand 2000;71:370–5.

83. Leunig M, Beck M, Woo A, et al. Acetabular rim degeneration: a constant finding in the aged hip. Clin Orthop Relat Res 2003;413:201–7.

84. Beck M, Kalhor M, Leunig M, et al. Hip morphology influences the pattern of damage to the acetabular cartilage: femoroacetabular impingement as a cause of early osteoarthritis of the hip. J Bone Joint Surg Br 2005;87:1012–8.

85. Pfirrmann CW, Mengiardi B, Dora C, et al. Cam and pincer femoroacetabular impingement: characteristic MR arthrographic findings in 50 patients. Radiology 2006;240:778–85 [erratum appears in Radiology. 2007 Aug;244(2):626].

86. Ito K, Leunig M, Ganz R. Histopathologic features of the acetabular labrum in femoroacetabular impingement. Clin Orthop Relat Res 2004;429: 262–71.

87. Wagner S, Hofstetter W, Chiquet M, et al. Early osteoarthritic changes of human femoral head cartilage subsequent to femoro-acetabular impingement. Osteoarthritis Cartilage 2003;11:508–18.

88. Leunig M, Beck M, Kalhor M, et al. Fibrocystic changes at anterosuperior femoral neck: prevalence in hips with femoroacetabular impingement. Radiology 2005;236:237–46.

89. Wilson DR, Apreleva MV, Eichler MJ, et al. Accuracy and repeatability of a pressure measurement system in the patellofemoral joint. J Biomech 2003;36:1909–15.

90. Radin EL, Ehrlich MG, Chernack R, et al. Effect of repetitive impulsive loading on the knee joints of rabbits. Clin Orthop Relat Res 1978;131:288–93.

91. Song Y, Greve JM, Carter DR, et al. Articular cartilage MR imaging and thickness mapping of a loaded knee joint before and after meniscectomy. Osteoarthritis Cartilage 2006;14:728–37.

92. Andherst W, Tashman S. The association between velocity of the center of closest proximity on subchondral bones and osteoarthritis progression. J Orthop Res 2009;27:71–7.

93. Ahmed AM, Burke DL, Yu A. In-vitro measurement of static pressure distribution in synovial joints–part II: retropatellar surface. J Biomech Eng 1983;105: 226–36.

94. Ahmed AM, Duncan NA, Tanzer M. In vitro measurement of the tracking pattern of the human patella. J Biomech Eng 1999;121:222–8.

95. Ahmed AM, Duncan NA. Correlation of patellar tracking pattern with trochlear and retropatellar surface topographies. J Biomech Eng 2000;122: 652–60.

96. Huberti HH, Hayes WC. Patellofemoral contact pressures. The influence of q-angle and tendofemoral contact. J Bone Joint Surg Am 1984;66: 715–24.

97. Huberti HH, Hayes WC. Contact pressures in chondromalacia patellae and the effects of capsular reconstructive procedures. J Orthop Res 1988;6: 499–508.

98. Ateshian GA, Kwak SD, Soslowsky LJ, et al. A stereophotogrammetric method for determining in situ contact areas in diarthrodial joints, and a comparison with other methods. J Biomech 1994;27:111–24.

99. Brown TD, Shaw DT. In vitro contact stress distributions in the natural human hip. J Biomech 1983;16: 373–84.

100. Apreleva M, Hasselman CT, Debski RE, et al. A dynamic analysis of glenohumeral motion after simulated capsulolabral injury. A cadaver model. J Bone Joint Surg Am 1998;80:474–80.

101. Blankevoort L, Kuiper JH, Huiskes R, et al. Articular contact in a three-dimensional model of the knee. J Biomech 1991;24:1019–31.

102. Blankevoort L, Huiskes R. Validation of a three-dimensional model of the knee. J Biomech 1996; 29:955–61.

103. Elias JJ, Wilson DR, Adamson R, et al. Evaluation of a computational model used to predict the patellofemoral contact pressure distribution. J Biomech 2004;37:295–302.

104. Wismans J, Veldpaus F, Janssen J, et al. A three-dimensional mathematical model of the knee-joint. J Biomech 1980;13:677–85.

105. van der Helm FC. A finite element musculoskeletal model of the shoulder mechanism. J Biomech 1994;27:551–69.

106. Brown TD, DiGioia AM III. A contact-coupled finite element analysis of the natural adult hip. J Biomech 1984;17:437–48.

107. Ahmad CS, Kwak SD, Ateshian GA, et al. Effects of patellar tendon adhesion to the anterior tibia on knee mechanics. Am J Sports Med 1998;26:715–24.

108. Kwak SD, Ahmad CS, Gardner TR, et al. Hamstrings and iliotibial band forces affect knee kinematics and contact pattern. J Orthop Res 2000;18:101–8.

109. Cohen ZA, Roglic H, Grelsamer RP, et al. Patellofemoral stresses during open and closed kinetic chain exercises. An analysis using computer simulation. Am J Sports Med 2001;29:480–7.

110. Cohen ZA, Henry JH, McCarthy DM, et al. Computer simulations of patellofemoral joint surgery. Patient-specific models for tuberosity transfer. Am J Sports Med 2003;31:87–98.

111. Kanamiya T, Naito M, Hara M, et al. The influences of biomechanical factors on cartilage regeneration after high tibial osteotomy for knees with medial compartment osteoarthritis: clinical and arthroscopic observations. Arthroscopy 2002;18:725–9.

112. Morrison JB. The mechanics of the knee joint in relation to normal walking. J Biomech 1970;3: 51–61.

113. Andriacchi TP, Alexander EJ, Toney MK, et al. A point cluster method for in vivo motion analysis: applied to a study of knee kinematics. J Biomech Eng 1998;120:743–9.

114. Delport HP, Banks SA, De SJ, et al. A kinematic comparison of fixed- and mobile-bearing knee replacements. J Bone Joint Surg Br 2006;88: 1016–21.

115. Komistek RD, Dennis DA, Mahfouz M. In vivo fluoroscopic analysis of the normal human knee. Clin Orthop Relat Res 2003;410:69–81.

116. Karrholm J, Brandsson S, Freeman MA. Tibiofemoral movement 4: changes of axial tibial rotation caused by forced rotation at the weight-bearing knee studied by RSA. J Bone Joint Surg Br 2000; 82:1201–3.

117. Fleming BC, Peura GD, Abate JA, et al. Accuracy and repeatability of Roentgen stereophotogrammetric analysis (RSA) for measuring knee laxity in longitudinal studies. J Biomech 2001;34:1355–9.

118. You BM, Siy P, Anderst W, et al. In vivo measurement of 3-D skeletal kinematics from sequences of biplane radiographs: application to knee kinematics. IEEE Trans Med Imaging 2001;20:514–25.

119. Anderst WJ, Tashman S. A method to estimate in vivo dynamic articular surface interaction. J Biomech 2003;36:1291–9.

120. Powers CM, Ward SR, Fredericson M, et al. Patellofemoral kinematics during weight-bearing and non-weight-bearing knee extension in persons with lateral subluxation of the patella: a preliminary study. J Orthop Sports Phys Ther 2003;33:677–85.

121. Muhle C, Brossmann J, Heller M. Kinematic CT and MR imaging of the patellofemoral joint. Eur Radiol 1999;9:508–18.

122. Sheehan FT, Zajac FE, Drace JE. Using cine phase contrast magnetic resonance imaging to non-invasively study in vivo knee dynamics. J Biomech 1998;31:21–6.

123. Sheehan FT, Zajac FE, Drace JE. In vivo tracking of the human patella using cine phase contrast magnetic resonance imaging. J Biomech Eng 1999;121:650–6.

124. Sheehan FT, Drace JE. Quantitative MR measures of three-dimensional patellar kinematics as a research and diagnostic tool. Med Sci Sports Exerc 1999;31:1399–405.

125. Barrance PJ, Williams GN, Novotny JE, et al. A method for measurement of joint kinematics in vivo by registration of 3-D geometric models with cine phase contrast magnetic resonance imaging data. J Biomech Eng 2005;127:829–37.

126. Barrance PJ, Williams GN, Snyder-Mackler L, et al. Altered knee kinematics in ACL-deficient non-copers: a comparison using dynamic MRI. J Orthop Res 2006;24:132–40.

127. Barrance PJ, Williams GN, Snyder-Mackler L, et al. Do ACL-injured copers exhibit differences in knee kinematics? An MRI study. Clin Orthop Relat Res 2007;454:74–80.

128. Rebmann AJ, Sheehan FT. Precise 3D skeletal kinematics using fast phase contrast magnetic resonance imaging. J Magn Reson Imaging 2003; 17:206–13.

129. Patel VV, Hall K, Ries M, et al. A three-dimensional MRI analysis of knee kinematics. J Orthop Res 2004;22:283–92.

130. Patel VV, Hall K, Ries M, et al. Magnetic resonance imaging of patellofemoral kinematics with weight-bearing. J Bone Joint Surg Am 2003;85: 2419–24.

131. Fellows RA, Hill NA, Macintyre NJ, et al. Repeatability of a novel technique for in vivo measurement of three-dimensional patellar tracking using magnetic resonance imaging. J Magn Reson Imaging 2005;22:145–53.

132. Fellows RA, Hill NA, Gill HS, et al. Magnetic resonance imaging for in vivo assessment of three-dimensional patellar tracking. J Biomech 2005;38: 1643–52.

133. Lerner AL, Tamez-Pena JG, Houck JR, et al. The use of sequential MR image sets for determining tibiofemoral motion: reliability of coordinate systems and accuracy of motion tracking algorithm. J Biomech Eng 2003;125:246–53.

134. McWalter E, Wilson D, Kacher D, et al. Three dimensional patellar kinematics in weightbearing flexion. Institut fur Biotechnik, Germany: World Congress of Biomechanics; 2006.

135. Ronsky JL, Herzog W, Brown TD, et al. In vivo quantification of the cat patellofemoral joint contact stresses and areas. J Biomech 1995;28:977–83.

136. Tashman S, Anderst W. In-vivo measurement of dynamic joint motion using high speed biplane radiography and CT: application to canine ACL deficiency. J Biomech Eng 2003;125:238–45.

137. Brechter JH, Powers CM. Patellofemoral joint stress during stair ascent and descent in persons with and without patellofemoral pain. Gait Posture 2002;16:115–23.

138. Heino BJ, Powers CM, Terk MR, et al. Quantification of patellofemoral joint contact area using magnetic resonance imaging. Magn Reson Imaging 2003;21:955–9.

139. Powers CM, Ward SR, Chan LD, et al. The effect of bracing on patella alignment and patellofemoral joint contact area. Med Sci Sports Exerc 2004;36: 1226–32.

140. Salsich GB, Ward SR, Terk MR, et al. In vivo assessment of patellofemoral joint contact area in individuals who are pain free. Clin Orthop Relat Res 2003;417:277–84.

141. Gold GE, Besier TF, Draper CE, et al. Weight-bearing MRI of patellofemoral joint cartilage contact area. J Magn Reson Imaging 2004;20:526–30.

142. Besier TF, Draper CE, Gold GE, et al. Patellofemoral joint contact area increases with knee flexion and weight-bearing. J Orthop Res 2005;23: 345–50.

143. von Eisenhart-Rothe R, Siebert M, Bringmann C, et al. A new in vivo technique for determination of 3D kinematics and contact areas of the patellofemoral and tibio-femoral joint. J Biomech 2004; 37:927–34.

144. Goto A, Moritomo H, Murase T, et al. In vivo elbow biomechanical analysis during flexion: three-dimensional motion analysis using magnetic resonance imaging. J Shoulder Elbow Surg 2004;13:441–7.

145. Hunter DJ, Zhang Y, Niu J, et al. Structural factors associated with malalignment in knee osteoarthritis: the Boston osteoarthritis knee study. J Rheumatol 2005;32:2192–9.

Radiographic-Based Grading Methods and Radiographic Measurement of Joint Space Width in Osteoarthritis

Marie-Pierre Hellio Le Graverand, MD, DSc, PhD[a],*,
Steve Mazzuca, PhD[b], Jeff Duryea, PhD[c], Alan Brett, PhD[d]

KEYWORDS
- Radiograph • Joint space width
- Joint space narrowing • Osteoarthritis

Osteoarthritis (OA) is the most common and costly form of arthritis. The disease is a slowly progressive, ultimately degenerative disorder confined to movable joints. OA occurs when the equilibrium between breakdown and repair of the joint tissues becomes unbalanced. Clinically, OA is mainly characterized by joint pain and functional limitation; however, many subjects with definite structural changes consistent with OA are asymptomatic.

OA remains a condition that is poorly understood and for which few effective therapeutic options are available. Modifying structural progression has become a focus of drug development in OA. Therapeutic development is constrained, however, by its heterogeneous clinical manifestations, the unclear relationship between structural progression and clinical endpoints, and the need for long-term follow-up to observe changes in structure. Therefore, accurate and highly reproducible measurements of the rate of progression is a prerequisite for assessing structural change for clinical trials and subsequently for patients in clinical practice.

Traditionally, measurement of OA structural change has been performed using radiographs. Conventional radiography is the simplest and least expensive method for imaging joints affected by OA. Radiography is used in clinical practice in patients to establish the diagnosis of OA and to monitor the progression of the disease. Radiographs clearly visualize bony features, including marginal osteophytes, subchondral sclerosis, and subchondral cysts that are associated with OA and provide an estimate of cartilage thickness and meniscal integrity by the interbone distance or joint space width (JSW). The radiographic definition of OA mainly relies on the evaluation of both osteophytes and joint space narrowing (JSN) (ie, the loss of JSW). Because osteophytes are considered specific to OA, develop at an earlier stage than JSN, are more correlated with knee pain, and are easier to ascertain than other radiographic features, they represent the widely applied criterion to define the presence of OA.[1–3] However, assessment of OA severity mainly relies on JSN and subchondral bone lesions. In addition,

[a] Clinical Development and Medical Affairs, Inflammation, Specialty Care Business Unit, Pfizer Inc., 50 Pequot Avenue, New London, CT 06320, USA
[b] Indiana University School of Medicine, Indianapolis, IN, USA
[c] Brigham and Women's Hospital, Harvard Medical School, Boston, MA, USA
[d] Optasia Medical, Manchester, UK
* Corresponding author.
E-mail address: helliomp@pfizer.com (M.P. Hellio Le Graverand).

Radiol Clin N Am 47 (2009) 567–579
doi:10.1016/j.rcl.2009.04.004

progression of JSN is the most commonly used criterion for the assessment of OA progression and the complete loss of JSW, characterized by bone-on-bone contact, is one of the factors considered in the decision for joint replacement.

The severity of OA can be estimated using semi-quantitative scoring systems. Published atlases provide images that represent specific grades.[4,5] Several grading scales incorporating combinations of features also have been developed, including the most widely employed Kellgren and Lawrence grade (KLG) classification.[6] The KLG scoring system suffers from limitations based on the invalid assumptions that changes in radiographic features (eg, osteophytes, JSN) are linear over the course of the disease and that the relationship between these features is constant. In contrast, the Osteoarthritis Research Society International (OARSI) atlas classification grades separately the tibiofemoral JSN and osteophytes in each compartment of the knee.[4]

Current clinical research tends to focus on knee OA due to the prevalence of the disease in this joint; therefore, this review focuses on the assessment of OA in the femorotibial compartment of the knee. Traditionally, the progression of knee OA in clinical trials has been assessed by measuring changes in JSW between the medial femoral condyle and medial tibial plateau on plain radiographs,[7] as the medial femorotibial compartment is the most common site of involvement in knee OA. Both a reduction in cartilage thickness and meniscal integrity are inferred from a reduction in JSW.[7–9]

RADIOANATOMIC ALIGNMENT OF THE TIBIOFEMORAL JOINT

The *sine qua non* for accurate measurement of radiographic JSW is a reproducible image of the joint space. A reproducible radiographic image of the tibiofemoral joint space requires adherence to exacting standards of positioning of the knee, which include specifications for flexion and rotation of the joint, and angulation of the x-ray beam.[10] In a majority of patients, the anatomy of the knee is such that full extension of the joint (as is required for a conventional weight-bearing extended-knee radiograph) tilts the tibial plateau to an angle that is skew (ie, not parallel) to a horizontally directed x-ray beam (Fig. 1).[11] Skewed radioanatomic alignment of the tibial plateau in an anteroposterior (AP) or posteroanterior (PA) knee radiograph is apparent in the displacement of the anterior and posterior margins of the medial plateau (Fig. 2). Reproducibility of positioning notwithstanding, when the alignment of the

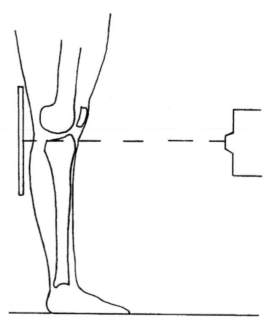

Fig. 1. Positioning for the conventional extended-knee radiograph.

plateau is notably skewed, the floor of the joint space can become indistinct, and a key reference point for the measurement of minimum JSW (minJSW) (ie, the shortest distance between femoral condyle and tibial plateau) is less reliably ascertained.

In their groundbreaking work on standardized knee radiography, Buckland-Wright and colleagues[12] demonstrated that individualized

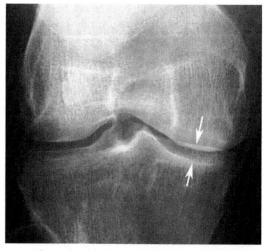

Fig. 2. Skewed radioanatomic alignment of the medial tibial plateau alignment, apparent in the displacement of anterior and posterior margins of the plateau (*arrows*).

flexion of the knee to achieve superimposition ($\pm$1 mm) of the anterior and posterior margins of the medial tibial plateau (Fig. 3) that was confirmed under fluoroscopy before image acquisition resulted in measurements of medial tibiofemoral JSW in repeat AP radiographs that were significantly more reproducible than those obtained from concurrent extended-knee radiographs. Since then, so-called "parallel radioanatomic alignment" of the medial tibial plateau, which affords a distinct reference point for measurement of tibiofemoral JSW, has been a goal of developers of alternative protocols for standardized knee radiography.

Protocols for Standardized Radiographic Examination of the Knee

For 40 years, the extended-knee radiograph (ie, a bilateral weight-bearing AP view of both knees in full extension) has been the conventional plain radiograph employed to image the tibiofemoral joint.[13,14] It was the procedure used to acquire reference images for contemporary pictorial atlases of the radiographic severity of tibiofemoral OA[4,6,15] and remains an accepted radiographic technique for characterizing the bony changes of OA (eg, osteophytosis, subchondral sclerosis). Although the diagnostic utility of the extended-knee radiograph is established, this technique is severely limited as a means by which to visualize reproducibly the radiographic joint space.[16] This limitation stems from numerous technical shortcomings of the examination with respect to variability in the positioning of the knee in serial examinations. For example, longitudinal changes in weight-bearing (for example, due to weight gain or loss) may affect the extent of voluntary knee extension. Changes in the distance between

the knee and radiographic cassette may alter the degree of radiographic magnification in the image. Whereas the above sources of variation in knee position are likely to contribute random measurement error to estimates of tibiofemoral JSW, changes in knee pain from examination to examination (as may occur in a clinical trial of a purported disease-modifying OA drug) may introduce systematic measurement error. This discrepancy was demonstrated by Mazzuca and colleagues,[17] who detected significant increases in tibiofemoral JSW in extended-knee radiographs taken 7–14 days apart of OA subjects who had undergone relief of an induced flare of knee OA pain. These sources of error seriously limit the utility of the extended-knee radiograph to detect true JSN, the cardinal indicator of progression of knee OA.[6]

Over the past 15 years, several teams of investigators have developed alternative protocols for standardized positioning of the knee for a radiographic examination of the tibiofemoral joint. Common to all of the techniques described in this article is a standard for knee flexion, rather than extension, that provides contact between the tibia and the posterior aspect of the femoral condyle (ie, the region in which cartilage damage in OA is often most prominent).[18] The protocols differ, however, with respect to the degree of flexion required, angulation of the x-ray beam, and the parameter that is adjusted to meet the examination's positioning standards (Table 1). A key distinction among current positioning protocols is the use (or not) of fluoroscopy to confirm satisfactory radioanatomical positioning of the medial tibial plateau (ie, parallel or near-parallel alignment with the central x-ray beam) before acquisition of the radiograph.

Fluoroscopically assisted protocols
Semiflexed anteroposterior view Buckland-Wright and colleagues[12] were one of several teams that pioneered the use of fluoroscopy to standardize the radioanatomic positioning of the knee. Their semiflexed AP knee examination uses fluoroscopy to guide knee flexion and rotation to achieve reproducible anatomic markers of parallel alignment of the medial tibial plateau relative to a horizontal x-ray beam. Under fluoroscopy, small degrees of flexion (7–10°) are evaluated in terms of the resulting distance between anterior and posterior margins of the medial tibial plateau (Fig. 4A). When semiflexion affords an intermargin distance (IMD) of 1 mm or less, the foot is rotated internally or externally, as needed, to center the tibial spines beneath the femoral notch. When both markers are apparent in the fluoroscope, the AP radiograph is acquired.

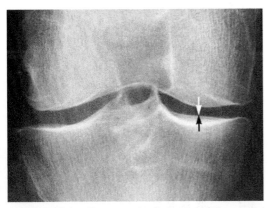

Fig. 3. Parallel radioanatomic alignment of the medial tibial plateau, apparent in superimposition of the anterior and posterior margins of the plateau.

Table 1
Comparison of technical specifications for alternative protocols for standardized knee radiography

	Buckland-Wright Semiflexed[3]	Lyon Schuss[14]	Semiflexed Metatarsophalangeal[18]	Fixed Flexion[21]
Fluoroscopically assisted	Yes	Yes	No	No
Orientation of knee	Anteroposterior	Posteroanterior	Posteroanterior	Posteroanterior
Degree of flexion	Variable (7–10°)	Fixed (20–35°)	Fixed (7–10°)	Fixed (20–35°)
Standard for knee flexion	Flex to superimpose the anterior and posterior margins of the medial tibial plateau	Schuss position[a]	Coplanar alignment of the patella, first MTP joint and radiographic cassette	Schuss position[a]
Standard for foot rotation	Rotate to center the tibial spines beneath the femoral notch	10°	15°	10°
Standard for x-ray beam angulation	Horizontal	Adjust to bring the medial tibial plateau into sharpest focus	Horizontal	10° caudal
Adjustment for radiographic magnification	Required	Optional	Optional	Optional

[a] Coplanar alignment of front surface of radiographic cassette with the hip, patella, and tip of the great toe.

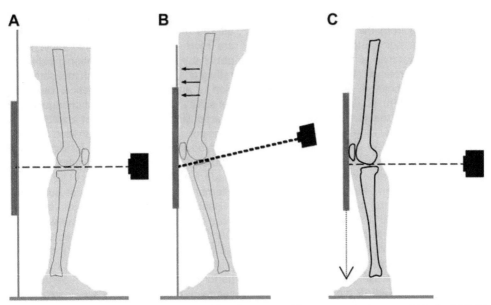

Fig. 4. Positioning of the subject for (A) the semiflexed AP view, (B) LS or FF PA views, and (C) the MTP PA view.

Horizontality of the beam prevents parallax distortion of the joint space. However, semiflexion of the AP knee draws the joint away from the radiographic film and introduces radiographic magnification, a potential obstacle to accurate JSW measurement. Therefore, the semiflexed AP protocol requires use of a foot map to reproduce the joint-to-film distance and a magnification marker (ie, a small steel ball of known diameter affixed to the skin over the head of the fibula) to permit correction of JSW estimates for longitudinal variations in radiographic magnification, which may be as great as 35%.[12] Although magnification correction poses several challenges to accurate measurement of tibiofemoral JSW,[8] the semiflexed AP view has been shown to afford estimates of JSW that are more precise than those obtained from the conventional extended-knee view[12,19,20] and less subject to the confounding effects of longitudinal changes in knee pain.[17]

Lyon schuss view Vignon and colleagues have developed an alternative protocol that uses PA schuss position of the subject (ie, placement of the anterior aspect of the hip, the patella, and tip of the great toe against the radiographic cassette or surface of the vertical radiographic table). Lyon schuss (LS) positioning requires a greater degree of flexion than that seen in semiflexed AP views (see Table 1). Coplanar alignment of the hip, patella, and great toe fixes the degree of flexion for repeat examinations (20–35°, depending on the relative lengths of the tibia and foot). This element of positioning is not guaranteed to be reproduced with the semiflexed AP protocol.

To compensate for the effect of knee flexion on the orientation of the medial tibial plateau relative to the horizontal plane, fluoroscopy is used to adjust the angle of the x-ray beam caudally to bring the tibial plateau into sharpest focus (Fig. 4B).

Early data derived from the LS radiograph confirmed that it afforded reproducibility of measurement of medial tibiofemoral JSW superior to that of the conventional extended-knee view.[20] A recent modification of the LS protocol has incorporated use of the SynaFlexer (Synarc, Inc., San Francisco, California), an acrylic positioning frame in which subjects stand and position themselves to fix knee flexion and external foot rotation in schuss position. Recent applications of the protocol have also adopted the IMD as the standard for evaluating radioanatomic alignment of the medial tibial plateau.[21–23]

Nonfluoroscopically assisted protocols

Semiflexed metatarsophalangeal view In an effort to develop a more exportable, nonfluoroscopically assisted alternative to their semiflexed AP view, Buckland-Wright and colleagues[24] have disseminated procedures for the semiflexed metatarsophalangeal (MTP) view. The MTP protocol provides a PA radiograph of both knees with the subject standing so that the MTP joints of both great toes are directly beneath the front surface of the radiographic cassette, with knees flexed slightly until the patellae are in contact with the cassette directly above the MTP joints (see Table 1). Positioning for the MTP view resembles that for the semiflexed view with respect to knee flexion and foot rotation. JSW measurements from the MTP view do not require correction for radioanatomic magnification. However, use of a foot map is advised to facilitate reproducibility of foot rotation (15°) and placement of first MTP joints beneath the front of the radiographic cassette (Fig. 4C).

The reproducibility of the semiflexed MTP view has been demonstrated with respect to measurements of tibiofemoral JSW and radioanatomic alignment of the medial tibial plateau in examinations repeated on the same day.[24,25] However, several cross-sectional and longitudinal analyses of the performance of the MTP protocol have noted that as many as 70% of MTP radiographs exhibit skewed alignment of the medial tibial plateau.[26,27] Moreover, alignment in MTP views is notably less reproducible over time than in the short-term, resulting in lesser sensitivity to JSN than concurrent semiflexed AP radiographs.[26]

Fixed-flexion view Peterfy and colleagues[28] have developed an empirically derived set of positioning standards for standardized knee radiography. Based on fluoroscopically guided measurements of beam angulation that produce parallel radioanatomic alignment of the medial tibial plateau in samples of normal and OA knees in schuss position (9.0 ± 3.6°), they designed positioning standards for the PA fixed-flexion (FF) view. As with the LS technique, both knees are in contact with the cassette and coplanar with the hips, patellae, and tips of the great toes (see Table 1). However, whereas the beam angle in the LS view is varied with each examination in an attempt to align the beam with the medial tibial plateau, the FF view requires that the x-ray beam be directed 10° caudally. Positioning of the knee and foot for the FF view is facilitated by use of the SynaFlexer positioning frame.

Like other standardization protocols, the FF PA view permits highly precise measurements of JSW.[28] However, because of biologic variability in the anatomy of the tibial plateau, the FF technique often produces a radiograph with skewed radioanatomic alignment of the medial tibial plateau.[26] This problem has led investigators to explore a modification of the FF protocol that entails ascertainment of the quality of alignment produced by 10° caudal angulation and reacquisition of the radiograph with small adjustments of the angle (cranially or caudally) until satisfactory alignment is achieved.[22,29]

Sensitivity to Joint Space Narrowing

The developers of the standardized knee radiography protocols described above have each offered evidence to indicate that their protocol affords measurements of tibiofemoral JSW that are more precise and reproducible than those obtainable from the conventional extended-knee radiograph.[12,20,24–28] Although measurement precision is an important theoretical determinant of sensitivity to the detection of change (eg, thinning of articular cartilage), it is not a sufficient basis to conclude that one standardized technique is more advisable than another for use in longitudinal studies of OA progression. Such choices are best made on the basis of direct comparisons of alternative protocols in the same subjects.

Head-to-head comparisons of alternative positioning protocols are rare in the OA literature. One such study compared the semiflexed AP view with its nonfluoroscopically assisted counterpart (MTP view) in examinations of 52 OA knees performed 14 months apart.[26] Serial MTP views suggested a small average *increase* in mean minJSW over 14 months that was not significantly greater than zero (mean ± SD = +0.09 ± 0.66 mm). In contrast, concurrent semiflexed AP examinations showed a marginally significant *decrease* in mean minJSW (−0.09 ± 0.31 mm; $P = .10$) in the same knees. Also important was the observation that the SD of JSN in serial LS views was less than half the magnitude of that in measurements from MTP views. This result suggests a notably smaller level of random measurement error in JSW estimates from semiflexed AP radiographs than from MTP views. The relative insensitivity of the MTP view to JSN in OA knees was attributed, at least in part, to longitudinal changes in the radioanatomic position of the medial plateau despite adherence to positioning standards for the examination. IMDs measured in repeat baseline MTP radiographs were very highly correlated (+0.88), whereas IMDs in the MTP views taken 14 months apart were only moderately correlated (+0.45).[26]

A recent study compared the LS view with its nonfluoroscopically assisted counterpart (FF view) in examinations of 62 OA and 99 non–OA knees taken 12 months apart.[21] In radiographically normal knees, mean minJSW did not change over 12 months in either view. In the OA knees, mean change in medial minJSW was −0.22 ± 0.43 mm in LS views and +0.01 ± 0.46 mm in FF views ($P = .0002$ and $P = .92$, respectively). At both time points the mean IMD in LS views was only half as large as that in FF views (approximately 0.9 ± 0.5 mm versus 1.9 ± 1.2 mm, $P<.0001$).[21]

Investigators from the same study have also evaluated the performance of a nonfluoroscopically guided variation on the LS radiograph, in which an initial PA radiograph of the knee in schuss position was acquired with 10° caudal angulation (ie, as in the FF view).[22] If the IMD in the initial radiograph exhibited skewed alignment, the examination was repeated up to three more times. Each iteration of the examination occurred with a small (1–2°) adjustment of beam angulation until parallel MTP alignment was achieved. The performance of original and modified LS radiographs was compared with that of standard FF radiographs in serial examinations of 74 OA knees performed 12 months apart. Compared to FF, modified LS radiographs afforded a smaller mean IMD at baseline (0.89 versus 2.06 mm, $P = .002$), more reproducible alignment over 12 months (mean IMD change = 0.49 versus 0.91 mm, $P = .007$) and more rapid JSN (mean change in minJSW = −0.25 versus −0.02 mm/yr, $P = .005$). These differences paralleled those observed between original LS and FF procedures with respect to baseline alignment (0.96 versus 1.94 mm, $P<.001$), reproducibility of alignment (0.49 versus 1.00 mm, $P<.001$) and sensitivity to JSN (−0.16 versus 0.01 mm/yr, $P = .007$).[22]

Although the above comparisons indicate clearly that sensitivity to radiographic JSN is enhanced by fluoroscopically assisted joint positioning and/or beam angulation, it should be acknowledged that the nonfluoroscopically assisted methods described above can detect disease progression in knee OA. A report from the Health, Aging, and Body Composition Study offered evidence that the FF radiograph exhibits noteworthy sensitivity to JSN in OA knees over a 3-year interval (mean JSN ± SD = 0.43 ± 0.66 mm).[30] Sensitivity of this view to JSN over shorter intervals is uncertain. The semiflexed MTP view was the source of primary outcome data for the Glucosamine/Chondroitin Arthritis Intervention Trial (GAIT). A recent report suggests that the MTP view detected loss of JSW over 2 years in treatment and control groups of the GAIT Study (eg, mean JSN in the placebo group = 0.166 mm); however, the failure of the trial to detect significant differences between treatment groups with respect to JSN was attributed in part to "increased variability of measurement."[31]

TIBIOFEMORAL JOINT SPACE WIDTH AND PROGRESSION OF OSTEOARTHRITIS
Manual Methods

Before the development of the automated and semiautomated methods of the early 1990s, JSW measurement was conducted using purely manual methods in which the site of measurement within the compartment and the locations of the landmarks for measurement were judged purely by eye. Various methods have been employed to obtain measurements from a radiograph laid on a light box, including applying a ruler to the radiograph and reading the distance directly from the ruler; direct measurement from the radiograph using a magnifying lens with an internal measurement scale; direct measurement using a set of dial calipers; and a method developed by Lequesne[32] that involved applying a set of simple calipers to the distance to be measured before transferring its points to a ruler[33] to measure the distance between them. A modified version of the last of these methods was introduced by Laoussadi and Menkes[34] in which the points were transferred to a sheet of paper to make prick marks, the distance between which could then be measured using a 1/10 mm graduated magnifying glass. In this modified form, the method has become a standard for performing manual measurements from radiographs, often referred to as chondrometry or "Lequesne's method."

Although these manual methods benefit from simplicity of equipment and application, and from the fact that the same method could be used to measure any linear distance, they are time consuming, subjective, and labor intensive, even for trained staff.

Semiautomated and Automated Methods

The purpose of the development of automated and semiautomated techniques for use in clinical trials was to develop more rapid, objective, and precise measurements of JSW. Software algorithms have been used to evaluate digital radiographic images for well over 2 decades. Initially, much of this work was in fields such as mammography and the purpose of the software was to provide a computer-aided diagnosis of potentially malignant structures.[35] This work has culminated in the creation of clinically used commercial software that attempts to provide a surrogate for the judgment of the physician. The goal of image processing software applied to knee radiography for OA assessment is generally to provide quantitative measures of structural changes over time rather than a one-time diagnosis. Most of the work has been aimed at quantifying radiographic JSW to replace semiquantitative scoring, or the need for a reader to make measurements manually. Fig. 5 shows an example of a cropped image of the knee, where the image analysis software has delineated both margins of the joint and determined the location of minJSW in the medial tibiofemoral compartment.

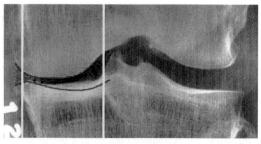

Fig. 5. Delineation of the tibiofemoral joint space and identification of minJSW by semiautomated measurement software. The vertical yellow lines are delineated by the operator to define the regions of interest where minJSW is to be measured. These regions are drawn to limit measurement to weight-bearing areas and to avoid bony changes (ie, osteophytes) at the extreme margins of the joint space that may bias measurement. Within each region, the software delineates the femoral and tibial margins of the joint space (*red lines*) and identifies the shortest distance between each pair of margins (*blue line*).

An early study by Dacre and colleagues[36] examined radiographic images of the knee using a video capture of the films illuminated by a light box. This technique produced 512 × 512–pixel images that were presented on a screen along with a mouse tool with which the reader could use to trace the joint margins and allow for the measurement of the joint space width and area at selected locations along the joint. The study demonstrated improved reproducibility compared with manual readings and a good correlation to qualitative scoring. A subsequent paper by this group[37] used a more direct capture method to convert the image into a digital file that was stored on the local computer for further analysis. For this second study the researchers used automated edge detection software algorithms provided by a commercial software package to delineate the joint margins and make the measurements of JSW. A 1996 study by Conrozier and Vignon[38] also demonstrated improved reproducibility of a digital assessment over manual methods. The study used a modified digital caliper and the viewing of images on a back-lighted table to make measurements of radiographic JSW.

In 1993, Lynch and colleagues[39] described a study using a new custom-designed software algorithm[40] written in the C programming language by the researchers in their laboratory. The software functioned by delineating both margins of the knee joint aided by the placement of seed points on the image by the reader. The software was validated by measuring the reproducibility on duplicate films, digitized using

a 1280 × 1024–pixel CCD camera, of in vivo subjects as well as post mortem knees. The study demonstrated an improved reproducibility of the minJSW compared with the manual technique. A subsequent publication confirmed these results on macroradiographs of the knee.[12]

Duryea and colleagues[41] described a different "rule-based" custom-written software algorithm used to delineate the joints of the knee and make a measurement of minJSW. The method is trainable, meaning that the core algorithm can be optimized for different data sets by applying the software to a representative subset of the data in a study. Validation of the software was made using duplicate films digitized with a commercial radiographic film digitizer. Comparisons with a manual reading using a graduated hand-held lens demonstrated a twofold improvement in reproducibility over the manual method. The study also validated the software-delineated joint margins through a comparison to gold standard hand-delineated contours performed by an expert reader using a mouse tool on the digital images. Conrozier and colleagues[42] described an "edge-based algorithm" to perform joint delineation to examine the effect of tibial plateau alignment and different patient positioning protocols on the sensitivity to change for JSW.

More recently, a class of technologies known as statistical shape models[43] has been used to segment the anatomy of the knee joint in radiographs. This approach uses multivariate statistics to derive the allowable shape of an object from a set of examples. Seise and colleagues[44] describe an adaptation of the original "Active Shape Model"[45] approach to the automated segmentation of the tibia and the rims of the tibial plateaus in digitized radiographs. Although segmentation of the femoral condyles is also described, the extension of the method to a measurement of JSW is not. A different, but related, statistical modeling approach is described by Lacey and colleagues[46] for the determination of JSW and other measurements. This approach requires the operator to initialize the statistical model using a set of six approximate landmarks. The result is an annotation of the femoral condyles and the tibial plateaus from the tibial spines to the outer margin of the joint in each compartment. A software application based on this approach was tested as a workflow tool in which no manual correction of the resulting annotation was performed on 640 knee radiographs from the Osteoarthritis Initiative (OAI)[47] database. In this study, 10% of the radiographs were not analyzed because they were either of poor quality or significant manual correction to the annotation was required; average time to perform JSW measurement was approximately 50 seconds.

An interactive analysis system termed "Knee Images Digital Analysis" is described by Marijnissen and colleagues.[48] The authors state that images must be acquired using the weight-bearing semiflexed MTP protocol of Buckland-Wright and colleagues[24] and an aluminium step-wedge is required for calibration. The software determines a range of parameters including medial and lateral JSW, subchondral bone density, knee alignment, and size of osteophytes. The analysis begins with a suggestion by the software of a framework of four lines that define the position of the joint, which may be repositioned by the user. This framework is then used to support the interactive placement of circles marking positions at which to measure JSW and the other parameters. The entire interactive process takes approximately 10 minutes. The system was tested by two operators using radiographs of 20 healthy knees and 55 showing signs of OA and demonstrated a small interoperator variation in the measurements made.

Minimum Joint Space Width Versus Mean Joint Space Width and Joint Space Width at Specific Locations

Because the current software-based methods delineate the full extent of the joint, a logical next step was to make a systematic study of JSW. The determination of a mean JSW or a joint space area has been studied in either a constant area or a region of interest and its performance compared with that of minJSW. MinJSW was found to be more reproducible and more sensitive to change than mean JSW or a joint space area.[49,50] Although some reports suggest that mean JSW performs better, minJSW remains the most generally used and accepted outcome measurement for OA progression.[33,51,52]

Another approach more recently described is the determination of JSW at more general positions along the joint interface (**Figs. 6** and **7**). This method generally requires the use of robust anatomic landmarks so that consistent locations can be established both cross-sectionally and longitudinally. (In **Fig. 5** the inner landmarks are the tips of the tibial spines.) For each compartment, the outer landmark is defined as being midway between a landmark at the outer extent of the tibial fossa and the edge of the tibial plateau, which is usually found as the point of maximum curvature at the edge of the compartment. Duryea and colleagues[52] found improved reproducibility of location-specific JSW compared with software measurements of minJSW. More recent

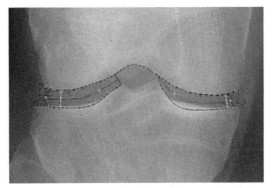

Fig. 6. Delineation of femoral and tibial margins allows the calculation of medial JSW along a normalized distance across the medial and lateral compartments from the tibial spine to the medial and lateral margins of the tibia (*in pink*). The minJSW is also shown (*in yellow*).

publications have also shown an improved responsiveness over minJSW for more severely diseased knees imaged using an FF protocol.[53–55] There has also been a study undertaken to compare fixed-position JSW as measured in radiographs to a similar measure derived from magnetic resonance (MR) imaging data from the same subject, again using images from the OAI database.[56] In this comparative study, measurements from both modalities showed statistically significant progression of OA but in different populations. This may be because the radiographs, unlike MR imaging, are weight-bearing and measure changes due to structures other than the cartilage, but it is unclear whether the two approaches quantify the same progression in pathology but with poor agreement, or are sensitive to different manifestations of the disease. A recent study has also examined location-specific JSW in the lateral compartment and found improved responsiveness in a subset of OA knees exhibiting valgus malalignment.[57]

IMPLICATIONS FOR RESEARCH AND PRACTICE

A fair appraisal of alternative protocols for standardized knee radiography must take into account several practical limitations of fluoroscopically assisted techniques when they are exported for use in medical centers active in clinical research. Many established clinical research centers do not support the fluoroscopic equipment required for a weight-bearing knee examination. Even in the United States, where such equipment is available, a staffing shortage among radiology technologists makes maintenance of quality control of radiographs with respect to positioning

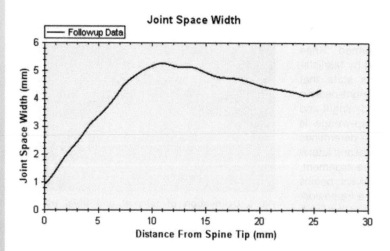

Fig. 7. The corresponding JSW plot for Fig. 6 from which can be derived fixed-position JSW at any position in the compartment.

criteria difficult. Ethical and practical considerations (eg, cumulative radiation exposure, willingness of subjects) may limit the capacity of investigators to attain uniformly high technical quality by precluding repetition of substandard examinations. Finally, fluoroscopic positioning increases the cost of a radiographic knee examination threefold to fourfold. These reservations notwithstanding, the benefits associated with fluoroscopically assisted knee radiography, with respect to quality and reproducibility of radioanatomic positioning of the tibiofemoral joint space and resulting sensitivity to JSN, are commensurate with the costs. However, where fluoroscopy is unavailable, an FF protocol modified to include iterative acquisitions with small adjustments of beam angle to achieve parallel radioanatomic alignment of the medial tibial plateau[22,29] is recommended.

The advances in standardized knee radiography that have made clinical trials of purported disease-modifying OA drugs feasible can also benefit clinical practice. As noted, the conventional extended-view knee radiograph is still used by clinicians to document evidence of marginal tibiofemoral osteophytes on which the diagnosis of knee OA is based. Continued use of this view for diagnostic purposes is not contraindicated by the information presented in this analysis. However, the clinician should know that the extended-knee radiograph cannot be relied upon to afford an accurate or reliable representation of the tibiofemoral joint space. Therefore, the radiographic *severity* of knee OA (ie, the extent of JSN in the presence of marginal osteophytes) may not be apparent in the extended-knee view.[58]

Most clinical radiology departments are capable of producing a PA radiograph of the knee in LS position with 10° caudal angulation of the x-ray beam (ie, an FF radiograph, with or without use of a positioning frame). A radiograph satisfying these standards would offer two distinct advantages over the conventional extended-knee view. First, knee flexion is more likely to reveal cartilage loss that is common to the posterior aspect of the femur. Second, the FF view is more likely than the extended-knee view, albeit not certain, to represent the joint space in parallel or near-parallel alignment with the x-ray beam. These strengths should result in greater accuracy in the evaluation of the severity of structural changes of tibiofemoral OA. They should also provide an image of the knee that will be more reliably reproduced in future assessments of disease progression.

As in other fields, software techniques to evaluate knee radiography have become increasingly more advanced. Earlier approaches used simple digital calipers or modifications to commercial image processing software. Later attempts used a targeted approach based on low-level programming algorithms specially designed for the task of delineating the joint margins. This process had been aided by the advent of more powerful processors and research into more sophisticated algorithms. Computer-aided diagnosis in areas such as mammography, chest, and neurologic imaging continues to be a very active field. It is likely that the future development of image processing software to assess knee radiography for OA will draw from work in these other areas. Some of the systems described here already include software to assess additional structural features such as osteophytes, bone alignment, and subchondral sclerosis, and will likely begin to include more abstract analysis of the shape and appearance or bone texture of the joint.

Before the advent of fully digital modalities such as computed radiography and digital radiography

(DR), digitized radiographic images were created by capturing the illuminated image with a digital camera or using a specialized radiographic film digitizer. The new fully digital modalities have the potential to integrate seamlessly with these software approaches through hospital PACS (picture archiving and communications system) infrastructure for research studies and for patient care once these methods reach the clinic. This may be particularly true for DR, which produces an image file directly on the hard disk of a computer without the need for any intermediate steps. However, many clinical DR systems designed for chest or abdominal imaging use detectors with inferior spatial resolution compared with the traditional digitized film–screen system. Given the similarity in size of the breast and knee, and the need for high spatial resolution for both imaging tasks, it may be advisable to design future digital imaging systems for skeletal radiography using mammography detectors.

SUMMARY

Osteoarthritis is the most common form of arthritis and one of the leading causes of disability in elders. With little currently available in the treatment of this disease, better understanding of responsive and valid endpoints is essential to identifying potential new interventions. Over the past 2 decades, numerous knee radiography protocols have been developed with various levels of complexity and performance as they relate to detecting change. Sensitivity to JSN is improved when radioanatomic alignment of the medial tibial plateau is achieved. The development of a fully automated algorithm where no reader interaction is used to make the assessment could be considered the ultimate goal of these efforts. However, it is unlikely that a 100% accurate software approach will ever be achieved, particularly for knees that are poorly positioned or more advanced in severity. The use of a reader as a quality assurance and correction step using a graphical user interface permits a method to evaluate all images in a study. There are currently a large number of epidemiologic and clinical trials underway in OA collecting both plain radiographic and MR imaging data, with ongoing investigations to identify the most valid and responsive set of endpoints. Before recommending the widespread use of one particular imaging construct in structure modifying clinical trials, it is essential that we have this information as well as an established relationship with clinical endpoints, such as pain, function, and need for joint replacement.

REFERENCES

1. Altman R, Asch E, Bloch D, et al. Development of criteria for the classification and reporting of osteoarthritis. Arthritis Rheum 1986;29:1039–49.
2. Altman R, Alarcon D, Appelrouth D, The American College of Rheumatology Subcommitee on criteria for osteoarthritis. The American College of Rheumatology criteria for the classification and reporting of osteoarthritis of the hip. Arthritis Rheum 1991;34:505–11.
3. Spector TD, Hart DJ, Byrne J, et al. Definition of osteoarthritis of the knee for epidemiological studies. Ann Rheum Dis 1993;52:790–4.
4. Altman R, Hochberg M, Murphy W, et al. Atlas of individual radiographic features in osteoarthritis. Osteoarthritis Cartilage 1995;3(Suppl A):3–70.
5. Scott WW Jr, Lethbridge-Cejku M, Reichle R, et al. Reliability of grading scales for individual radiographic features of osteoarthritis of the knee. The Baltimore Longitudinal Study of Aging atlas of knee osteoarthritis. Invest Radiol 1993;28:497–501.
6. Kellgren JH, Lawrence JS. Radiographic assessment of osteoarthritis. Ann Rheum Dis 1957;16:494–502.
7. Mazzuca SA, Brandt KD. Is knee radiography useful for studying the efficacy of a disease-modifying osteoarthritis drug in humans? Rheum Dis Clin North Am 2003;29:819–30.
8. Mazzuca SA, Brandt KD, Buckwalter KA, et al. Pitfalls in the accurate measurement of joint space narrowing in semiflexed, anteroposterior radiographic imaging of the knee. Arthritis Rheum 2004;50:2508–15.
9. Hunter DJ, Zhang YQ, Tu X, et al. Change in joint space width: hyaline articular cartilage loss or alteration in meniscus? Arthritis Rheum 2006;54(8):2488–95.
10. Brandt KD, Mazzuca SA, Conrozier T, et al. Which is the best radiologic/radiographic protocol for a clinical trial of a structure-modifying drug in patients with knee osteoarthritis? Proceedings of January 17–18, 2002 workshop in Toussus-le-Noble, France. J Rheumatol 2002;29:1308–20.
11. Mazzuca SA, Brandt KD, Dieppe PA, et al. Effect of alignment of the medial tibial plateau and x-ray beam on apparent progression of osteoarthritis in the standing anteroposterior knee radiograph. Arthritis Rheum 2001;44:1786–94.
12. Buckland-Wright JC, Macfarlane DG, Williams SA, et al. Accuracy and precision of joint space width measurements in standard and macroradiographs of osteoarthritic knees. Ann Rheum Dis 1995;54:872–80.
13. Ahlback S. Osteoarthritis of the knee. A radiographic investigation. Acta Radiol Diagn (Stockh) 1968;(Suppl 277):7–72.

14. Leach RE, Gregg T, Siber FJ. Weight bearing radiography in osteoarthritis of the knee. Radiology 1970;97:265–8.

15. Burnett S, Hart DJ, Cooper C, et al. A radiographic atlas of osteoarthritis. London: Springer-Verlag; 1994.

16. Mazzuca SA, Brandt KD, Katz BP. Is conventional radiography suitable for evaluation of a disease-modifying drug in patients with knee osteoarthritis? Osteoarthritis Cartilage 1997;5:217–26.

17. Mazzuca SA, Brandt KD, Buckwalter KA, et al. Knee pain reduces joint space width in conventional standing anteroposterior radiographs of osteoarthritic knees. Arthritis Rheum 2002;46:1223–7.

18. Messieh SS, Fowler PJ, Munro T. Anteroposterior radiographs of the osteoarthritic knee. J Bone Joint Surg Br 1990;72:639–40.

19. Mazzuca SA, Brandt KD, Buckland-Wright JC, et al. Field test of the reproducibility of automated measurements of medial tibiofemoral joint space width derived from standardized knee radiographs. J Rheumatol 1999;26:1359–65.

20. Piperno M, Hellio Le Graverand M-P, Conrozier T, et al. Quantitative evaluation of joint space width in femorotibial osteoarthritis: comparison of three radiographic views. Osteoarthritis Cartilage 1998;6: 252–9.

21. Hellio Le Graverand M-P, Brandt KD, Mazzuca SA, et al. Head-to-head comparison of the Lyon schuss and fixed flexion radiographic techniques. Long-term reproducibility in normal knees and sensitivity to change in osteoarthritic knees. Ann Rheum Dis 2008;67:1562–6.

22. Mazzuca SA, Hellio Le Graverand M-P, Vignon E, et al. Performance of a non-fluoroscopically assisted substitute for the Lyon schuss knee radiograph: quality and reproducibility of positioning and sensitivity to joint space narrowing in osteoarthritic knees. Osteoarthritis Cartilage 2008;16:1555–9.

23. Hellio Le Graverand M-P, Buck RJ, Wyman BT, et al. Change in regional cartilage morphology and joint space width in osteoarthritis participants versus healthy controls – a multicenter study using 3.0 Tesla MRI and Lyon schuss radiography. Ann Rheum Dis 2008; [Epub ahead of print].

24. Buckland-Wright JC, Wolfe F, Ward RJ, et al. Substantial superiority of semiflexed (MTP) views in knee osteoarthritis: a comparative radiographic study, without fluoroscopy, of standing extended, semiflexed (MTP), and schuss views. J Rheumatol 1999;26:2664–74.

25. Mazzuca SA, Brandt KD, Buckwalter KA, et al. Field test of the reproducibility of the semiflexed metatarsophalangeal (MTP) view in repeated radiographic examinations of subjects with osteoarthritis of the knee. Arthritis Rheum 2002;46:109–13.

26. Mazzuca SA, Brandt KD, Buckwalter KA. Longitudinal comparison of the metatarsophalangeal and semiflexed anteroposterior views: detection of radiographic joint space narrowing in osteoarthritic knees. Arthritis Rheum 2002;46(Suppl 9):S150.

27. Hellio Le Graverand MP, Mazzuca S, Lassere M, et al. Radiography Working Group of the OARSI-OMERACT Imaging Workshop. Assessment of the radioanatomic positioning of the osteoarthritic knee in serial radiographs: comparison of three acquisition techniques. Osteoarthritis Cartilage 2006; 14(Suppl A):A37–43.

28. Peterfy C, Li J, Zaim S, et al. Comparison of fixed-flexion positioning with fluoroscopic semi-flexed positioning for quantifying radiographic joint-space width in the knee: test-retest reproducibility. Skeletal Radiol 2003;32:128–32.

29. Charles HC, Kraus VB, Ainslie M, et al. Optimization of the fixed-flexion radiograph. Osteoarthritis Cartilage 2007;15:1221–4.

30. Nevitt MC, Peterfy C, Guermazi A, et al. Longitudinal performance evaluation and validation of fixed-flexion radiography of the knee for detection of joint space loss. Arthritis Rheum 2007;56(5):1512–20.

31. Sawitzke AD, Shi H, Finco MF, et al. The effect of glucosamine and/or chondroitin sulfate on the progression of knee osteoarthritis: a report from the Glucosamine/Chondroitin Arthritis Intervention Trial. Arthritis Rheum 2008;58(10):3183–91.

32. Lequesne M. Chondrometry. Quantitative evaluation of joint space width and rate of joint space loss in osteoarthritis of the hip. Rev Rhum Engl Ed 1995; 62(3):155–8.

33. Ravaud P, Chastang C, Auleley GR, et al. Assessment of joint space width in patients with osteoarthritis of the knee: a comparison of 4 measuring instruments. J Rheumatol 1996;23(10):1749–55.

34. Laoussadi S, Menkes CJ. [Amelioration de la precision de la mesure visuelle de la hauteur del l'interligne articulaire du genou et de la hanche a l'aide d'une loupe graduee]. Rev Rhum Mal Osteoartic 1991;58:678.

35. Vyborny CJ, Giger ML, Nishikawa RM. Computer-aided detection and diagnosis of breast cancer. Radiol Clin North Am 2000;38(4):725–40.

36. Dacre JE, Coppock JS, Herbert KE, et al. Development of a new radiographic scoring system using digital image analysis. Ann Rheum Dis 1989;48(3): 194–200.

37. Dacre JE, Huskisson EC. The automatic assessment of knee radiographs in osteoarthritis using digital image analysis. Br J Rheumatol 1989;28(6):506–10.

38. Conrozier T, Vignon E. Quantitative radiography in osteoarthritis: computerized measurement of radiographic knee and hip joint space. Baillieres Clin Rheumatol 1996;10(3):429–33.

39. Lynch JA, Buckland-Wright JC, Macfarlane DG. Precision of joint space width measurement in knee osteoarthritis from digital image analysis of high definition macroradiographs. Osteoarthritis Cartilage 1993;1(4):209–18.

40. Lynch JA. Textural and geometric measurement of changes in joint structure from high definition macroradiographs of osteoarthritic knees. London: University of London (UMDS); 1993.

41. Duryea J, Li J, Peterfy CG, et al. Trainable rule-based algorithm for the measurement of joint space width in digital radiographic images of the knee. Med Phys 2000;27(3):580–91.

42. Conrozier T, Favret H, Mathieu P, et al. Influence of the quality of tibial plateau alignment on the reproducibility of computer joint space measurement from Lyon schuss radiographic views of the knee in patients with knee osteoarthritis. Osteoarthritis Cartilage 2004;12(10):765–70.

43. Cootes TF, Taylor CJ. Anatomical statistical models and their role in feature extraction. Br J Radiol 2004;77(Spec No 2):S133–9.

44. Seise M, McKenna SJ, Ricketts IW, et al. Learning active shape models for bifurcating contours. IEEE Trans Med Imaging 2007;26(5):666–77.

45. Cootes TF. Active shape models - their training and application. Comput Vis Image Underst 1995;61(1):38–59.

46. Lacey T, et al. Performance of workflow software for the assessment of knee x-ray parameters on baseline and 12-month data for the Osteoarthritis Initiative (OAI). Osteoarthritis Cartilage 2007;15(Suppl C):C176.

47. Osteoarthritis Initiative (OAI). Available at: http://www.oai.ucsf.edu/.

48. Marijnissen AC, Vincken KL, Vos PA, et al. Knee Images Digital Analysis (KIDA): a novel method to quantify individual radiographic features of knee osteoarthritis in detail. Osteoarthritis Cartilage 2008;16(2):234–43.

49. Conrozier T, Lequesne M, Favret H, et al. Measurement of the radiological hip joint space width. An evaluation of various methods of measurement. Osteoarthritis Cartilage 2001;9:281–6.

50. Vignon E. Radiographic issues in imaging the progression of hip and knee osteoarthritis. J Rheumatol Suppl 2004;70:36–44.

51. Bruyere O, Henrotin YE, Honore A, et al. Impact of the joint space width measurement method on the design of knee osteoarthritis studies. Aging Clin Exp Res 2003;15:136–41.

52. Duryea J, Zaim S, Genant HK. New radiographic-based surrogate outcome measures for osteoarthritis of the knee. Osteoarthritis Cartilage 2003;11:102–10.

53. Chu E, DiCarlo JC, Peterfy C, et al. Fixed-location joint space width measurement increases sensitivity to change in osteoarthritis. Osteoarthritis Cartilage 2007;15:S192.

54. Neumann G, Hunter D, Nevitt M, et al. Location specific radiographic joint space width for osteoarthritis progression. Osteoarthritis Cartilage 2008; [Epub ahead of print].

55. Wyman B, Buck R, Vignon E, et al. Comparison of one year change in minimum joint space width to fixed location joint space measurements in Lyon Schuss X-rays from the A9001140 study. Osteoarthritis Cartilage 2008;16(Suppl 4):S164.

56. Lacey T, Brett A, Williams TG, et al. Comparison of x-ray and MRI in the determination of OA progression in the knee measured at a fixed-load-bearing position in the medical compartment. Osteoarthritis Cartilage 2008;16(Suppl 4):S176.

57. Duryea J, Hunter DJ, Nevitt MC, et al. Study of location specific lateral compartment radiographic joint space width for knee osteoarthritis progression: analysis of longitudinal data from the Osteoarthritis Initiative (OAI). Osteoarthritis Cartilage 2008;16:S168.

58. Merle-Vincent F, Vignon E, Brandt K, et al. Superiority of the Lyon-schuss view over the standing anteroposterior view for detecting joint space narrowing, especially in the lateral tibiofemoral compartment, in early knee osteoarthritis. Ann Rheum Dis 2007;66(6):747–55.

Ultrasonography in Osteoarthritis

Helen I. Keen, MBBS, FRACP[a],
Philip G. Conaghan, MBBS, PhD, FRACP, FRCP[b],*

KEYWORDS

- Ultrasonography • Osteoarthritis • Synovitis
- Osteophytes • Cartilage

Osteoarthritis (OA) refers to a group of joint disorders with a variety of causes but common clinical and pathologic features. The disease is difficult to define in a succinct phrase because of its complex pathologic nature and heterogeneous clinical presentation. For OA epidemiologic studies, OA is usually defined according to radiographic changes. These changes can be graded according to existing criteria, which generally focus on the presence of joint space narrowing, osteophytes, subchondral bone sclerosis, subchondral bone cysts, and bone end deformity.[1] Radiographic features of OA do not correlate with symptoms of OA at the individual patient level, however,[2–6] and the value of conventional radiography (CR) has limitations in the clinical setting. The use of radiographs in the clinical trials setting also has limitations.[7] For these reasons, novel imaging techniques are being tested and used as an adjuvant to CR in the investigation and management of OA in the clinical setting and investigational studies. Ultrasonography, which is one of these techniques, is the focus of this article.

ULTRASONOGRAPHY IN PRACTICE

Ultrasonography of joints is well developed and has become part of mainstream practice, thanks largely to the development of modern ultrasonographic technologies. For superficial joints, higher frequency probes are appropriate (> 7.5 MHz), whereas deeper placed joints, such as the hip, may require the use of lower frequency probes.

Modern machines can use beam steering and compound imaging technologies to allow wider fields of view. Many machines also permit extended field of view scanning. Although the larger field of view offers no additional diagnostic information, it can make anatomic demonstration of the larger joints easier, and it offers advantages when trying to demonstrate findings on hard copy images to colleagues. Ultrasonography has limitations for assessing joint disease, particularly for assessing OA. Fundamental to this is the inability of ultrasonography to visualize moat articular surface in most joints because of a limited sonographic window. In many joints it is not possible to usefully visualize most articular cartilage lesions seen in OA. The second limitation is the inability of ultrasonography to demonstrate intrinsic bone abnormalities, such as marrow lesions, cysts, and sclerosis.

ULTRASONOGRAPHY OF SYNOVIAL JOINT PATHOLOGY

Synovial joints affected by OA display common pathologic features on imaging. Although anatomic differences exist with respect to the site of pathology or what can be visualized by ultrasonography because of the physical limitations of the modality, it is first worth considering the generic structures and pathology of the synovial joint that can be imaged in OA. Definitions of synovial pathologies demonstrable by ultrasonography in OA of synovial joints are reviewed, as is evidence

[a] School of Medicine and Pharmacology, Medical Research Foundation Building, Level 3, Rear 50 Murray Street, Perth, Western Australia 6000
[b] Section of Musculoskeletal Disease, Leeds Institute of Molecular Medicine, University of Leeds, Chapel Allerton Hospital, Chapeltown Road, Leeds LS7 4SA, Leeds, UK
* Corresponding author.
E-mail address: p.conaghan@leeds.ac.uk (P.G. Conaghan).

Radiol Clin N Am 47 (2009) 581–594
doi:10.1016/j.rcl.2009.04.007

regarding the validity of ultrasonography in assessing each of these pathologies. Although pathologic conditions detectable by ultrasonography presented in this article occasionally require the lesion to be imaged in two planes, imaging in two planes should be considered in all examinations to minimize potential effects of artifact and confirm pathology (**Fig. 1**).

Synovium

Normal synovium is between 1 and 3 cells thick; however, it becomes hypertrophied as a result of inflammation, which allows detection by current generation ultrasonographic technology.[8,9] An ultrasonographic definition of synovial hypertrophy was developed by the Outcome Measures in Rheumatoid Arthritis Clinical Trials (OMERACT) Ultrasonography Taskforce:

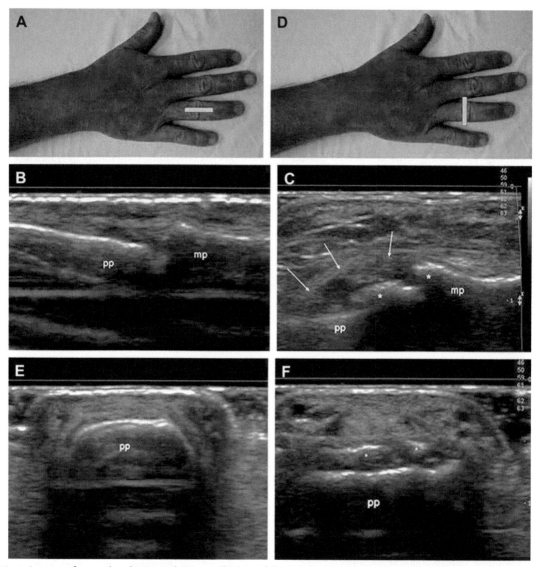

Fig. 1. Images of normal and osteoarthritic small joints of the hand with appearance of osteophytes in two planes. (*A*) Position of probe footprint, longitudinal. (*B*) Longitudinal ultrasonographic image shows the cortical bone of the proximal (pp) and middle (mp) phalanx. (*C*) Longitudinal ultrasonographic image demonstrates the cortical bone of the proximal (pp) and middle (mp) phalanx, with osteophyte (*) proximal and distal to the joint. (*D*) Position of probe footprint, transverse. (*E*) Transverse ultrasonographic image shows the cortical bone of the proximal (pp) phalanx. (*F*) Transverse ultrasonographic image demonstrates the cortical bone of the proximal (pp) phalanx, with osteophytes marked (*).

"Abnormal hypoechoic (relative to subdermal fat, but sometimes may be isoechoic or hyperechoic) intraarticular tissue that is non displaceable and poorly compressible and which may exhibit Doppler" (**Figs. 2** and **3**).[10]

Although this definition was developed for application to rheumatoid arthritis (RA), it may be generalizable to other forms of arthritis, particularly because OA and RA synovial inflammation types largely differ quantitatively rather than qualitatively.[11,12]

Ultrasonography has been demonstrated to have criterion and construct validity in detecting synovial hypertrophy. The criterion validity of ultrasonographically detected gray scale synovial morphology has been demonstrated compared with direct visualization by arthroscopy.[8,9,13] Construct validity has been demonstrated against MR imaging of the knee, acromioclavicular joint, and small joints of the hands and feet.[14–21] Research also has demonstrated convincingly that ultrasonography is better able to detect synovitis than clinical examination. This has been demonstrated in the knee and the small joints of the hands and feet using MR imaging as the

comparator.[8,21–24] Of clinical relevance, ultrasonography is able to detect gray scale synovitis in joints thought to be clinically quiescent.[25–27] In addition to morphologic changes, synovial vascularity as detected by Doppler signal also has validity.[28–30] Intra-articular Doppler signal demonstrated in knee and hip joints has been shown to correlate with histologic vascularity and inflammatory infiltrates.[28–30]

Most of the validity data referred to previously is derived from the literature on inflammatory arthritis, with a paucity of information specific to the validity of ultrasonography in detecting synovitis in OA. It has been demonstrated to correlate moderately with MR imaging and direct visualization by arthroscopy at the knee joint[18,31] and detect more synovial hypertrophy than clinical examination in knees and hands with OA.[24,32] Doppler signal in OA correlates with histologic evidence of vascularity in knees and hips with OA.[29,30] When using Doppler imaging to assess synovial vascularity in any joint, it is important to realize that the vessels detected in synovium are compressible; the lightest transducer pressure possible must be used to avoid obliterating any evidence of vascular flow. A gel stand-off or water

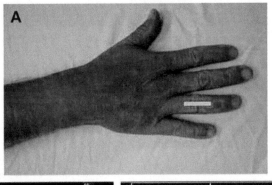

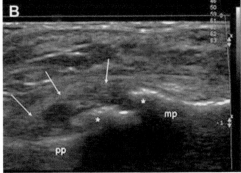
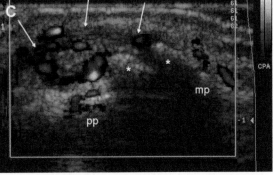

Fig. 2. Dorsal longitudinal ultrasonographic images of the proximal interphalangeal joint. (*A*) Position of probe footprint. (*B*) Gray scale ultrasonographic image of an osteoarthritic proximal interphalangeal joint demonstrates the proximal phalanx (pp), middle phalanx (mp) with associated synovial hypertrophy (*arrows*), and osteophytes (***). (*C*) Power Doppler image of the same osteoarthritic proximal interphalangeal joint demonstrates the vascularity within the region of synovial hypertrophy (*arrows*) as indicated by the flash of color.

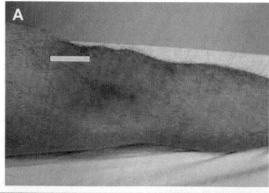

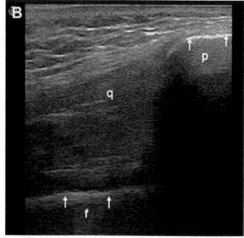 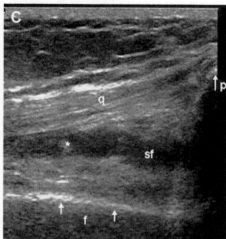

Fig. 3. Sagittal ultrasonographic image of the suprapatellar pouch. (A) Position of probe footprint. (B) Longitudinal ultrasonographic appearance of a normal knee demonstrates the cortical (arrows) bone of the patella (p) and distal femur (f) and quadriceps tendon. (C) Longitudinal ultrasonographic image of an osteoarthritic knee shows hypoechoic collection of synovial fluid in the suprapatellar sac (sf) and villous synovial hypertrophy extending into the fluid collection (*).

bath can be used, but generally liberal use of acoustic jelly is sufficient to avoid excess transducer pressure.

Synovial Fluid

Fluid collections within the joint are readily detected by ultrasonography. The OMERACT Ultrasonography Taskforce defined synovial fluid as

> "Abnormal hypoechoic or anechoic (relative to subdermal fat, but sometimes may be isoechoic or hyperechoic) intra-articular material that is displaceable and compressible, but does not exhibit Doppler signal" (see Fig. 3).[10]

Few studies have focused on the validity of ultrasonography in detecting synovial fluid in isolation from synovial hypertrophy; they are often considered together in published studies. Studies have demonstrated that ultrasonographically detected hypoechoic collections can be

demonstrated to be synovial fluid on aspiration, however.[33,34] Ultrasonographically detected synovial fluid has been validated against MR imaging in the small joints of the hands, wrists,[35] and ankles, although more fluid was required to detect effusions by ultrasonography than MR imaging.[36] This may partly be caused by the ability of fluid to pool in sonographically inaccessible recesses within the joint. One way to improve visualization of subtle effusions is to ensure that the joint is moved into different positions as it is examined, which may move any fluid to areas where it can be visualized.

A further problem can be distinguishing joint fluid from synovium, which is of low reflectivity itself. Clues are that Doppler signal may be detected in synovium but not effusion and that the fluid appears compressible because it can be displaced into other areas of the joint in contrast to synovium. This is why the compressibility and absence of Doppler signal are important elements of the definition of an effusion. In deep joints, such as the hip, where Doppler signal may be difficult to detect and compression is not possible, it can be difficult to make the distinction. In cases in which distinction is critical, such as the need to exclude infection, attempted joint aspiration may be required. Ultrasonography is certainly better able to detect effusions than clinical examination, although most of this evidence arises from studies of the knee joint.[8,24,37–42]

BONE CORTEX

The highly echogenic cortical bone surface is readily demonstrated with ultrasonography, although the internal structure of the bone is not seen. Normally it appears as a continuous smooth bright line that allows easy visualization of any abnormalities,[43] such as erosions,[44,45] irregularities,[45,46] osteophytes,[43,45,47–49] and enthesophytes.[50] Little is known about the validity of ultrasonographically detected cortical changes in OA, and most of the evidence relates to pathologic

and structures changes seen in inflammatory arthritis.

Osteophytes are one of the cardinal features of OA and are commonly described in the ultrasonography OA literature.[43,45,47–49] There are no published consensus statements regarding ultrasound definitions, however, perhaps because osteophytes are so frequently recognized on ultrasonography and their appearances are not considered as controversial as other features of arthropathy. Recently used definitions include

> "A single or multiple characteristic irregularities of the bone profile, located at the edges of the joint surfaces"[43]
> "Cortical protrusions seen in 2 planes" (see **Figs. 1, 2,** and **4**)[51]

There is also little evidence of the validity of ultrasonography in detecting osteophytes. Given the sensitivity and specificity of ultrasonography in detecting cortical erosions in RA, it is likely to have a similar ability to detect osteophytes. In

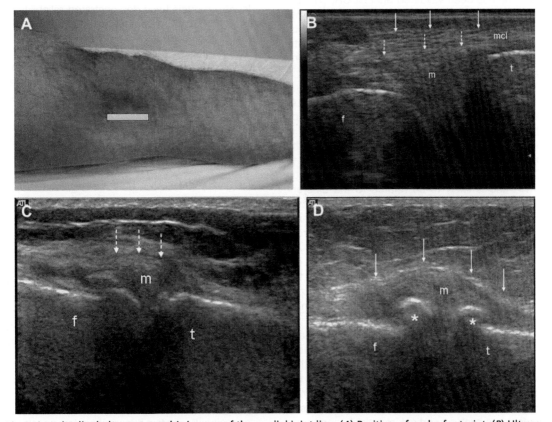

Fig. 4. Longitudinal ultrasonographic images of the medial joint line. (*A*) Position of probe footprint. (*B*) Ultrasonographic image of a normal knee shows distal femur (f), proximal tibia (t), triangular outline of the medial meniscus (m, *dashed arrows*), and the linear echoes produced by the medial collateral ligament (mcl, *solid arrows*). (*C*) Ultrasonographic image shows medial meniscal extrusion (m, *dashed arrows*). (*D*) Ultrasonographic image in knee OA demonstrates medial meniscal extrusion (m) with resulting displacement of the medial collateral ligament (*arrows*) and obvious osteophytes (*) proximal and distal to the joint line.

a recently published study that examined small joint OA in the hand, ultrasonography detected more osteophytes than CR.[52] This is most likely a reflection of the multiplanar imaging capability of ultrasonography, particularly its ability to image joints in the dorsal longitudinal plane, which is not routinely done with CR.

Erosions are the most commonly studied ultrasonographically detected cortical abnormality in the rheumatologic ultrasonography literature. Although they are a feature of a subtype of hand OA and MR imaging studies suggest that they may be more frequently seen in OA than CR suggests,[53] they are much less commonly appreciated than in RA. The OMERACT Ultrasonography Taskforce published a definition of rheumatoid erosion, which is defined as

> "An intra-articular discontinuity of the bone surface that is visible in 2 perpendicular planes."[10]

The ability of ultrasonography to detect RA erosions has been validated against CR, CT, and MR imaging, largely focusing on the small joints of the hands and feet but also focusing on wrists, knees, and shoulder joints.[17,21,22,54–56] Importantly in RA, ultrasonography can detect small erosions earlier in the disease process than CR.[21,54,56] This advantage may have implications for studying cortical changes in OA before development of radiographic evidence of disease. The only study that examined the validity of ultrasonography in detecting erosions in OA of the small joints of the hand found ultrasonography to be inferior to CR.[44] This finding was in contrast to the findings in RA and is likely to be related to the different pathologic processes involved in the two diseases. The presence of osteophyte formation at the joint margins may shield erosions from view because they can hide other periarticular features normally well visualized.[42] Although RA erosions are characteristically juxta-articular, the location of erosions in OA is classically recognized as being central, and the central area of the joint is poorly visualized using ultrasonography.

Other cortical abnormalities in OA that have been described as being detectable by ultrasonography, such as cortical irregularities and enthesophytes, are not well reported in the literature.[45,46,50] Two studies addressed the sensitivity of ultrasonography in diagnosing OA based on features such as cortical irregularity compared with CT and MR imaging. In these studies, although ultrasonography was sensitive to the detection of OA, the use of bone remodeling as a diagnostic tool had poor specificity.[19,57]

CARTILAGE

Hyaline cartilage is readily identified on ultrasonography if an acoustic window is available. In some joints, particular maneuvers can be made to improve the area of articular cartilage visualized. For instance, a larger proportion of the femoral trochlear cartilage can be identified with the knee maximally flexed, and plantar flexion of the ankle exposes more of the cartilage over the talus for examination. Flexion of the small joints of fingers, including the metacarpophalangeal joints allows a more extensive assessment of the cartilage over proximal joint surface. Normal hyaline cartilage appears as a homogenous low reflective layer closely paralleling the subchondral bone (Fig. 5). Abnormalities described in OA seen on ultrasonography include[43,47,58]

- Loss of the sharpness of the cartilage margins
- Heterogeneity
- Irregularities in thickness

In vitro models have demonstrated reliability of ultrasonography in detecting cartilage thickness[59,60] compared with histologic examination. Ultrasonography compares reasonably to MR imaging in detecting femoral condylar cartilage thickness in in vivo studies.[18,31,61] The clinical relevance of noninvasive ultrasonographically detected cartilage changes is uncertain. Generally only peripheral, non–load-bearing regions of cartilage can be visualized using noninvasive B-mode ultrasonography.

TENDONS AND LIGAMENTS

The ultrasound appearances of tendons and ligaments are well described.[62] Ultrasonographically detected ligamentous abnormalities have been described in arthritis,[63] and tendon tears resulting from attrition of the tendon on osteophyte or bony irregularity may be associated with OA and identified by ultrasonography.[64] Perhaps of most relevance to OA is inflammation of the tendon or ligament enthesis (enthesitis). Although not specific to OA, enthesitis has been defined by the OMERACT Ultrasonography Taskforce as

> "Abnormally hypoechoic(loss of normal fibrillar architecture) and/or thickened tendon or ligament at it's bony attachment (may occasionally contain hyperechoic foci consistent with calcification), seen in 2 perpendicular planes that may exhibit Doppler signal and/or bony changes including enthesophytes, erosions, or irregularity."[10]

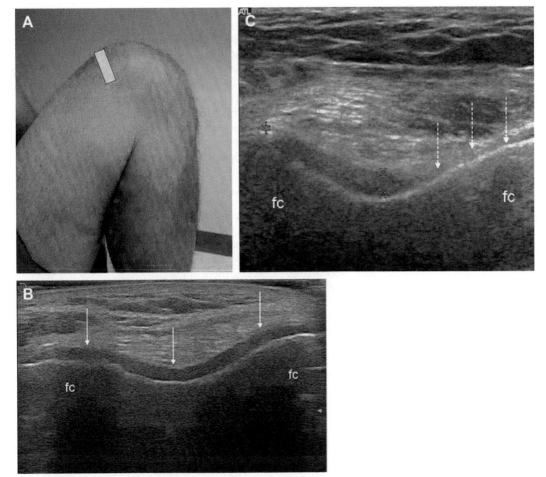

Fig. 5. Coronal images over the distal femur in full flexion. (*A*) Position of probe footprint. (*B*) Ultrasonographic image demonstrates a smooth regular homogenous band of cartilage (*arrows*) overlying the distal femoral condyles (fc). (*C*) Ultrasonographic image shows pathologic cartilage band, with irregular thickness, increased echogenicity, and loss of clarity of the cartilage margins (*dashed arrows*).

There is a paucity of published information about the validity of ultrasonography in detecting enthesitis, with little investigation in OA specifically, although ultrasonography has been demonstrated to detect more sites of entheseal disease in OA than CR in the foot[65] and more than CR or clinical examination at the shoulder.[46]

IMAGING SPECIFIC JOINTS

Guidelines for the acquisition of ultrasonography images of synovial joints for rheumatology have been published by the European League Against Rheumatism (EULAR) Ultrasonography Taskforce[66] and are reviewed here by joint, along with changes commonly detected in OA by ultrasonography and, where available, the relative frequency of the changes.

SHOULDER

The capabilities of ultrasonography in the diagnosis of shoulder pathology, specifically rotator cuff disease, are well recognized. The various positions in which the shoulder should be examined, along with appropriate dynamic maneuvers, are well described.[67] A comprehensive examination includes examination of the glenohumeral joint from its posterior aspect and from the axilla.[66] Because the shoulder joint is considered to include also the acromioclavicular joint and the sternoclavicular joint, they also can be imaged.

OA of the glenohumeral joint is often a result of long-standing rotator cuff condition, particularly tears that allow superior migration of the humeral head and subsequent contact with the inferior surface of the acromion. The ultrasonographic appearance of these changes include thinning and tears of the rotator cuff, irregularity of the bony cortex of the humeral head, particularly superiorly, and inferior osteophytes.[64] There also may be fluid within the subacromial bursa and glenohumeral joint.[64] The glenoid labrum can be appreciated as a homogenous but slightly hyperechoic appearance, akin to the menisci of the knee. Because of the normal anatomic structure of the labrum, identifying different portions of the labrum requires maneuvers and use of probes of varying frequencies. The posterior labrum is most superficial and most easily visualized, and identification is further aided by the presence of a glenohumeral joint effusion. Pathology such as tears can be visualized by ultrasonography, although superior lesions are difficult to appreciate with ultrasonography because of acoustic shadowing by the acromion.[64]

OA of the acromioclavicular joint appears as narrowing of the joint space between the acromion and the clavicle, irregularity and bony prominence of the juxta-articular cortical bones, including osteophyte formation, and synovial hypertrophy with low levels of Doppler signal within the joint capsule (Fig. 6). Inferior osteophytes on the acromioclavicular joint can cause trauma to the supraspinatus tendon, and although these injuries are not seen on ultrasonography, the tendon damage may be visible.[64] Imaging of the sternoclavicular joint is a common request to investigate the cause of a localized mass over this joint. OA is common at this joint, particularly in middle-aged women; it is characterized by joint space narrowing, cortical osteophytosis, and cysts.[64]

HAND

The palmar and dorsal surfaces of the hand and wrist joints should be imaged in longitudinal and transverse planes; medial and lateral longitudinal views of the small joints also should be obtained. In OA, most of the pathologic cases are seen over the small joints of the hand and base of thumb rather than the thenar and hypothenar eminences. The most commonly affected regions (as detected by ultrasonography) in OA of the small

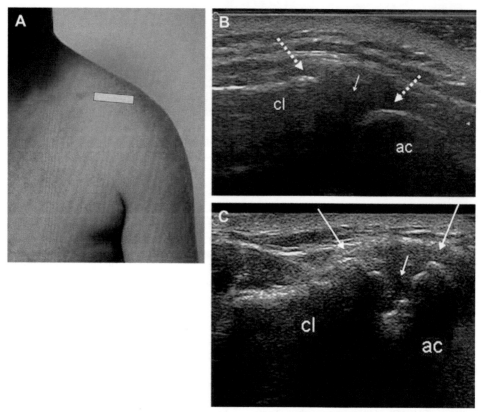

Fig. 6. Longitudinal image of the acromioclavicular joint. (A) Position of probe footprint. (B) Ultrasonographic image shows normal acromioclavicular joint. There is a smooth uniform appearance of the cortical bone (*dashed arrows*) at the joint line (*small arrow*). (C) Ultrasonographic image shows osteoarthritic acromioclavicular joint. There are raised cortical bone (*arrows*) and irregularities surrounding the joint line (*small arrow*). Clavicle (cl), acromion (ac).

joints of the hand are the base of thumb and distal and proximal interphalangeal joints, as would be expected from epidemiologic studies of the distribution of OA of the hand.[52] Involvement of metacarpophalangeal joints may be more common than appreciated by assessing CR images of OA, however.[52]

Ultrasonographically detected osteophytes are commonly seen on the dorsal aspect of the hand in the midline protruding along the longitudinal plane of the phalanx (see **Fig. 2**).[52] This is not well appreciated on CR because the standard dorsiplanar and dorsiplanar oblique planes do not allow imaging of this region. Erosive changes in OA of the small joints of the hand have been described with ultrasonography; however, the only study that assessed the validity of ultrasonographically detected erosions in OA of the small joints of the hand found ultrasonography inferior to CR.[44] Qualitative or quantitative changes in cartilage in the small joints of the hand are often appreciated with ultrasonography. The prevalence of osteophytes in OA that produces acoustic shadows can hamper this and make accurate quantification impossible. A surrogate of joint space loss was examined with ultrasonography in the small joints of the hand and found to be problematic.[52]

Synovial hypertrophy and fluid are commonly seen in association with osteophytes in OA of the hand (see **Fig. 2**), with Doppler signal being less often appreciated and generally in low levels.[32] Occasionally florid Doppler signal in a distal interphalangeal joint or proximal interphalangeal joint may mimic a more inflammatory process, such as psoriatic arthritis. Researchers recently hypothesized that ligamentous pathologic conditions may play a pathogenic role in OA of the small joints of the hand,[68] and although the collateral ligament complexes can be visualized on ultrasonography, the reliability and clinical and pathologic significance of ultrasonographically detected changes are yet to be established.

HIP

The deep anatomic location and physical structure of the hip joint mean that clinical examination is not reliably able to detect synovial pathology or the bone changes of OA.[66] Similarly, visualization by ultrasonography is somewhat limited, particularly because of the acoustic shadow created by the acetabulum.[64] Changes that have been described in OA of the hip include synovial hypertrophy or effusion causing distension of the hip joint capsule, osteophytes (most commonly arising from the anterior inferior margin of the femoral head), and flattening of the profile of the normal curved, visible portion of the femoral head.[48,64] Just deep to the joint capsule, where the capsule inserts into the acetabulum, the labrum can be visualized as a homogenous hyperechoic structure. Pathologic conditions, such as labral tears, can be detected with ultrasonography, and cystic, mucoid degeneration of labral fissures can be appreciated as circumscribed, hypoechoic lesions with a lobulated appearance that are not easily compressible.[64]

KNEE

At the knee joint, the typical features of synovial hypertrophy, effusion, osteophytes, and cartilage thinning have been described. Meniscal extrusion and tears may be visualized, with associated displacement of the collateral ligaments. Recommendations for acquisition of images of the knee joint have been described by EULAR.[66] It is recommended that the knee initially be imaged with the patient supine in the neutral or slightly flexed position (30°) for lateral and anterior images, then in the prone position for posterior images. Slight flexion with quadriceps contraction aids visualization of the suprapatellar pouch, and maximal flexion aids visualization of the trochlear cartilage. Standard scans should include imaging in the transverse and longitudinal plane of the suprapatellar region, infrapatellar region, and posterior knee (both medial and lateral). The knee also should be imaged longitudinally over the medial and lateral aspects of the joint.[66]

In cases of OA, synovial hypertrophy in the suprapatellar pouch can be readily visualized as either flattened, thickened synovium or frond-like protrusions into the pouch.[8] Ultrasonographically detected synovial hypertrophy is common in OA of the knee, but the prevalence ranges depend on the definition used and study population examined (see **Fig. 3**). Synovial fluid is easily detected in the suprapatellar pouch, especially with the aid of dynamic maneuvers, and can aid visualization of synovial hypertrophy through transmitting sound to the underlying sac wall (see **Fig. 3**). In addition to imaging the suprapatellar pouch in the midline, it is important to image the lateral and medial recesses because they may be the only sites of synovial hypertrophy or effusion.[69,70] Synovial hypertrophy and small amounts of fluid also can be found in the lateral and medial longitudinal planes surrounding the medial and lateral joint lines. Enthesophytes extending into the quadriceps and patellar tendons also can be identified by ultrasonography.

Imaging of the popliteal fossa can allow identification of popliteal cysts associated with OA. They appear as a hypoechoic or anechoic mass arising between the semimembranous and medial head of gastrocnemius tendons.[64] They may have a heterogeneous echoic appearance because they can be filled with debris from the communicating knee joint.[64] Leakage of fluid from the cyst is characterized by fluid within the surrounding tissue and a beaked appearance of the cyst distally. Complete rupture and emptying of the cyst may be indicated only by the detection of residual fluid between the heads of the semimembranous tendon and medial gastrocnemius.[64]

Cartilage pathology can be appreciated in the trochlea of the distal femur with the knee in full flexion (see Fig. 5).[64] Changes such as thinning, heterogeneity, and loss of clarity can be seen. The changes, particularly thinning, are generally more pronounced in OA than in inflammatory arthritis.[64] The clinical significance of these ultrasonographically detected changes in the hyaline cartilage of the knee are uncertain, however. The peripheral superficial aspects of menisci also can be visualized with ultrasonography, allowing some meniscal pathologic conditions such as cysts, extrusion, or horizontal tears to be visualized.[63,64] Meniscal extrusion is a significant component of the joint space narrowing as seen radiographically in OA of the knee and has been demonstrated to be associated with ultrasonographically detectable displacement of the medial collateral ligament and some pain parameters in OA of the knee (see Fig. 4).[63]

Ultrasonographically detected osteophytes are a common feature of OA of the knee, commonly seen around the medial and lateral joint line, either originating from the distal femur or proximal tibia (see Fig. 4). The other relatively common place to detect osteophytes by ultrasonography is over the distal femoral condyles with the knee fully flexed to distally displace the patella. Enthesophytes can be seen protruding from the patella into the quadriceps or patellar tendons.

ANKLE

Because of the anatomy of the ankle joint, imaging of the joint cavity is somewhat limited by ultrasonography.[64] Dynamic imaging of the ankle joint while the patient dorsi- and plantarflexes the foot aids detection of pathology.[64] Synovial hypertrophy and fluid in OA can be detected anteriorly assuming the pathology is of sufficient severity.[36] Large effusions displace the anterior capsular fat pad inferiorly, aiding diagnosis.[36] Large effusions also can be visualized posteriorly and may be

seen to surround the flexor hallucis tendon as the tendon sheath communicates with the ankle joint in most cases. The chondral surface of the talus can be visualized by plantar flexing the ankle joint, which allows cartilaginous pathologic conditions to be identified.[64] Osteophytes are most commonly seen extending from the distal tibia or talus and can result in anterior impingement of the ankle.[64] Osteophytes also may result in tendon impingement about the ankle.

FOREFOOT

OA in the forefoot is most commonly found in the first metatarsophalangeal joint (Fig. 7).[64] Typical ultrasound findings include cortical irregularity (including osteophytes), synovial hypertrophy, and effusion (although a small amount of fluid or synovial hypertrophy is considered within the normal range in this load-bearing joint).[64] Changes in cartilage also can be appreciated in the first metatarsophalangeal joint, although as with other joints, the reliability and significance of changes are not yet established.

FUTURE RESEARCH ENDEAVORS

Ultrasonography offers several advantages in the assessment of OA in clinical practice. As an adjuvant to conventional methods of assessing joints, it allows sensitive and specific identification of soft tissue and bone changes (including vascularity). In contrast to radiographs, it does not require ionizing radiation, can image the joint in multiple planes, and allows dynamic assessment of moving structures.[71] In the hands of a clinician skilled in image acquisition and interpretation, ultrasonography can be performed in the clinical setting, making it part of the clinical assessment.[71] This fact, in addition to its relative patient friendliness and low cost compared with CT and MR imaging, make it a useful clinical tool.[71] Acquisition of ultrasonography skills takes time and practice and ongoing maintenance of competency.[71] It can be time consuming to perform in the clinical setting. The quality of the images obtained and the interpretation of the images depend on the skills and experience of the technician.[71] Visualization of certain structures is limited by the intrinsic properties of the technique and current technology (discussed later).

Another important consideration is that ultrasonography should be used as an adjuvant to routine clinical assessment and investigations to aid the diagnosis and management of disease rather than as a stand-alone diagnostic test.[71] Although there is a lot of published data regarding the

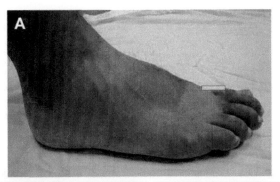

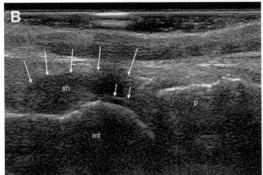
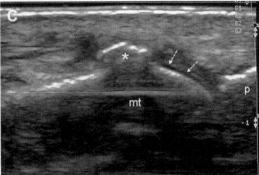

Fig. 7. Dorsal longitudinal images of the first metatarsophalangeal joint. (A) Position of probe footprint. (B) Ultrasonographic image shows metatarsal (mt) and proximal phalanx (p) joint with associated synovial hypertrophy (sh) considered to be within normal range (arrows). The metatarsal articular cartilage is indicated by the small dashed arrows. (C) Ultrasonographic image shows osteoarthritic metatarsophalangeal joint with osteophyte (*) and cartilage thinning (dashed arrows).

validity of ultrasonography in inflammatory arthritis,[72,73] the validity of ultrasonography OA requires further work, with particular focus on the pathology that can be detected.[74] Areas that need refinement and confirmation include definitions of pathology in OA, assessment of the criterion and construct validity of these definitions, development of standardized, universally applicable scoring systems with good reliability, and demonstrable sensitivity to change. The benefits of ultrasonography over CR include the ability to image soft tissue structures and the potential to detect small or early structural lesions. These types of pathologic conditions should be the focus of investigation by ultrasonography. Perhaps there will be a role for studying preradiographic OA.

The significance of ultrasonographically detected pathologic conditions in OA needs further investigation. Because there is a discordance between radiographic structural changes and symptoms in OA, the clinical importance of ultrasonographically detected structural changes with regards to symptoms, prognosis, outcome, and response to therapy needs investigation.[2–6] If ultrasonographically detected structural changes bear no relationship to any of these domains,

then the use of ultrasonography in cases of OA is likely to be limited. In reality, such endeavors likely will increase use of ultrasonography in the clinical setting and clinical trial setting in cases that involve OA.

REFERENCES

1. Zhang Y, Jordan JM. Epidemiology of osteoarthritis. Rheum Dis Clin North Am 2008;34(3):515–29.
2. Hart D, Spector T, Egger P, et al. Defining osteoarthritis of the hand for epidemiological studies: the Chingford study. Ann Rheum Dis 1994;53(4):220–3.
3. Spector TD, Hart DJ, Byrne J, et al. Definition of osteoarthritis of the knee for epidemiological studies. Ann Rheum Dis 1993;52(11):790–4.
4. Felson DT, Naimark A, Anderson J, et al. The prevalence of knee osteoarthritis in the elderly: the Framingham Osteoarthritis Study. Arthritis Rheum 1987;30(8):914–8.
5. Felson DT. An update on the pathogenesis and epidemiology of osteoarthritis. Radiol Clin North Am 2004;42(1):1–9.
6. Sonne-Holm S, Jacobsen S. Osteoarthritis of the first carpometacarpal joint: a study of radiology and

clinical epidemiology. Results from the Copenhagen Osteoarthritis Study. Osteoarthr Cartil 2006;14(5): 496–500.

7. Guermazi A, Eckstein F, Hellio Le Graverand-Gastineau MP, et al. Osteoarthritis: current role of imaging. Med Clin North Am 2009;93(1):101–26.

8. Karim Z, Wakefield R, Quinn M, et al. Validation and reproducibility of ultrasonography in the detection of synovitis in the knee: a comparison with arthroscopy and clinical examination. Arthritis Rheum 2004; 50(2):387–94.

9. Fiocco U, Cozzi L, Rubaltelli L, et al. Long-term sonographic follow-up of rheumatoid and psoriatic proliferative knee joint synovitis. Br J Rheumatol 1996;35(2):155–63.

10. Wakefield RJ, Balint PV, Szkudlarek M, et al. Musculoskeletal ultrasound including definitions for ultrasonographic pathology. J Rheumatol 2005;32(12): 2485–7 [erratum appears in J Rheumatol 2006 Feb;33(2):440].

11. Haraoui B, Pelletier JP, Cloutier JM, et al. Synovial membrane histology and immunopathology in rheumatoid arthritis and osteoarthritis: in vivo effects of antirheumatic drugs. Arthritis Rheum 1991;34(2): 153–63.

12. Peter JB, Pearson CM, Marmor L. Erosive osteoarthritis of the hands. Arthritis Rheum 1966;IX(3): 365–88.

13. Rubaltelli L, Fiocco U, Cozzi L, et al. Prospective sonographic and arthroscopic evaluation of proliferative knee joint synovitis. J Ultrasound Med 1994; 13(11):855–62.

14. Scheel A. A novel ultrasonographic synovitis scoring system suitable for analyzing finger joint inflammation in rheumatoid arthritis. Arthritis Rheum 2005; 52(3):733–43.

15. Backhaus M, Kamradt T, Sandrock D, et al. Arthritis of the finger joints: a comprehensive approach comparing conventional radiography, scintigraphy, ultrasound, and contrast-enhanced magnetic resonance imaging. Arthritis Rheum 1999;42(6): 1232–45.

16. Beckers C, Jeukens X, Ribbens C, et al. (18)F-FDG PET imaging of rheumatoid knee synovitis correlates with dynamic magnetic resonance and sonographic assessments as well as with the serum level of metalloproteinase-3. Eur J Nucl Med Mol Imaging 2006; 33(3):275–80, Epub 2005 Oct 25.

17. Scheel AK, Schmidt WA, Hermann KG, et al. Interobserver reliability of rheumatologists performing musculoskeletal ultrasonography: results from a EULAR "train the trainers" course. Ann Rheum Dis 2005;64(7):1043–9.

18. Tarhan S, Unlu Z. Magnetic resonance imaging and ultrasonographic evaluation of the patients with knee osteoarthritis: a comparative study. Clin Rheumatol 2003;22(3):181–8.

19. Alasaarela E, Tervonen O, Takalo R, et al. Ultrasound evaluation of the acromioclavicular joint. J Rheumatol 1997;24(10):1959–63.

20. Eich G, Halle F, Hodler J, et al. Juvenile chronic arthritis: imaging of the knees and hips before and after intraarticular steroid injection. Pediatr Radiol 1994;24(8):558–63.

21. Szkudlarek M, Narvestad E, Klarlund M, et al. Ultrasonography of the metatarsophalangeal joints in rheumatoid arthritis: comparison with magnetic resonance imaging, conventional radiography, and clinical examination. Arthritis Rheum 2004;50(7): 2103–12.

22. Szkudlarek M. Ultrasonography of the metacarpophalangeal and proximal interphalangeal joints in rheumatoid arthritis: a comparison with magnetic resonance imaging, conventional radiography and clinical examination. Arthritis Res Ther 2006;8(2):R52.

23. Cellerini M, Salti S, Trapani S, et al. Correlation between clinical and ultrasound assessment of the knee in children with mono-articular or pauci-articular juvenile rheumatoid arthritis. Pediatr Radiol 1999;29(2):117–23.

24. D'Agostino M. EULAR report on the use of ultrasonography in painful knee osteoarthritis. Part 1: prevalence of inflammation in osteoarthritis. Ann Rheum Dis 2005;64(12):1703–9, Epub 2005 May 5.

25. Hau M, Schultz H, Tony HP, et al. Evaluation of pannus and vascularization of the metacarpophalangeal and proximal interphalangeal joints in rheumatoid arthritis by high-resolution ultrasound (multidimensional linear array). Arthritis Rheum 1999;42(11): 2303–8.

26. Bajaj S, Lopez-Ben R, Oster R, et al. Ultrasound detects rapid progression of erosive disease in early rheumatoid arthritis: a prospective longitudinal study. Skeletal Radiol 2007;36(2):123–8, Epub 2006 Oct 11.

27. Wakefield RJ, Green MJ, Marzo-Ortega H, et al. Should oligoarthritis be reclassified? Ultrasound reveals a high prevalence of subclinical disease. Ann Rheum Dis 2004;63(4):382–5 [see comment].

28. Schmidt WA, Volker L, Zacher J, et al. Colour Doppler ultrasonography to detect pannus in knee joint synovitis. Clin Exp Rheumatol 2000;18(4):439–44.

29. Walther M, Harms H, Krenn V, et al. Synovial tissue of the hip at power Doppler US: correlation between vascularity and power Doppler US signal. Radiology 2002;225(1):225–31.

30. Walther M, Harms H, Krenn V, et al. Correlation of power Doppler sonography with vascularity of the synovial tissue of the knee joint in patients with osteoarthritis and rheumatoid arthritis. Arthritis Rheum 2001;44(2):331–8.

31. Ostergaard M, Court-Payen M, Gideon P, et al. Ultrasonography in arthritis of the knee: a comparison with MR imaging. Acta Radiol 1995;36(1):19–26.

32. Keen HI, Wakefield RJ, Grainger AJ, et al. An ultra-sonographic study of osteoarthritis of the hand: synovitis and its relationship to structural pathology and symptoms. Arthritis Rheum 2008;59(12): 1756–63.

33. Iagnocco A, Coari G. Usefulness of high resolution US in the evaluation of effusion in osteoarthritic first carpometacarpal joint. Scand J Rheumatol 2000; 29(3):170–3.

34. Balint PV, Kane D, Hunter J, et al. Ultrasound guided versus conventional joint and soft tissue fluid aspiration in rheumatology practice: a pilot study. J Rheumatol 2002;29(10):2209–13.

35. Hoving J, Buchbinder R, Hall S, et al. A comparison of magnetic resonance imaging, sonography, and radiography of the hand in patients with early rheumatoid arthritis. J Rheumatol 2004;31(4):663–75.

36. Jacobson JA, Andresen R, Jaovisidha S, et al. Detection of ankle effusions: comparison study in cadavers using radiography, sonography, and MR imaging. AJR Am J Roentgenol 1998;170(5):1231–8.

37. van Holsbeeck M, van Holsbeeck K, Gevers G, et al. Staging and follow-up of rheumatoid arthritis of the knee: comparison of sonography, thermography, and clinical assessment. J Ultrasound Med 1988; 7(10):561–6.

38. Kane D. Ultrasonography is superior to clinical examination in the detection and localization of knee joint effusion in rheumatoid arthritis. J Rheumatol 2003;30(5):966–71.

39. Toolanen G, Lorentzon R, Friberg S, et al. Sonography of popliteal masses. Acta Orthop Scand 1988;59(3):294–6.

40. Fam AG, Wilson SR, Holmberg S. Ultrasound evaluation of popliteal cysts on osteoarthritis of the knee. J Rheumatol 1982;9(3):428–34.

41. Andonopoulos A, Yarmenitis S, Sfountouris H, et al. Baker's cyst in rheumatoid arthritis: an ultrasonographic study with a high resolution technique. Clin Exp Rheumatol 1995;13(5):633–6.

42. Gompels B, Darlington L. Evaluation of popliteal cysts and painful calves with ultrasonography: comparison with arthrography. Ann Rheum Dis 1982;41(4):355–9.

43. Delle Sedie A, Riente L, Bombardieri S. Limits and perspectives of ultrasound in the diagnosis and management of rheumatic diseases. Mod Rheumatol 2008;18:125–31.

44. Iagnocco A, Filippucci E, Ossandon A, et al. High resolution ultrasonography in detection of bone erosions in patients with hand osteoarthritis. J Rheumatol 2005;32(12):2381–3.

45. Grassi W. Sonographic imaging of the distal phalanx. Semin Arthritis Rheum 2000;29(6):379–84.

46. Falsetti P, Frediani B, Filippou G, et al. Enthesitis of proximal insertion of the deltoid in the course of seronegative spondyloarthritis: an atypical enthesitis that can mime impingement syndrome. Scand J Rheumatol 2002;31(3):158–62.

47. Grassi W, Filippucci E, Farina A. Ultrasonography in osteoarthritis. Semin Arthritis Rheum 2005;34(6 Suppl 2):19–23.

48. Qvistgaard E, Torp-Pedersen S, Christensen R, et al. Reproducibility and inter-reader agreement of a scoring system for ultrasound evaluation of hip osteoarthritis. Ann Rheum Dis 2006;65(12):1613–9.

49. Robinson P, Keenan AM, Conaghan PG. Clinical effectiveness and dose response of image-guided intra-articular corticosteroid injection for hip osteoarthritis. Rheumatology (Oxford) 2007;46(2): 285–91.

50. Frediani B, Falsetti P, Storri L, et al. Ultrasound and clinical evaluation of quadricipital tendon enthesitis in patients with psoriatic arthritis and rheumatoid arthritis. Clin Rheumatol 2002;21(4):294–8.

51. Keen HI, Lavie F, Wakefield RJ, et al. The development of a preliminary ultrasonographic scoring system for features of hand osteoarthritis. Ann Rheum Dis 2008;67(5):651–5.

52. Keen HI, Wakefield RJ, Grainger A, et al. Can ultrasonography improve on radiographic assessment in osteoarthritis of the hands? A comparison between radiographic and ultrasonographic detected pathology. Ann Rheum Dis 2008;67(8): 1116–20.

53. Grainger AJ, Farrant JM, O'connor PJ, et al. MR imaging of erosions in interphalangeal joint osteoarthritis: is all osteoarthritis erosive? Skeletal Radiol 2007;36(8):737–45.

54. Wakefield R, Gibbon W, Conaghan P, et al. The value of sonography in the detection of bone erosions in patients with rheumatoid arthritis: a comparison with conventional radiography. Arthritis Rheum 2000;43(12):2762–70.

55. Magnani M, Salizzoni E, Mule R, et al. Ultrasonography detection of early bone erosions in the meta-carpophalangeal joints of patients with rheumatoid arthritis. Clin Exp Rheumatol 2004;22(6):743–8.

56. Lopez-Ben R, Bernreuter WK, Moreland LW, et al. Ultrasound detection of bone erosions in rheumatoid arthritis: a comparison to routine radiographs of the hands and feet. Skeletal Radiol 2004;33(2):80–4.

57. Brandlmaier I, Bertram S, Rudisch A, et al. Temporo-mandibular joint osteoarthrosis diagnosed with high resolution ultrasonography versus magnetic resonance imaging: how reliable is high resolution ultrasonography? J Oral Rehabil 2003;30(8):812–7.

58. Grassi W. Sonographic imaging of normal and osteoarthritic cartilage. Semin Arthritis Rheum 1999; 28(6):398–403.

59. Myers SL, Dines K, Brandt DA, et al. Experimental assessment by high frequency ultrasound of articular cartilage thickness and osteoarthritic changes. J Rheumatol 1995;22(1):109–16.

60. Jurvelin JS, Rasanen T, Kolmonen P, et al. Comparison of optical, needle probe and ultrasonic techniques for the measurement of articular cartilage thickness. J Biomech 1995;28(2):231–5.

61. Jonsson K, Buckwalter K, Helvie M, et al. Precision of hyaline cartilage thickness measurements. Acta Radiol 1992;33(3):234–9.

62. Grobbelaar N, Bouffard JA. Sonography of the knee: a pictorial review. Semin Ultrasound CT MR 2000; 21(3):231–74.

63. Naredo E, Cabero F, Palop MJ, et al. Ultrasonographic findings in knee osteoarthritis: a comparative study with clinical and radiographic assessment. Osteoarthr Cartil 2005;13:568–74.

64. Bianchi S, Martinoli C. Ultrasound of the musculoskeletal system. Berlin: Springer; 2007.

65. Falsetti P, Frediani B, Fioravanti A, et al. Sonographic study of calcaneal entheses in erosive osteoarthritis, nodal osteoarthritis, rheumatoid arthritis and psoriatic arthritis. Scand J Rheumatol 2003;32(4):229–34.

66. Backhaus M, Burmester GR, Gerber T, et al. Guidelines for musculoskeletal ultrasound in rheumatology. Ann Rheum Dis 2001;60(7):641–9.

67. Allen GM, Wilson DJ. Ultrasound of the shoulder. Eur J Ultrasound 2001;14(1):3–9.

68. Tan AL, Toumi H, Benjamin M, et al. Combined high-resolution magnetic resonance imaging and histological examination to explore the role of ligaments and tendons in the phenotypic expression of early hand osteoarthritis. Ann Rheum Dis 2006;65(10): 1267–72.

69. Song I-H, Hermann K-G, Scheel AK, et al. Comparison of the efficacy of contrast-enhanced ultrasonography and magnetic resonance imaging in detecting synovial process in patients with knee osteoarthritis compared to healthy subjects [abstract]. Arthritis Rheum 2006;54(Suppl):s262.

70. Song IH, Althoff CE, Hermann KG, et al. Knee osteoarthritis efficacy of a new method of contrast-enhanced musculoskeletal ultrasonography in detection of synovitis in patients with knee osteoarthritis in comparison with magnetic resonance imaging. Ann Rheum Dis 2008;67(1):19–25.

71. Wakefield RJ, Gibbon WW, Emery P. The current status of ultrasonography in rheumatology. Rheumatology 1999;38(3):195–8.

72. Joshua F, Edmonds J, Lassere M. Power Doppler ultrasound in musculoskeletal disease: a systematic review. Semin Arthritis Rheum 2006;36(2):99–108.

73. Joshua F, Lassere M, Bruyn G, et al. Summary findings of a systematic review of the ultrasound assessment of synovitis. J Rheumatol 2007;34(4): 839–47.

74. Keen HI, Wakefield RJ, Conaghan PG, et al. A systematic review of ultrasonography in osteoarthritis. Ann Rheum Dis 2009;68(5):611–9.

CT Arthrography, MR Arthrography, PET, and Scintigraphy in Osteoarthritis

Patrick Omoumi, MD[a,b], Gustavo A. Mercier, MD, PhD[c],
Frédéric Lecouvet, MD, PhD[a], Paolo Simoni, MD[a],
Bruno C. Vande Berg, MD, PhD[a,*]

KEYWORDS

- CT arthrography • MR arthrography • PET • PET-CT
- Scintigraphy • Osteoarthritis • Cartilage

Damage to articular cartilage is considered to be the hallmark of osteoarthritis (OA), even if other factors are involved in the pathogenesis of the disease. The radiological assessment of OA has been based mostly on the radiographic grading of the joint space width, an indicator of cartilage thickness, and on indirect signs such as osteophytes.[1–3] Attempts have been made to better delineate cartilage lesions by using intraarticular contrast material in arthrography,[4] which has inherent limitations due to the projection of three-dimensional structures on a plane. The advent of cross-sectional imaging enabled arthrography to develop further.[5–7] Indeed, arthrographic techniques such as computed tomography (CT) arthrography and magnetic resonance (MR) arthrography, thanks to their high resolution and the possibility of multiplanar imaging, remain superior to conventional MR imaging for the delineation of surface lesions of all cartilage areas. However, MR imaging is the only technique enabling the analysis of the internal structure of cartilage, and many recent developments include biochemical qualitative assessment.[2]

The development of nuclear medicine techniques have focused mainly on the subchondral changes associated with OA, because there are no radiopharmaceuticals to image the articular cartilage in clinical practice.

We review technical aspects of CT arthrography and MR arthrography of various joints, compare both methods, and report on their most common and useful indications, as well as their pitfalls and limitations. We also describe in detail the nuclear medicine methods that might be relevant for OA research and clinical application.

CT ARTHROGRAPHY AND MR ARTHROGRAPHY
Technical Considerations

Type of contrast material with CT arthrography
CT arthrography can be performed using either a single (iodine) or double-contrast (iodine and air) technique. In the past, air was used with conventional arthrography to distend the joints, which is not necessary when using CT, because the penetration of the air into cartilage lesions is poor when compared with that of fluid. Nowadays, there is a general consensus in using a single-contrast technique, which is easier to perform[8,9] and probably less painful.[10]

Dilution of the contrast material can be achieved with local anesthetics or saline to avoid beam-hardening artifacts. Nevertheless, the dilution

[a] Department of Radiology, Cliniques Universitaires Saint-Luc, Université Catholique de Louvain, Brussels, Belgium
[b] Department of Radiology, Centre Hospitalo-Universitaire de Tours, Tours, France
[c] Department of Radiology, Nuclear Medicine and Molecular Imaging, Boston University Center, Boston, MA, USA
* Corresponding author.
E-mail address: vandeberg@rdgn.ucl.ac.be (B.C. Vande Berg).

Radiol Clin N Am 47 (2009) 595–615
doi:10.1016/j.rcl.2009.04.005
0033-8389/09/$ – see front matter © 2009 Published by Elsevier Inc.

radiologic.theclinics.com

mainly depends on the radiologist preference and investigated joint.[11–17]

Type of contrast material with MR arthrography

The contrast material of choice for MR arthrography is gadolinium-based (gadolinium-DTPA). It is possible to perform either indirect (less invasive, intravenous gadolinium-DTPA injection) or direct MR arthrography (intraarticular gadolinium injection). For the study of cartilage, the intraarticular injection of contrast material is favored because it allows joint repletion, thus, better delineation of superficial cartilage defects.[18] Other types of contrast material have also been tested, such as saline combined with T2-weighted MR imaging, but gadolinium provides the best contrast-to-noise ratios.[19–21] A metaanalysis of 112 published studies found gadolinium-DTPA to be a safe and efficient technique for diagnosing internal derangement of joints.[22]

Many studies have focused on determining the best gadolinium-DTPA concentration and temporal behavior of intraarticular contrast after injection. At 1.5 T, a concentration of 2–2.5 mmol/L is considered best for imaging to be performed within about an hour after injection.[22,23] At 3.0 T, a slightly greater dilution may be useful.[24] Aspiration of joint effusion before injection can prevent excessive dilution of contrast material, but this is usually not a problem in clinical practice.[24,25]

It has been shown that iodinated and gadolinium-based contrast material can safely be mixed, and combined MR arthrography and CT arthrography examinations have successfully been obtained for comparison of both studies (Fig. 1).[26–29] However, at 3.0 T, the presence of iodinated contrast agents has to be minimized, because signal-to-noise peak levels are lower at 3.0 T than at 1.5 T.[24]

Volume of contrast material

The volume of injected contrast material necessary for proper capsular distention varies according to the joint and is the same for all arthrographic techniques. As a rule, adequate distention is indicated by increased resistance to injection or retrograde flow of contrast material into the needle after disconnection of the syringe.[30] The injection should be stopped if the patient has pain.

Injection technique

The injection is usually performed under fluoroscopic guidance,[16,30] but other injection techniques have been described, using CT,[16,31] ultrasound,[32–34] MR[35] guidance, or even by using surface landmarks.[36–38] The choice relies on the radiologist's preference and on the equipment available. The injection technique follows standard arthrographic procedures, which have been widely described in the literature.[39–41]

Time delay between the injection of contrast material and imaging

Once injected in the joint, the concentration of contrast materials rapidly decreases by diffusion into the cartilage and synovium, resorption, and fluid influx into the joint.[42] It is recommended to perform the CT within 30 minutes and the MR within an hour after the contrast injection.[23,29,43,44] The time delay, however, varies according to the joint. The use of epinephrine in adjunction to the injected material (for instance by mixing 1 mL of a 0.1% solution containing 1 mg of epinephrine with 10 mL of contrast material[45]) slows down the resorption of the latter.[46,47] However, the use of epinephrine may increase postarthrographic morbidity.[10] Use of epinephrine is usually not necessary with MR arthrography.[48]

It has been shown for the shoulder that exercise has no beneficial or detrimental effect for MR arthrography.[49] However, in our experience, active and passive full-range articular motion after the injection allows the contrast material to completely cover cartilage surfaces.[50]

Acquisition parameters

CT arthrography exposes the patient to ionizing radiation. Radiation doses should be kept to a minimum, especially in regions close to sensitive areas such as the shoulder (Fig. 2) (thyroid) and the hip (gonads), at the expense of signal-to-noise ratio. The minimal field-of-view should be selected. In knee CT arthrography, for instance, the suprapatellar recess should not be imaged (Fig. 3). Synovial and intraarticular pathologies are depicted on conventional radiographs obtained early after intraarticular injection, before imbibition occurs and masks synovial masses. These radiographs in the case of the knee will cover the suprapatellar recess not imaged by CT.

The CT acquisition parameters include narrow collimation, low-pitch values, and a high milliampere–second value to obtain high resolution isotropic multiplanar reformats.[51] The reconstructions use bone algorithms, providing high spatial resolution images, and bone windowing is used to view the images. Posttreatment of these high-resolution isotropic images may include curved and maximum-intensity projection reformatting (Fig. 4). Metallic artifacts can be diminished and, more generally, signal-to-noise ratio can be

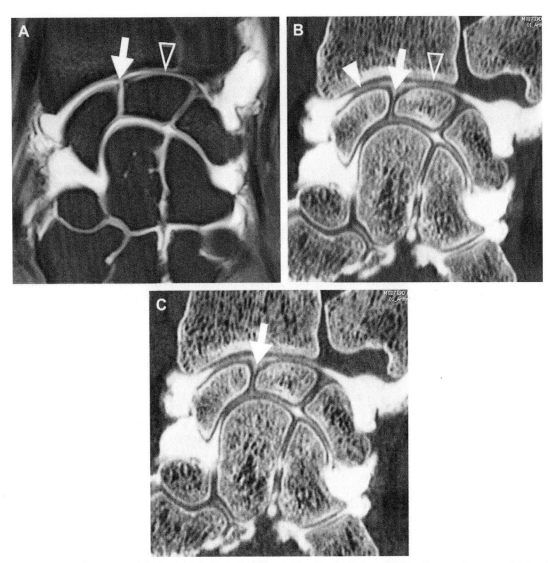

Fig. 1. 34-year-old man with history of trauma. Combined CT arthrography and MR arthrography were obtained after intraarticular injection of gadolinium and iodine. Normal aspect of cartilage (*white arrowheads*) and partial tear of central portion of scapholunate ligament (*arrow*). (*A*) Coronal fat-suppressed spin-echo T1-weighted MR arthrography image (669/11 ms, TR/TE) shows normal wrist cartilage with intermediate signal intensity (*arrowhead*). Its surface is smooth and regular. (*B*) 2.4 mm-thick coronal CT arthrography reformatted image shows normal hypodense cartilage, well delimited by the underlying subchondral bone and the intraarticular contrast material at its surface. (*C*) A 0.6 mm thick coronal CT arthrography reformatted image obtained from same examination demonstrates the same findings. Retrospectively increasing the reformat thickness [from (*C*) to (*B*)] leads to an increase of the signal-to-noise ratio. Note that the thickness of the cartilage is easier to evaluate at CT arthrography than at MR arthrography, with better coverage of cartilage surface areas by the contrast material at CT arthrography (*open arrowheads*).

increased by retrospectively increasing the thickness of the reformats and, at the expense of spatial resolution, by using soft tissue algorithms[52,53] (see **Fig. 1**). Metallic artifacts usually remain mild on new generation CT scanners compared with MR imaging, which makes CT arthrography more suitable for postoperative patients who have metallic hardware near the joint (**Fig. 5**).[8,54]

MR arthrography typically includes fat-suppressed spin-echo T1-weighted sequences in three planes, associated to at least one fluid-sensitive sequence for bone marrow edema and extraarticular fluid collections.[55]

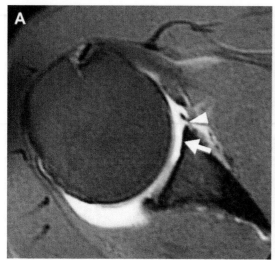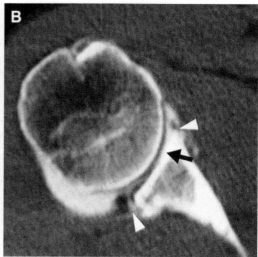

Fig. 2. 40-year-old man with shoulder instability. (*A*) Axial fat-suppressed spin-echo T1-weighted MR arthrography image (786/12 ms, TR/TE) shows cartilage abrasion (grade 4 cartilage loss) of the anterior part of the glenoid (*arrow*). (*B*) Axial CT arthrography reformat shows the same chondral lesion (*arrow*). However, the use of low radiation doses as in this image lead to low signal-to-noise ratio. Note the presence of labral lesions (*arrowheads*).

Three-dimensional gradient-echo sequences can also be performed and allow multiplanar reformatting.[56]

Risks

As with any other arthrographic procedure, CT arthrography and MR arthrography present risks related to the puncture (infection) and to the injected contrast material (allergic reaction).[57] However, the risk of infection is quite low (with one infection out of 25,000 arthrograms, according to Berquist,[58] and three cases of iatrogenic septic arthritis out of 126,000 arthrographic procedures, according to Newberg and colleagues[57]). The risk of severe systemic allergic reactions is also low, although minor reactions can occur.[58]

Moreover, as with other invasive techniques, there is a risk for vasovagal reactions and pain. The best prevention for vasovagal reactions is good communication with the patient and preparation of the injection material out of the patient's sight.[59] In a recent study evaluating pain and other side-effects of MR arthrography, Saupe and colleagues[60] concluded that mild postarthrographic pain is most pronounced 4 hours after the procedure, and disappears within 1 week. The origin of postarthrographic pain is debated.[61] It may depend on the nature of the iodinated contrast material for CT arthrography (higher with double contrast CT arthrography,[10] ionic contrast material (probably due to a higher sodium content),[10,12,62] and the use of epinephrine[10,63]).

The arthrographic procedure is generally well-tolerated by patients. In a study by Binkert and colleagues,[61] the arthrographic procedure was better tolerated than the MR imaging examination itself.

In addition to those risks, there is patient radiation exposure with CT arthrography but not with MR arthrography.

Role in Osteoarthritis

Internal structure and cartilage thickness

At CT arthrography, the normal hyaline cartilage appears as a low attenuating structure. The internal contrast of cartilage does not present any variation in its density at CT arthrography, and purely intrachondral lesions, without communication with the surface, cannot be detected (**Fig. 6**).[3] On spin-echo T1-weighted MR imaging, cartilage demonstrates low-to-intermediate signal intensity. Purely intrachondral lesions are barely seen on those sequences. However, fluid-sensitive sequences such as fast spin-echo T2-weighted images acquired during MR arthrography allow detection of concealed lesions of cartilage.

Cartilage loss and thinning are one of the hallmarks of OA. CT arthrography is the most accurate method for the evaluation of cartilage thickness, thanks to its spatial resolution and high contrast between the low attenuating cartilage and its high attenuating deep (subchondral bone) and superficial (contrast material filling the joint) boundaries (see **Fig. 1**). Indeed, CT arthrography is more accurate than MR imaging even when using cartilage sensitive sequences such as

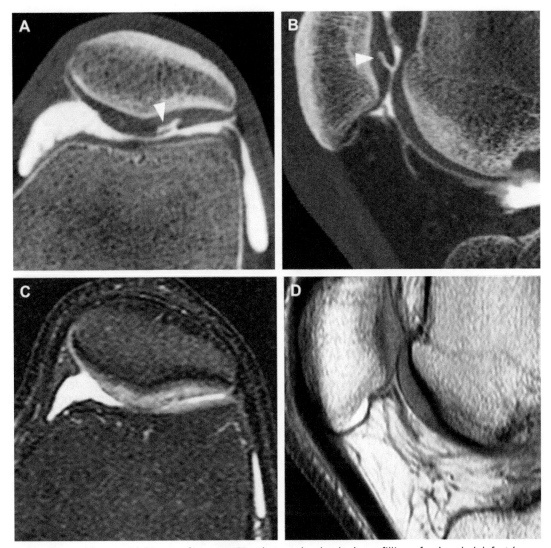

Fig. 3. 23-year-old man with history of trauma. CT arthrography clearly shows filling of a chondral defect (*arrowhead*) by contrast material in lateral patellar facet on axial (*A*) and sagittal (*B*) reformats. This defect is underestimated by MR imaging on the corresponding (*C*) axial fat-suppressed intermediate-weighted fast spin-echo image (2200/45 ms, TR/TE) and (*D*) sagittal proton density-weighted spin-echo image (2200/18 ms, TR/TE).

SPGR as shown by cadaveric studies on the ankle.[64] CT arthrography is also more accurate than MR arthrography for the assessment of cartilage thickness in cadaver hip joints (**Figs. 7** and **8**).[17] CT arthrography has been used as a reference in studies evaluating the accuracy of noninvasive MR imaging sequences for the assessment of cartilage thickness.[65] However, CT arthrography measurements can be influenced by some technical factors as recently shown by Anderson and colleagues[66] in a phantom study. The authors suggest the use of lower contrast agent concentrations and the maximization of joint space by completely filling the joint capsule with diluted contrast and/or by applying traction to the joint. A more recent study concluded that multidetector CT arthrography and MR arthrography are equally accurate in measuring hip cartilage thickness as far as the coronal plane is concerned.[67]

The thickness of cartilage is highly variable from one individual to another, from one joint to another, and from one area of the joint to another. This is particularly true for the knee, where the cartilage is usually thicker in areas with concave subchondral bone and thinner in areas adjacent to the menisci.[50] In the hips, a cartilage thickness gradient exists from the periphery to the center of the femoral head and from the medial to the lateral edge of the acetabulum (see **Figs. 7**

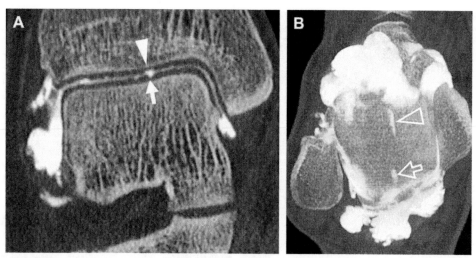

Fig. 4. CT arthrography in a 43-year-old man with history of trauma. (*A*) Coronal reformat shows a grade 3 (more than 50% in depth) cartilage defect in talar dome (*arrow*) and a grade 2 (less than 50% in depth) defect in the tibial plafond (*arrowhead*). (*B*) Curved axial maximum-intensity projection image shows the spatial orientation of the cartilage fissure, whose long axis is parallel to the axis of the talar dome (*arrowhead*). Another cartilage defect is seen more posteriorly (*arrow*).

and 8).[17] The inversion of that thickness gradient is an early sign of degenerative OA. In shoulders, glenoid cartilage is physiologically thinner at the center.

Cartilage surface

The normal cartilage surface appears smooth and continuous (see **Fig. 1**). Some focal physiologic defects, such as the glenoid central defect, the trochlear notch at the elbow, and the stellate lesion in the acetabulum (see **Fig. 8**), may exist and should not be mistaken with cartilage lesions. In addition to those focal physiologic defects, some epiphyseal areas are physiologically not covered by cartilage (bare areas).

Focal surface lesions of the cartilage are well depicted with both techniques and appear as areas filled with the intraarticular contrast material (see **Figs. 2–4, 9**). However, the contrast between the cartilage and the intraarticular contrast material,

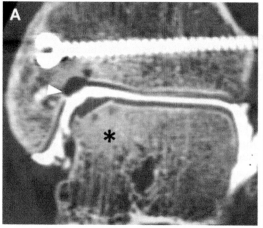
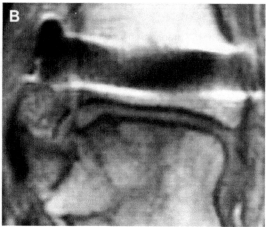

Fig. 5. 40-year-old man with history of traumatic osteochondral lesion of the talus dome, treated with osteochondral grafting. (*A*) Coronal CT arthrography reformat shows the well-incorporated osteochondral graft (*). Cartilage surface shows minor irregularities and its thickness is acceptable. The graft is well incorporated with no contrast at the interface between the graft and the adjacent talar cartilage. A focal chondral lesion is visualized on the opposite tibial surface (*arrowhead*). (*B*) Coronal proton density-weighted MR imaging (920/12 ms, TR/TE) shows the cartilage surface is poorly defined in comparison to the CT arthrography image. Note that metal-related artifact is milder on CT arthrography (*A*) than on MR imaging (*B*).

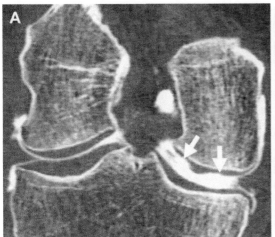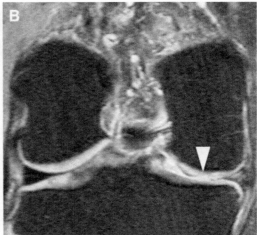

Fig. 6. 46-year-old woman with osteoarthritis. (*A*) Coronal CT arthrography reformat shows extensive grade 3 chondral loss at the medial femoral condyle (*arrows*), associated with thinning of the medial tibial plateau carti-lage, well delineated by the intraarticular contrast material. (*B*) Coronal fat-suppressed fast spin-echo interme-diate-weighted MR imaging shows irregularity of the chondral surface and chondral signal intensity changes in the medial compartment. The normal variations in cartilage signal intensity of the lateral tibial plateau seen with MR imaging (*B*) are not detected on the CT arthrography (*A*). Injection of intraarticular contrast allows distention of the joint space (*A*) and good delineation of cartilage surface compared with the nonenhanced MR imaging. This allows better characterization of femoral and tibial chondral lesions.

as well as the image resolution, are higher with CT arthrography compared with MR arthrography, leading to a higher degree of confidence in depict-ing those lesions, and a higher interobserver reproducibility.[68]

Cartilage loss can be either focal or extensive and different terms are used to characterize either the shape or the depth of the defects. Fissures have a linear shape with one diameter being much smaller than the other (see Fig. 4). Cartilage ulcers have a more round shape on en face view (see Fig. 9). This classification system, based on the shape of the surface defect, has barely been validated. Numerous grading systems of cartilage lesions are derived from the grading systems used at arthroscopy and are mainly based on the following parameters: integrity of cartilage surface and depth of cartilage defects (Table 1).[15,69–71]

Sensitivities and specificities at chondral lesions depiction are good for thin or thick cartilage.[9,72] However, CT arthrography is more accurate for thinner cartilage lesions compared with MR ar-thrography (see Fig. 1).[11]

CT arthrography and MR arthrography have significantly better sensitivity and specificity for high grade lesions (3 and above) for various joints, such as patellar,[3] knee,[72] elbow,[68] and shoulder,[11] than for more superficial lesions (see Figs. 2, 6–9).

The coverage of the cartilage surface and delin-eation of opposite cartilage surfaces is poor with

certain joints such as the ankle and hip, and is usually better at CT arthrography than at MR arthrography (see Fig. 1) [68,73], leading some authors to propose traction maneuvers.[64,74]

Subchondral changes

Both CT arthrography and MR arthrography can show subchondral bone changes. CT arthrogra-phy is better at depicting subchondral bone scle-rosis and osteophytes (see Figs. 7 and 8). Both techniques can show central (nonmarginal) osteo-phytes, associated with more severe changes of OA than marginal osteophytes.[75,76] MR arthrogra-phy is the only technique allowing depiction of subchondral bone marrow edema-like lesions on the fluid-sensitive sequences usually acquired along the T1-weighted sequences. This depiction is usually a sign of high-grade cartilage lesions (see Fig. 9).[72]

PET AND SCINTIGRAPHY
Tracers and Imaging Technologies

Even though it may not be the first step in the pathology of OA, damage to the articular cartilage remains the hallmark of the disease.[77] In clinical practice there are no radiopharmaceuticals to image articular cartilage, but selenium-based tracers are under development for this purpose.[78–80] Radiopharmaceuticals that are available for clinical imaging target secondary

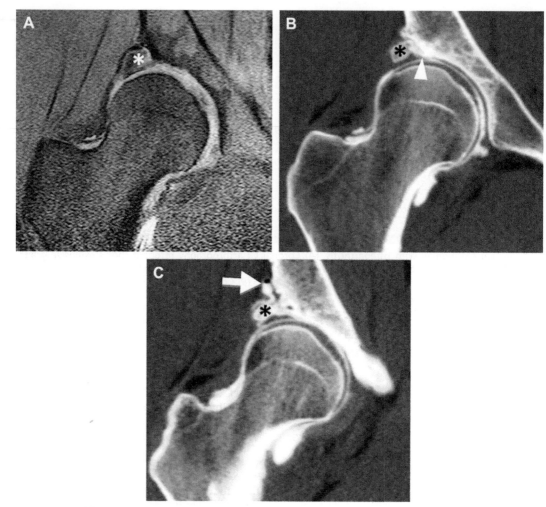

Fig. 7. 39-year-old woman with dysplastic hip. (A) Coronal fat-suppressed spin-echo T1-weighted MR arthrography image (489/12 ms, TR/TE) shows acetabular chondropathy and bony fragment (*) separated from the acetabular margin by contrast material. (B,C) Coronal CT arthrography reformats clearly show a down-to-bone cartilage defect (arrowhead) on the lateral margin of acetabulum and acetabular bony fragment (*). On CT arthrography image, the bone fragment is easily recognized but the contrast material at the bone–acetabular interface is less well depicted than at MR arthrography. The contrast material between the acetabulum and the femoral head is better seen at CT arthrography than at MR arthrography. Accumulation of contrast material at the margins of the acetabulum (arrow) is well seen in (C). Femoral head cartilage is normal, with a preserved gradient of cartilage thickness from the periphery to the center of the femoral head.

features of OA that are associated with damage to the articular cartilage, primarily bone turnover changes seen with osteophyte formation, subchondral sclerosis, and subchondral cyst formation.[81,82] Inflammation is a minor element of OA with the exception of the erosive OA seen in the hands, and this has also been the target of imaging with radiopharmaceuticals.[81]

Strategies that focus on bone imaging are more widespread, and diphosphonate derivatives radiolabeled with Tc-99m are the primary agents for this imaging. They have the added value that a modicum of soft tissue imaging is still possible

with these agents when a radionuclide angiogram and blood pool acquisition is added to the routine delayed views (ie, imaging done in three phases).

Two diphosphonates are in common use: Tc-99 methylene diphosphonate (Tc-99m MDP; Tc-99 medronate) and Tc-99 hydroxymethylene diphosphonate (Tc-99m HDP; Tc-99m oxidronate). These radiopharmaceuticals have a proven track record since their introduction in the 1970s, and are readily prepared from kits available from suppliers around the world. The agents have significant affinity to bone, with nearly 50% of the tracer binding to the bone trabeculae through the

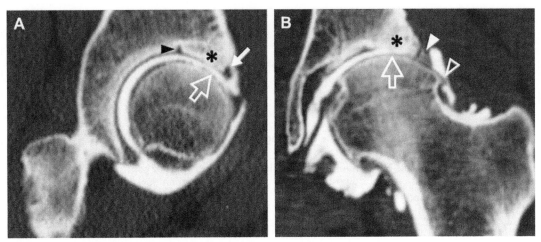

Fig. 8. 45-year-old woman with left hip osteoarthritis. (A) Sagittal and (B) coronal CT arthrography reformats clearly depict typical changes of osteoarthritis in the superolateral and anterior aspects of the hip joint: femoral head and acetabular cartilage thinning (*open arrows*), marginal femoral osteophytes (*open arrowhead*), acetabular osteophytes (*white arrowhead*), subchondral bone sclerosis (*), and subchondral cystic changes (*arrow*). Note the presence of a physiologic stellate defect of the subchondral bone plate at the apex of the acetabular bone (*black arrowhead, A*).

process of chemisorption. They have an excellent safety profile and the standard adult dose of 20–25 mCi results in excellent imaging with acceptable radiation exposure to the patient (approximately 5 mSv/25mCi dose).[83] They are readily excreted in the urine. The bladder is the critical organ so frequent voiding minimizes the exposure to radiation. Delayed imaging starts 2–3 hours after

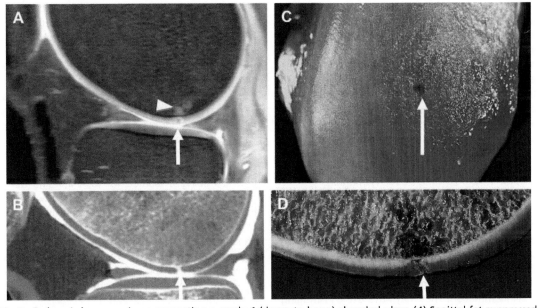

Fig. 9. Cadaveric knee specimen presenting a grade 4 (down-to-bone) chondral ulcer. (A) Sagittal fat-suppressed fast spin-echo intermediate-weighted MR imaging (3400/29 ms, TR/TE) shows grade 4 down-to-bone chondral ulcer (*arrow*) associated with subchondral bone edema (*arrowhead*) in the lateral femoral condyle. (B) Sagittal CT arthrography reformat shows the grade 4 chondral defect (*arrow*) filled with contrast material. Subchondral edema cannot be seen with CT. (C) En face photograph of the specimen shows the focal, round-shaped chondral defect (*arrow*). (D) Close-up photograph of the corresponding anatomic sagittal section shows the down-to-bone defect (*arrow*) in the lateral femoral condyle. Both MR imaging and CT arthrography are accurate for the evaluation of high-grade chondral lesions (grade 3 and above) but CT arthrography cannot demonstrate bone marrow changes.

Table 1
Grading systems for cartilage lesions at arthroscopy and CT and MR arthrography

Grade	Arthroscopic Findings	CT and MR Arthrography
Grade 0	Normal	Smooth surface and normal thickness of cartilage
Grade 1	Fibrillation without cartilage loss and cartilage softening	Smooth surface and normal thickness of cartilage
Grade 2	Substance loss less than 50% of cartilage thickness	Penetration of contrast in cartilage to less than 50% in depth
Grade 3	Substance loss more than 50% of cartilage thickness but not down-to-bone	Penetration of contrast in cartilage to more than 50% in depth
Grade 4	Down-to-bone cartilage loss	Penetration of contrast down to subchondral bone

injection to allow for clearance from the soft tissues. Imaging is earlier with Tc-99m HDP, given its higher affinity for bone. However, Tc-99m HDP is more expensive than Tc-99m MDP.

Another bone imaging agent is 18-Fluoride (18-F⁻), a positron-emitting radioisotope that predates the diphosphonates compounds.[84] However, it is only now, with the widespread acceptance of positron emission tomography (PET) and PET-CT technologies, that it is possible to exploit this agent in clinical imaging.[84] This radioisotope is readily produced in a cyclotron, and has high affinity to bone through the process of anion substitution in the hydroxyapatite complex. Bone images of high quality are readily obtained using modern PET-CT scanners as early as 30 minutes after injection of 5–10 mCi of tracer. Excretion is through the urine, and nearly 50% of the tracer binds bone.[83,84] The estimated whole body dose is 10 mSv/10 mCi dose. As of January 1, 2008, changes to the clinical procedural terminology of the American Medical Association in the United States allows physicians to bill insurance companies for 18-F⁻ PET (and PET-CT) imaging.[85]

Radiopharmaceuticals that image soft tissue components and largely target the inflammatory component of OA include radiolabeled white blood cells, Gallium-67 citrate, and 18-fluorodeoxyglucose (18-FDG). White blood cells labeled with Tc-99m or In-111 and Gallium-67 citrate are gamma photon emitters that are used in detecting infection and inflammation. They may have a role in imaging of septic arthritis, and possibly inflammatory arthritides, but are not used in imaging OA, and therefore not discussed in this review.[86–88] 18-FDG is a positron-emitting radiopharmaceutical that accumulates at sites of increased glucose metabolism, particularly due to increase in glucose transporters, and to increase in aerobic glycolysis as seen in tumor cells and activated leukocytes.[89,90] Although

18-FDG is used primarily for imaging in oncology, it has also been applied to infection and inflammation imaging, including bone infections.[87,91] The PET in the 18-FDG PET-CT scans of subjects referred for cancer imaging shows uptake at sites of OA in the CT part of the examination. Recent reports suggest a possible role for 18-FDG to detect and possibly evaluate the inflammatory component of OA.[92–94]

To image the joints there are a variety of methods in nuclear medicine. In addition to three-phase bone scans, delayed views with planar scintigraphy or single-photon computed tomography (SPECT) are common (**Fig. 10**).[95] Magnification imaging with pinhole collimators (see **Fig. 10**) provides details in planar scintigraphy.[96] Today, PET imaging is done largely in whole body PET-CT scanners capable of hardware fusion of anatomic and physiologic images, as well as the attenuation correction necessary for quantitative imaging.[97] Similar hybrid imaging has been developed for SPECT, and, as expected, is labeled SPECT-CT.[98–101] There are new small part PET scanners designed for breast imaging[102] that are being evaluated for joint imaging using either 18-F⁻ and/or 18-FDG. An example is the PEM Flex Solo II PET scanner (Naviscan PET Systems, Inc., San Diego, California) (**Fig. 11**).[103] These scanners have exquisite sensitivity and higher resolution than whole body scanners. They promise to extend PET imaging into new areas, including joint imaging, but at this time remain the subject of research.

Applications

Diphosphonate imaging

Although the role of scintigraphy in the diagnosis of OA is not clear, rheumatologists find bone scans useful in their practice,[104] because bone scintigraphy is a simple examination that allows for

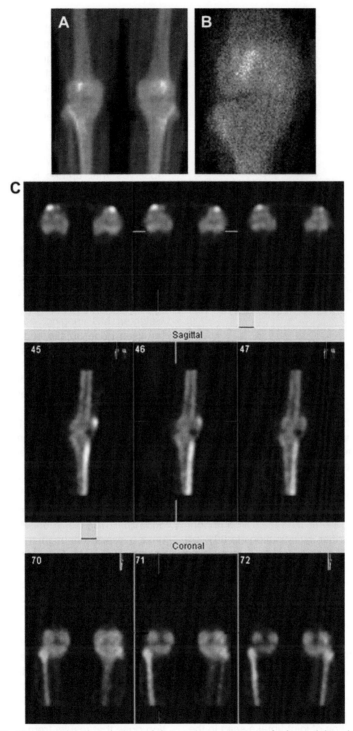

Fig. 10. Asymptomatic 48-year-old male volunteer. (A) Anterior projection of 5-hour delayed 25 mCi Tc-99m MDP scintigram. (B) Magnification pinhole image of the right knee in (A). (C) Selected nonattenuation corrected SPECT views in axial (upper row), sagittal (middle row), and coronal (lower row) planes through the right knee. There is no activity in the joint but uptake is seen in the anterior surface of both patellae, and the SPECT scans shows narrowing of the tibiofemoral joint on the left side with no increased uptake.

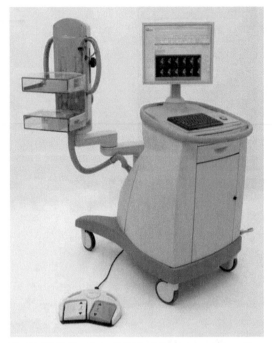

Fig. 11. PEM Flex Solo II Clinical System configuration. (*Courtesy of* Naviscan PET Systems, Inc., San Diego, CA; with permission.)

a full body survey that helps to discriminate between soft tissues versus bone/joint origin of pain, and to locate the site of pain in patients with complex symptoms. An analysis by Duncan and colleagues[104] of the practice of Australian rheumatologists found that bone scans altered clinical diagnosis and changed the course of management over 30% of the time. More important, it prevented further investigations in 60% of the cases.

In the specific case of "unclassified arthritis," Duer and colleagues[105] have shown that a combination of MR imaging of the hands and wrists and Tc-99m HDP whole body scintigraphy is useful to discriminate between the different arthritides. They evaluated a cohort of 41 subjects that remained unclassified after applying conventional clinical, biochemical, and radiographic methods, including the American College of Rheumatology criteria for rheumatoid arthritis (RA). Discrimination between the different RA and OA was done on the basis of the distribution of joint uptake seen in the bone scans, and the presence of synovitis and erosions in the MR imaging scans. The gold standard was specialist review 2 years after initial imaging and evaluation. The combination of MR imaging and scintigraphy was 95% accurate in discriminating between RA and non–RA. Although their intent was to help with the early diagnosis of

RA, none of the eight subjects originally classified as OA on the basis of their imaging algorithm were reclassified by the gold standard.

It is clear that scintigraphy has high sensitivity in detecting bone reaction to the pathology of OA.[82,106–108] It is important to recognize that bone scintigraphy with diphosphonates targets the bone response that results from the abnormal biomechanics of joint motion when the articular cartilage is damaged. The physiology of this uptake has been reviewed by Merrick,[82] who observes that uptake is related to osteophyte formation, subchondral sclerosis, and subchondral cyst formation that all result from abnormal loads on the joint. When osteophyte formation is successful in reducing the point forces that result from cartilage damage, tracer uptake may stop as the osteophyte matures and no new osteophytes are formed. It is noteworthy that uptake associated with subchondral sclerosis correlates well with increases in bone marrow signal in T2-weighted MR imaging, and that the agreement between bone uptake and MR imaging features of osteophytes or cartilage defects is less striking.[82,109]

Therefore, it is not surprising that bone scans show abnormal uptake before the detection of abnormal morphology in routine radiography (**Fig. 12**).[82,106,107] Also, activity in bone scintigraphy implies that abnormal stress persists and that the disease will progress.[82] For this reason, some advocate the use of scintigraphy to select candidates for clinical trials that evaluate disease-modifying drugs. In clinical practice, a negative bone scan may provide some reassurance that disease is unlikely to progress in the next 5 years, although the predictive power of scintigraphy is far from 100%.[110] Indeed, recent work by Mazzuca and colleagues[108,111] demonstrates that similar or better predictive power for progression of disease can be obtained by combining indices of clinical symptoms with radiographic methods that are common in the research setting, namely measurement of joint space narrowing using standard projections and computer-assisted measurements. His approach provides a simpler and safer alternative to scintigraphy in selecting patients that are likely to progress in their disease, because it avoids the whole body radiation dose that results from injecting a radiotracer. However, his radiographic methods are uncommon in routine clinical imaging departments.

In addition to assisting in the diagnosis and prognosis of OA, scintigraphy may also assist in therapy. Facet OA of the spine can lead to back pain that responds to the injection of

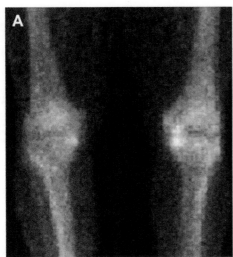

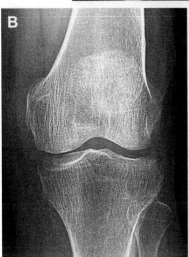

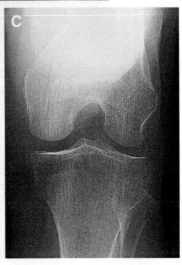

Fig. 12. Left knee pain in middle-aged woman. (*A*) 3-hour delayed 25 mCi Tc-99 MDP bone scan in the anterior projection shows uptake in the medial compartments is worse on the left side. This is compatible with osteoarthritis. However, (*B*) posteroanterior and (*C*) tunnel view radiographs show no significant findings.

steroids.[112,113] Early work by Dolan and colleagues[113] demonstrated that spine SPECT imaging with diphosphonates is able to select those facets that will respond to steroid injections (**Fig. 13**). In the authors' experience, this technology is most useful when studies are read in conjunction with CT myelograms or MR imaging that allow for evaluation of disc disease. Good physical examination is imperative to confirm that imaging findings are compatible with the patient's pain. Recently Kim and Park described a pattern of uptake in planar scintigraphy of the lumbar spine that is so characteristic of facet OA that it renders SPECT unnecessary.[114] In this pattern, bilateral facet uptake at the same axial level leads to a characteristic "V" shape to the uptake in the posterior view. However, it is likely that this pattern has low sensitivity and SPECT imaging is necessary when the pattern is not seen in a patient with back pain.

As of now, imaging with diphosphonates is dominated by planar scintigraphy. SPECT imaging has better sensitivity and improves anatomic localization. A recent study confirmed the ability of SPECT to detect early osteoarthritis of the knee with good correlation to clinical findings.[115] Due to its improved anatomic localization, SPECT of the knee has also proven useful in planning unicompartmental knee arthroplasty of the medial compartment of the tibiofemoral joint, because it is in this compartment that scintigraphic findings correlate best with those features of OA detected at the time of surgery.[116] SPECT-CT imaging allows for attenuation correction that may lead to quantification and improves specificity.[98,100,101] Recent literature illustrates how the hybrid technology improves bone imaging, because the CT not only improves the quality of the scintigraphic imaging, but also leads to the characterization of commonly nonspecific scintigraphic

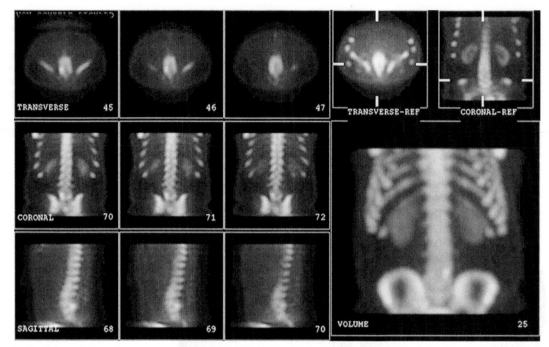

Fig. 13. Selected views from a nonattenuation corrected 3-hour delayed 25 mCi lumbar spine SPECT scan show uptake in the right facet joint at the L4-L5 level. The maximum intensity projection imaging on the right lower corner is seen from the posterior view.

uptake.[98,99,101,117] Resolution recovery methods allow for faster SPECT imaging or improved quality when the imaging time is unchanged.[118,119] This feature is already being offered by several manufacturers. Pinhole collimation is time-consuming, but it affords details seen more often in pediatric applications,[96] though seldom applied to adults with arthritis (see Fig. 10). For the most

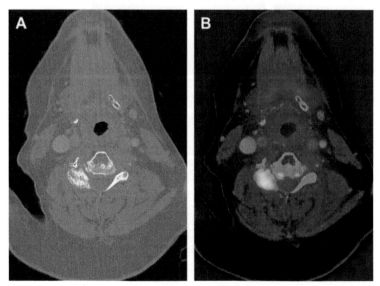

Fig. 14. 62-year-old man treated for hypopharyngeal cancer who presents to 18-FDG PET-CT for restaging. (A) Axial CT scan shows clear evidence of advanced OA in a right facet of the cervical spine. (B) Axial fused 18-FDG PET-CT scan (10 mCi 18-FDG with 60 minutes' incubation before imaging) shows the intense 18-FDG uptake of the osteoarthritic cervical facet.

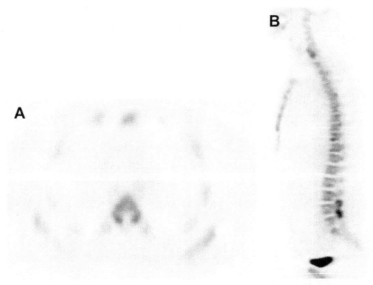

Fig. 15. Selected axial and sagittal views from a 90-minute delayed 10 mCi 18-Fluoride PET scan done in a whole body scanner with CT attenuation correction show facet uptake consistent with L3-L4 and L4-L5 osteoarthritis. Contrast the quality of these images with the SPECT scan in Fig. 13.

part, none of these methods have found their way into arthritis imaging.

Positron emitters

Musculoskeletal imaging with positron emitters and PET-CT technology is still in its infancy. The effort is largely confined to oncology imaging, but there is no reason to expect that these technologies will not play a role in imaging patients with arthritis. Anecdotal experience with 18-FDG in imaging patients with cancer and two early reports demonstrate that PET with this agent is able to detect OA (Fig. 14).[92,93] The uptake is seen in the synovitis associated with OA, and therefore is different from the imaging done with bone-seeking agents. Indeed, it is not surprising that 18-FDG is seen more often in joints affected by RA than OA.[94]

18-F⁻ PET and PET-CT imaging improves on the poor resolution of SPECT imaging with diphosphonates while retaining excellent sensitivity. Comparison of Figs. 13 and 15 makes it clear that images from the positron emitter are superior to those from the gamma emitter.

Hybrid technologies like PET-CT bring a new element to arthritis imaging and research, because they combine anatomic and functional imaging in ways that no other imaging technologies are able to do. The field would benefit from the development of cartilage-specific agents. Such a radiopharmaceutical combined with 18-FDG and 18-F⁻would bring a new dimension to arthritis imaging, because the applications of these three tracers would target three major elements in the pathology of OA and arthritis in general: cartilage, inflammation, and bone.

PET scanners to image small parts have been developed specifically to image the breast (see Fig. 11).[103] The scanner is noteworthy for its sensitivity and resolution, but lacks attenuation correction, so quantification is not possible as it is with whole body PET-CT scanners. Nevertheless, Figs. 16 and 17 show very preliminary images of a normal volunteer imaged using significantly lower doses than those used with whole body scanners. These images are far from optimal, but, using existing technology, they can be improved by tweaking the dose of radiotracer and time to image as illustrated by comparing Figs. 16 and 18. The unit is portable, and the cost and operational requirements are significantly less than those for whole body scanners. Time will tell if these units find their way into imaging of joints in a fashion similar to small-parts fixed-field specialty MR imaging units.

SUMMARY

MR imaging currently remains the method of choice for noninvasive diagnosis of chondral lesions. It is the only technique that allows the evaluation of surface lesions, subchondral changes, and the structure of cartilage. Whenever accurate evaluation of surface changes is needed, however, invasive arthrographic techniques are indicated. Compared with MR arthrography, CT

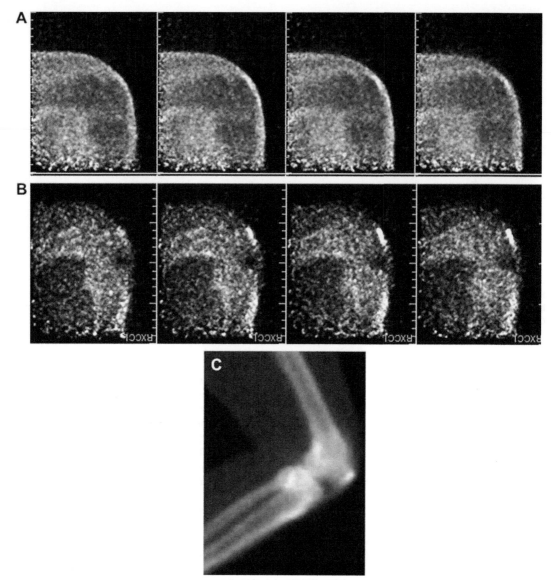

Fig. 16. Right knee of the same asymptomatic volunteer as in Fig. 10. (*A*) Selected sagittal views of 18-FDG PET scan (4 mCi with 60 minutes' incubation) done with small part scanner shown in Fig. 11 shows no activity in the joint and only apparent tracer uptake in the skin over the patella. (*B*) Selected sagittal views of 18-Fluoride scan (0.87 mCi with 90 minutes' incubation) using small parts PET scanner and (*C*) right lateral view of 25 mCi Tc-99m MDP 5-hour delayed scintigram demonstrate no activity in the joint, but uptake is seen in the anterior surface of the patella.

arthrography has the inconvenience of radiation exposure and the limitation to surface lesions only. CT arthrography is, however, a valuable technique whenever MR arthrography is not possible (eg, not available, contraindicated, or technically impossible, such as with obese or claustrophobic patients, or the presence of metallic hardware). The indications of the intraarticular injection of contrast material may evolve in the near future, with the development of new 3.0 T imaging techniques and three-dimentional acquisitions.

Radioisotope methods to image osteoarthritis suffer from the lack of agents that specifically target articular cartilage and the need to use ionizing radiation. However, bone scintigraphy is sensitive to the reaction of the underlying bone when the cartilage is damaged, and a negative bone scan may provide assurance that the disease is unlikely to progress. The advent of 18-FDG PET and PET-CT imaging brings the opportunity to explore the inflammatory component of osteoarthritis. 18-F⁻ PET and PET-CT and Tc-99m MDP/

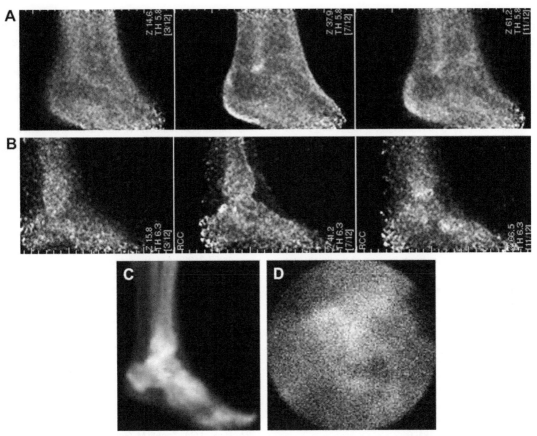

Fig. 17. Right ankle of the same asymptomatic volunteer as in Fig. 10. (*A*) Selected sagittal views of 18-FDG PET scan (4 mCi with 60 minutes' incubation) done with small part scanner shown in Fig. 11. (*B*) Selected sagittal views of 18-Fluoride scan (0.87 mCi with 90 minutes' incubation) using small parts PET scanner. (*C*) Right lateral view of 25 mCi Tc-99m MDP 5-hour delayed scintigram. (*D*) Magnification pinhole image of the right ankle focusing in the tibiotalar joint. An uptake is seen in the posterior aspect of the talotibial joint in both 18-FDG and bone imaging.

HDP imaging with SPECT and SPECT-CT bring added sensitivity and improved anatomic localization that has not been readily exploited in imaging osteoarthritis. They also bring the opportunity to combine molecular and anatomic imaging in one image. Small-part PET devices are already in clinical use in breast imaging, and in development for joint imaging. Their value stems from lower

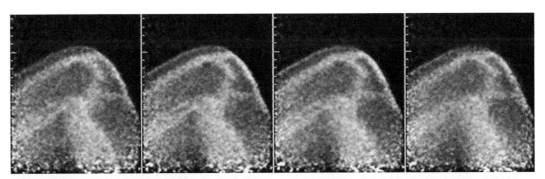

Fig. 18. 79-year-old woman with asymptomatic knee who underwent a restaging of ovarian cancer with 18-FDG PET-CT imaging. Selected sagittal views through one knee using small parts PET scanner (after whole body scan, 100 minutes after injection of 10.6 mCi of 18-FDG) show improved imaging with larger dose and longer incubation period.

operating costs, and lower radiation burden to the patient while still retaining significant resolution and sensitivity.

REFERENCES

1. Drapé JL, Pessis E, Sarazin L, et al. MRI and articular cartilage. J Radiol 1998;79(5):391–402.
2. Link TM, Stahl R, Woertler K. Cartilage imaging: motivation, techniques, current and future significance. Eur Radiol 2007;17(5):1135–46.
3. Rand T, Brossmann J, Pedowitz R, et al. Analysis of patellar cartilage. Comparison of conventional MR imaging and MR and CT arthrography in cadavers. Acta Radiol 2000;41(5):492–7.
4. Daniel E, Lajko P. Diagnostic significance of the positive arthrography in injuries of the knee cartilage. Magy Seb 1954;7(5):331–9.
5. Boven F, Bellemans MA, Geurts J, et al. The value of computed tomography scanning in chondromalacia patellae. Skeletal Radiol 1982;8(3):183–5.
6. Boven F, Bellemans MA, Geurts J, et al. A comparative study of the patello-femoral joint on axial roentgenogram, axial arthrogram, and computed tomography following arthrography. Skeletal Radiol 1982;8(3):179–81.
7. Reiser M, Karpf PM, Bernett P. Diagnosis of chondromalacia patellae using CT arthrography. Eur J Radiol 1982;2(3):181–6.
8. Buckwalter KA. CT arthrography. Clin Sports Med 2006;25(4):899–915.
9. Lecouvet FE, Simoni P, Koutaïssoff S, et al. Multidetector spiral CT arthrography of the shoulder: Clinical applications and limits, with MR arthrography and arthroscopic correlations. Eur J Radiol 2008;68(1):120–36.
10. Hall FM, Goldberg RP, Wyshak G, et al. Shoulder arthrography: comparison of morbidity after use of various contrast media. Radiology 1985;154(2):339–41.
11. Lecouvet F, Dorzée B, Dubuc J, et al. Cartilage lesions of the glenohumeral joint: diagnostic effectiveness of multidetector spiral CT arthrography and comparison with arthroscopy. Eur Radiol 2007;17(7):1763–71.
12. Railhac J. Iopentol (Imagopaque 300) compared with ioxaglate (Hexabrix 320) in knee arthrography. A clinical trial assessing immediate and late adverse events and diagnostic information. Eur Radiol 1997;7(4):S135–9.
13. Vande Berg BC, Lecouvet F, Malghem J. Frequency and topography of lesions of the femoro-tibial cartilage at spiral CT arthrography of the knee: a study in patients with normal knee radiographs and without history of trauma. Skeletal Radiol 2002;31(11):643–9.
14. Noël C, Campagna R, Minoui A, et al. Fissures of the posterior labrum and associated lesions: CT arthrogram evaluation. J Radiol 2008;89(4):487–93.
15. Daenen BR, Ferrara MA, Marcelis S, et al. Evaluation of patellar cartilage surface lesions: comparison of CT arthrography and fat-suppressed FLASH 3D MR imaging. Eur Radiol 1998;8(6):981–5.
16. Binkert CA, Verdun FR, Zanetti M, et al. Arthrography of the glenohumeral joint: CT fluoroscopy versus conventional CT and fluoroscopy–comparison of image-guidance techniques. Radiology 2003;229(1):153–8.
17. Wyler A, Bousson V, Bergot C, et al. Hyaline cartilage thickness in radiographically normal cadaveric hips: comparison of spiral CT arthrographic and macroscopic measurements. Radiology 2007;242(2):441–9.
18. Osinski T, Malfair D, Steinbach L. Magnetic resonance arthrography. Orthop Clin North Am 2006;37(3):299–319, vi.
19. Hajek PC, Sartoris DJ, Neumann CH, et al. Potential contrast agents for MR arthrography: in vitro evaluation and practical observations. Am J Roentgenol 1987;149(1):97–104.
20. Zanetti M, Hodler J. Contrast media in MR arthrography of the glenohumeral joint: intra-articular gadopentetate vs saline: preliminary results. Eur Radiol 1997;7(4):498–502.
21. Binkert CA, Zanetti M, Gerber C, et al. MR arthrography of the glenohumeral joint: two concentrations of gadoteridol versus ringer solution as the intraarticular contrast material. Radiology 2001;220(1):219–24.
22. Schulte-Altedorneburg G, Gebhard, et al. MR arthrography: pharmacology, efficacy and safety in clinical trials. Skeletal Radiol 2003;32(1):1–12.
23. Hodler J. Technical errors in MR arthrography. Skeletal Radiol 2008;37(1):9–18.
24. Masi JN, Newitt D, Sell CA, et al. Optimization of gadodiamide concentration for MR arthrography at 3 T. Am J Roentgenol 2005;184(6):1754–61.
25. Andreisek G, Froehlich JM, Hodler J, et al. Direct MR arthrography at 1.5 and 3.0 T: signal dependence on gadolinium and iodine concentrations–phantom study. Radiology 2008;247(3):706–16.
26. Detreille R, Sauer B, Zabel JP, et al. [Technical considerations for injection of a mixture of iodinated contrast material and Artirem for combined CT and MR arthrography]. J Radiol 2007;88(6):863–9.
27. Brown RR, Clarke DW, Daffner RH. Is a mixture of gadolinium and iodinated contrast material safe during MR arthrography? Am J Roentgenol 2000;175(4):1087–90.
28. Choi JY, Kang HS, Hong SH, et al. Optimization of the contrast mixture ratio for simultaneous direct MR and CT arthrography: an in vitro study. Korean J Radiol 2008;9(6):520–5.

29. Kopka L, Funke M, Fischer U, et al. MR arthrography of the shoulder with gadopentetate dimeglumine: influence of concentration, iodinated contrast material, and time on signal intensity. Am J Roentgenol 1994;163(3):621–3.

30. Jacobson JA, Lin J, Jamadar DA, et al. Aids to successful shoulder arthrography performed with a fluoroscopically guided anterior approach. Radiographics 2003;23(2):373–8.

31. Mulligan ME. CT-guided shoulder arthrography at the rotator cuff interval. Am J Roentgenol 2008; 191(2):W58–61.

32. Koivikko MP, Mustonen AO. Shoulder magnetic resonance arthrography: a prospective randomized study of anterior and posterior ultrasonography-guided contrast injections. Acta Radiol 2008; 49(8):912–7.

33. Lohman M, Vasenius J, Nieminen O. Ultrasound guidance for puncture and injection in the radiocarpal joint. Acta Radiol 2007;48(7):744–7.

34. Rutten M, Collins J, Maresch B, et al. Glenohumeral joint injection: a comparative study of ultrasound and fluoroscopically guided techniques before MR arthrography. Eur Radiol 2009;19(3):722–30.

35. Petersilge CA, Lewin JS, Duerk JL, et al. MR arthrography of the shoulder: rethinking traditional imaging procedures to meet the technical requirements of MR imaging guidance. Am J Roentgenol 1997;169(5):1453–7.

36. Berná-Serna JD, Redondo MV, Martínez F, et al. A simple technique for shoulder arthrography. Acta Radiol 2006;47(7):725–9.

37. Catalano OA, Manfredi R, Vanzulli A, et al. MR arthrography of the glenohumeral joint: modified posterior approach without imaging guidance. Radiology 2007;242(2):550–4.

38. DeMouy EH, Menendez CV, Bodin CJ. Palpation-directed (non-fluoroscopically guided) saline-enhanced MR arthrography of the shoulder. Am J Roentgenol 1997;169(1):229–31.

39. Freiberger RH. Arthrography. Upper Saddle River (NJ): Prentice Hall; 1979.

40. Chevrot A, Pallardy G. Arthrographies opaques. Masson; 1988.

41. Crim J. Arthrography: principles & practice in radiology. Lippincott Williams & Wilkins; 2008.

42. Obermann WR, Bloem JL, Hermans J. Knee arthrography: comparison of iotrolan and ioxaglate sodium meglumine. Radiology 1989;173(1):197–201.

43. Andreisek G, Duc SR, Froehlich JM, et al. MR arthrography of the shoulder, hip, and wrist: evaluation of contrast dynamics and image quality with increasing injection-to-imaging time. Am J Roentgenol 2007;188(4):1081–8.

44. Wagner SC, Schweitzer ME, Weishaupt D. Temporal behavior of intraarticular gadolinium. J Comput Assist Tomogr 2001;25(5):661–70.

45. Mutschler C, Vande Berg BC, Lecouvet FE, et al. Postoperative meniscus: assessment at dual-detector row spiral CT arthrography of the knee. Radiology 2003;228(3):635–41.

46. Spataro RF, Katzberg RW, Burgener FA, et al. Epinephrine enhanced knee arthrography. Invest Radiol 1978;13(4):286–90.

47. Hall FM. Epinephrine-enhanced knee arthrography. Radiology 1974;111(1):215–7.

48. Chung CB, Isaza IL, Angulo M, et al. MR arthrography of the knee: how, why, when. Radiol Clin North Am 2005;43(4):733–46, viii–ix.

49. Brenner ML, Morrison WB, Carrino JA, et al. Direct MR arthrography of the shoulder: is exercise prior to imaging beneficial or detrimental? Radiology 2000;215(2):491–6.

50. Vande Berg BC, Lecouvet FE, Poilvache P, et al. Spiral CT arthrography of the knee: technique and value in the assessment of internal derangement of the knee. Eur Radiol 2002;12(7):1800–10.

51. Rydberg J, Buckwalter KA, Caldemeyer KS, et al. Multisection CT: scanning techniques and clinical applications. Radiographics 2000;20(6):1787–806.

52. Baert A, Tack D, Gevenois P. Radiation dose from adult and pediatric multidetector computed tomography. Springer; 2007.

53. Lee M, Kim S, Lee S, et al. Overcoming artifacts from metallic orthopedic implants at high-field-strength MR imaging and multi-detector CT. Radiographics 2007;27(3):791–803.

54. Vande Berg B, Malghem J, Maldague B, et al. Multi-detector CT imaging in the postoperative orthopedic patient with metal hardware. Eur J Radiol 2006;60(3):470–9.

55. Elentuck D, Palmer WE. Direct magnetic resonance arthrography. Eur Radiol 2004;14(11):1956–67.

56. Wutke R, Fellner FA, Fellner C, et al. Direct MR arthrography of the shoulder: 2D vs. 3D gradient-echo imaging. Magn Reson Imaging 2001;19(9): 1183–91.

57. Newberg AH, Munn CS, Robbins AH. Complications of arthrography. Radiology 1985;155(3):605–6.

58. Berquist TH. Imaging of articular pathology: MRI, CT, arthrography. Clin Anat 1997;10(1):1–13.

59. Cerezal L, Abascal F, García-Valtuille R, et al. Ankle MR arthrography: how, why, when. Radiol Clin North Am 2005;43(4):693–707, viii.

60. Saupe N, Zanetti M, Pfirrmann CWA, et al. Pain and other side effects after MR arthrography: prospective evaluation in 1085 patients. Radiology 2009; 250(3):830–8.

61. Binkert CA, Zanetti M, Hodler J. Patient's assessment of discomfort during MR arthrography of the shoulder. Radiology 2001;221(3):775–8.

62. Blum AG, Simon JM, Cotten A, et al. Comparison of double-contrast CT arthrography image quality with nonionic contrast agents: isotonic dimeric iodixanol

270 mg I/mL and monomeric iohexol 300 mg I/mL. Invest Radiol 2000;35(5):304–10.

63. Corbetti F, Malatesta V, Camposampiero A, et al. Knee arthrography: effects of various contrast media and epinephrine on synovial fluid. Radiology 1986;161(1):195–8.

64. El-Khoury GY, Alliman KJ, Lundberg HJ, et al. Cartilage thickness in cadaveric ankles: measurement with double-contrast multi-detector row CT arthrography versus MR imaging. Radiology 2004;233(3):768–73.

65. Haubner M, Eckstein F, Schnier M, et al. A non-invasive technique for 3-dimensional assessment of articular cartilage thickness based on MRI part 2: validation using CT arthrography. Magn Reson Imaging 1997;15(7):805–13.

66. Anderson AE, Ellis BJ, Peters CL, et al. Cartilage thickness: factors influencing multidetector CT measurements in a phantom study. Radiology 2008;246(1):133–41.

67. Wyler A, Bousson V, Bergot C, et al. Comparison of MR-arthrography and CT-arthrography in hyaline cartilage-thickness measurement in radiographically normal cadaver hips with anatomy as gold standard. Osteoarthritis Cartilage 2009;17(1):19–25.

68. Schmid MR, Pfirrmann CWA, Hodler J, et al. Cartilage lesions in the ankle joint: comparison of MR arthrography and CT arthrography. Skeletal Radiol 2003;32(5):259–65.

69. Ihara H. Double-contrast CT arthrography of the cartilage of the patellofemoral joint. Clin Orthop Relat Res 1985;198:50–5.

70. Noyes FR, Stabler CL. A system for grading articular cartilage lesions at arthroscopy. Am J Sports Med 1989;17(4):505–13.

71. Outerbridge RE. The etiology of chondromalacia patellae. J Bone Joint Surg Br 1961;43-B: 752–7.

72. Vande Berg BC, Lecouvet FE, Poilvache P, et al. Assessment of knee cartilage in cadavers with dual-detector spiral CT arthrography and MR imaging. Radiology 2002;222(2):430–6.

73. Schmid MR, Notzli HP, Zanetti M, et al. Cartilage lesions in the hip: diagnostic effectiveness of MR arthrography. Radiology 2003;226(2):382–6.

74. Llopis E, Cerezal L, Kassarjian A, et al. Direct MR arthrography of the hip with leg traction: feasibility for assessing articular cartilage. Am J Roentgenol 2008;190(4):1124–8.

75. McCauley TR, Kornaat PR, Jee W. Central osteophytes in the knee: prevalence and association with cartilage defects on MR imaging. Am J Roentgenol 2001;176(2):359–64.

76. Guermazi A, Burstein D, Conaghan P, et al. Imaging in osteoarthritis. Rheum Dis Clin North Am 2008;34(3):645–87.

77. Brandt KD, Radin EL, Dieppe PA, et al. Yet more evidence that osteoarthritis is not a cartilage disease. Ann Rheum Dis 2006;65(10):1261–4.

78. Yu WK, Bartlett JM, van Sickle DC, et al. Biodistribution of bis-[beta-(N, N, N-trimethylamino)ethyl]-selenide-75Se diiodide, a potential articular cartilage imaging agent. Int J Rad Appl Instrum B 1988;15(2):229–30.

79. Yu SW, Shaw SM, Van Sickle DC. Radionuclide studies of articular cartilage in the early diagnosis of arthritis in the rabbit. Ann Acad Med Singapore 1999;28(1):44–8.

80. Yu WK, Shaw SM, Bartlett JM, et al. The biodistribution of [75Se]bis-[beta-(N, N, N-trimethylamino)ethyl]selenide diiodide in adult guinea pigs. Int J Rad Appl Instrum B 1989;16(3):255–9.

81. Etchebehere EC, Etchebehere M, Gamba R, et al. Orthopedic pathology of the lower extremities: scintigraphic evaluation in the thigh, knee, and leg. Semin Nucl Med 1998;28(1):41–61.

82. Merrick MV. Investigation of joint disease. Eur J Nucl Med Mol Imaging 1992;19(10):894–901.

83. Klingensmith W III, Eshima D, Goddard J. Nuclear medicine procedure manual. 2006th edition. Englewood (CO): Wick Publishing; 2006.

84. Grant FD, Fahey FH, Packard AB, et al. Skeletal PET with 18F-fluoride: applying new technology to an old tracer. J Nucl Med 2008;49(1):68–78.

85. Beebe M, Dalton J, Espronceda M. CPT 2009 professional edition. American Medical Association; 2009.

86. Rosenthall L. Nuclear medicine techniques in arthritis. Rheum Dis Clin North Am 1991;17(3): 585–97.

87. Love C, Tomas MB, Tronco GG, et al. FDG PET of infection and inflammation. Radiographics 2005; 25(5):1357–68.

88. Filippi L, Schillaci O. Usefulness of hybrid SPECT/CT in 99mTc-HMPAO-labeled leukocyte scintigraphy for bone and joint infections. J Nucl Med 2006;47(12):1908–13.

89. Elgazzar AH. The pathophysiologic basis of nuclear medicine. 2nd edition. Berlin, Germany: Springer-Verlag; 2006.

90. Frauwirth KA, Thompson CB. Regulation of T lymphocyte metabolism. J Immunol 2004;172(8): 4661–5.

91. Kostakoglu L, Agress H, Goldsmith SJ. Clinical role of FDG PET in evaluation of cancer patients. Radiographics 2003;23(2):315–40.

92. Nakamura H, Masuko K, Yudoh K, et al. Positron emission tomography with 18F-FDG in osteoarthritic knee. Osteoarthritis Cartilage 2007;15(6): 673–81.

93. Wandler E, Kramer EL, Sherman O, et al. Diffuse FDG shoulder uptake on PET is associated with

clinical findings of osteoarthritis. Am J Roentgenol 2005;185(3):797–803.

94. Elzinga E, van der Laken C, Comans E, et al. 2-Deoxy-2-[F-18]fluoro-D-glucose joint uptake on positron emission tomography images: rheumatoid arthritis versus osteoarthritis. Mol Imaging Biol 2007;9(6):357–60.

95. Sarikaya I, Sarikaya A, Holder LE. The role of single photon emission computed tomography in bone imaging. Semin Nucl Med 2001;31(1):3–16.

96. Bahk Y, Kim S, Chung S, et al. Dual-head pinhole bone scintigraphy. J Nucl Med 1998;39(8):1444–8.

97. Townsend DW, Carney JP, Yap JT, et al. PET/CT today and tomorrow. J Nucl Med 2004; 45(1 suppl):4S–14S.

98. Horger M, Eschmann SM, Pfannenberg C, et al. Evaluation of combined transmission and emission tomography for classification of skeletal lesions. Am J Roentgenol 2004;183(3):655–61.

99. Strobel K, Burger C, Seifert B, et al. Characterization of focal bone lesions in the axial skeleton: performance of planar bone scintigraphy compared with SPECT and SPECT fused with CT. Am J Roentgenol 2007;188(5):W467–74.

100. Buck AK, Nekolla S, Ziegler S, et al. SPECT/CT. J Nucl Med 2008;49(8):1305–19.

101. Even-Sapir E, Flusser G, Lerman H, et al. SPECT/ multislice low-dose CT: a clinically relevant constituent in the imaging algorithm of nononcologic patients referred for bone scintigraphy. J Nucl Med 2007;48(2):319–24.

102. Tafra L. Positron emission tomography (PET) and mammography (PEM) for breast cancer: importance to surgeons. Ann Surg Oncol 2007;14(1):3–13.

103. Naviscan - home. Available at: http://www.naviscan. com. Accessed January 27, 2009.

104. Duncan I, Dorai-Raj A, Khoo K, et al. The utility of bone scans in rheumatology. Clin Nucl Med 1999;24(1):9–14.

105. Duer A, Ostergaard M, Horslev-Petersen K, et al. Magnetic resonance imaging and bone scintigraphy in the differential diagnosis of unclassified arthritis. Ann Rheum Dis 2008;67(1):48–51.

106. Hutton CW, Higgs ER, Jackson PC, et al. 99mTc HMDP bone scanning in generalised nodal osteoarthritis. II. The four hour bone scan image predicts radiographic change. Ann Rheum Dis 1986;45(8):622–6.

107. Buckland-Wright C. Current status of imaging procedures in the diagnosis, prognosis and monitoring of osteoarthritis. Baillieres Clin Rheumatol 1997;11(4):727–48.

108. Mazzuca SA, Brandt KD, Schauwecker DS, et al. Bone scintigraphy is not a better predictor of

progression of knee osteoarthritis than Kellgren and Lawrence grade. J Rheumatol 2004;31(2): 329–32.

109. Boegård T. Radiography and bone scintigraphy in osteoarthritis of the knee–comparison with MR imaging. Acta Radiol Suppl 1998;418:7–37.

110. Dieppe P, Cushnaghan J, Young P, et al. Prediction of the progression of joint space narrowing in osteoarthritis of the knee by bone scintigraphy. Ann Rheum Dis 1993;52(8):557–63.

111. Mazzuca SA, Brandt KD, Schauwecker DS, et al. Severity of joint pain and Kellgren-Lawrence grade at baseline are better predictors of joint space narrowing than bone scintigraphy in obese women with knee osteoarthritis. J Rheumatol 2005;32(8): 1540–6.

112. De Maeseneer M, Lenchik L, Everaert H, et al. Evaluation of lower back pain with bone scintigraphy and SPECT. Radiographics 1999;19(4): 901–12.

113. Dolan AL, Ryan PJ, Arden NK, et al. The value of SPECT scans in identifying back pain likely to benefit from facet joint injection. Rheumatology 1996;35(12):1269–73.

114. Kim CK, Park KW. Characteristic appearance of facet osteoarthritis of the lower lumbar spine on planar bone scintigraphy with a high negative predictive value for metastasis. Clin Nucl Med 2008;33(4):251–4.

115. Kim H, So Y, Moon S, et al. Clinical value of 99mTc-methylene diphosphonate (MDP) bone single photon emission computed tomography (SPECT) in patients with knee osteoarthritis. Osteoarthritis Cartilage 2008;16(2):212–8.

116. Jeer PJ, Mahr CC, Keene GC, et al. Single photon emission computed tomography in planning unicompartmental knee arthroplasty. A prospective study examining the association between scan findings and intraoperative assessment of osteoarthritis. Knee 2006;13(1):19–25.

117. Van der Wall H, Fogelman I. Scintigraphy of benign bone disease. Semin Musculoskelet Radiol 2007; 11(4):281–300.

118. Vanhove C, Andreyev A, Defrise M, et al. Resolution recovery in pinhole SPECT based on multiray projections: a phantom study. Eur J Nucl Med Mol Imaging 2007;34(2):170–80.

119. Beekman FJ, Kamphuis C, King MA, et al. Improvement of image resolution and quantitative accuracy in clinical single photon emission computed tomography. Comput Med Imaging Graph 2001; 25(2):135–46.

MR Imaging in Osteoarthritis: Hardware, Coils, and Sequences

Thomas M. Link, MD

KEYWORDS
- Osteoarthritis • MR imaging • Sequences
- Hardware • Field strength

MR imaging must be tailored for imaging of osteo-arthritis (OA) by using scanners with adequate field strength, coils that allow imaging with high spatial resolution, and optimized imaging sequences that best visualize tissues involved by OA. These tissues encompass cartilage, menisci, ligaments, and bone marrow. Among these tissues, cartilage has an outstanding role, and imaging cartilage is particularly challenging in terms of the required signal-to-noise-ratio (SNR), spatial resolution, and contrast. The requirements for cartilage imaging dictate the overall requirements in hardware and in sequence profiles.

This article (1) outlines requirements concerning field strength, analyzing scanners with different field strengths from 0.2 T to 7 T, (2) investigates the potential of open and extremity MR imaging, (3) examines the role of weight-bearing MR imaging, (4) reviews coil technology, and (5) analyzes sequence protocols and their role in imaging the different tissues involved in OA.

FIELD STRENGTH

Considerations concerning field strength required for OA imaging always should take into account that cartilage imaging is critical for adequate whole-organ OA analysis. Previous studies have shown that imaging with low field strength clearly has limitations in assessing cartilage morphology and therefore is not recommended for OA imaging.[1–3] Woertler and colleagues[3] compared the diagnostic performance of a dedicated orthopedic MR imaging system (0.18 T) and a conventional MR imaging system (1.0 T) in the detection of articular cartilage lesions created in an animal model. Using receiver operating characteristics (ROC) analysis with three different radiologists, these investigators found that the high-field-strength system demonstrated a significantly better diagnostic performance than the low-field-stength system in the detection of less-than-full-thickness articular cartilage lesions ($P < .001$). Ahn and colleagues[4] studied cadaver patellae using a 0.2-T extremity-only magnet and found that high-grade cartilaginous lesions could be evaluated reliably with low-field-strength MR imaging by using a combination of imaging sequences. Limitations were encountered analyzing less-than-full-thickness cartilage lesions, however. Based on the results of these previous studies, the use of MR imaging scanners with a field strength of at least 1.0 T is recommended for imaging cartilage.

The current standard is 1.5-T imaging, and most of the studies establishing MR imaging for assessment of OA were conducted at this field strength.[5–8] Semiquantitative scores to grade OA and techniques to quantify cartilage volume were developed at 1.5 T.[6,9,10] The early studies analyzing quantitative parameters to characterize the biochemical composition of cartilage, such as T2 relaxation time and T1rho mapping, as well as delayed gadolinium-enhanced MR imaging of cartilage (dGEMRIC), also were performed at 1.5 T.[11–13]

Department of Radiology and Biomedical Imaging, University of California at San Francisco, 400 Parnassus Avenue, A-367, San Francisco, CA 94131, USA
E-mail address: tmlink@radiology.ucsf.edu

Radiol Clin N Am 47 (2009) 617–632
doi:10.1016/j.rcl.2009.04.002
0033-8389/09/$ – see front matter

Although 1.5-T imaging is standard, a number of studies have demonstrated that 3.0-T MR imaging allows better visualization of cartilage lesions[14–19] and therefore may be better suited for the overall assessment of OA. Using optimized high-resolution MR imaging sequences in an animal model, Link and colleagues showed that cartilage lesions were visualized better and diagnostic performance was improved at 3.0 T compared with 1.5 T. Interestingly, however, standard lower-spatial-resolution intermediate (IM)-weighted fast spin echo (FSE) sequences did not improve diagnostic performance at 3.0 T. Fig. 1 shows two corresponding IM-weighted fat-saturated MR images obtained at 1.5 and 3.0 T demonstrating a superficial cartilage defect at the patella in a pig knee, which is visualized better at 3.0 T.[18] Although this study was performed at the knee, additional studies performed at human cadaver ankles[14,15] also showed better diagnostic performance in assessing cartilage lesions and a higher sensitivity for assessing ligamentous and tendon pathology at 3.0 T than at 1.5 T.

Recently Kijowski and colleagues[17,20] performed a retrospective study comparing the diagnostic performance of 1.5-T and 3.0-T MR imaging protocols for evaluating the articular cartilage of the knee joint in symptomatic patients. Analyzing 241 knee MR images at 1.5 T and 226 MR images at 3.0 T, these investigators found that the sensitivity, specificity, and accuracy of MR imaging for detecting cartilage lesions were 69.3%, 78.0%, and 74.5%, respectively, at 1.5 T and were 70.5%, 85.9%, and 80.1%, respectively, at 3.0 T. The MR imaging protocol had significantly higher specificity and accuracy ($P < .05$) but not higher sensitivity ($P = .73$) for detecting cartilage lesions at 3.0 T than at 1.5 T. The investigators concluded that 3.0-T MR imaging protocols were superior to the 1.5-T protocol for evaluating the articular cartilage of the knee joint in symptomatic patients (Figs. 2 and 3).

Bauer and colleagues[16] compared the precision and accuracy of 3.0-T and 1.5-T MR imaging in the quantification of cartilage volume by using direct volumetric measurements as a reference standard in a cadaver model. These investigators calculated accuracy errors for MR imaging–based volume calculations of 3.0% at the femur for standard fat-suppressed spoiled gradient-echo (SPGR) sequences at 3.0 T, versus 16% for the standard fat-suppressed SPGR sequence at 1.5 T. Effective signal-to-noise ratio and effective contrast-to-noise ratio also were substantially improved at 3.0 T. This study provides evidence that cartilage volumetric measurements obtained at 3.0 T are more accurate than those obtained at 1.5 T. Eckstein and colleagues[21] performed an in vivo study in patients who had OA and normal volunteers to evaluate the precision of quantitative MR imaging assessments of human cartilage morphology at 3.0 T and to correlate the measurements at 3.0 T with validated measurements at 1.5 T. They found that with a slice thickness of 1.5 mm, measurements tended to be more reproducible at 3.0 T than at 1.5 T, and they concluded that imaging at

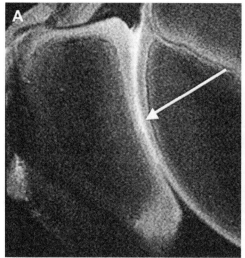 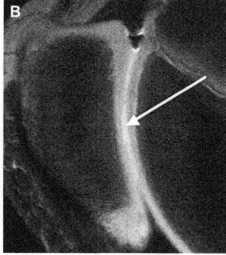

Fig. 1. Sagittal MR images of a pig knee with artificially created patellar cartilage defect obtained at (A) 1.5 T and (B) 3.0 T using fat-suppressed IM-weighted FSE sequences (4000/35 milliseconds; TR/TE for both 1.5; 3.0 T). Superficial cartilage defect at the patella (arrows) is well shown on the 3.0-T image (B) but is not well visualized on the 1.5-T image (A).

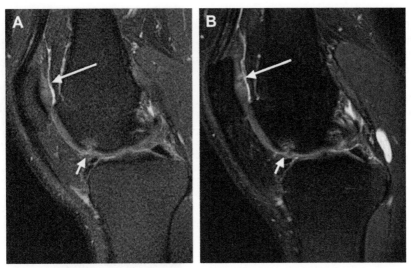

Fig. 2. Sagittal MR image of the knee obtained in a middle-aged runner with knee pain at (*A*) 1.5 T and (*B*) 3.0 T using fat-suppressed IM-weighted FSE sequences (3200/46 and 4300/51 milliseconds). Cartilage defects at the patella (*long arrow*) and osteochondral lesion at the trochlea (*short arrow*) are better visualized at 3.0 T than at 1.5 T.

3.0 T may provide superior ability to detect changes in cartilage status over time and to determine responses to treatment with structure-modifying drugs.

To achieve the best possible imaging technique for assessing OA, the National Institute of Health–sponsored Osteoarthritis Initiative (OAI) therefore adopted imaging at 3.0 T. The OAI is a nationwide, multicenter research study that provides a large dataset of clinical information, questionnaires, radiographs, and MR imaging studies obtained from nearly 5000 participants (4796 participants at baseline) who are followed up every 12 months for a period of 48 months. The overall aim of the OAI is to develop a public domain research resource to facilitate the scientific evaluation of biomarkers for OA as potential surrogate end points for disease onset and progression. The OAI recruits participants who have knee OA (the progression cohort) and participants who have risk factors but no symptoms of OA (the incidence cohort). The imaging protocol includes morphologic

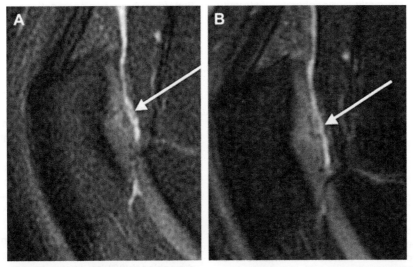

Fig. 3. (*A*) 1.5-T and (*B*) 3.0-T sagittal fat-suppressed IM-weighted FSE MRI of the patella (3200/46 and 4300/51 milliseconds). Fissures at the patella (*arrow*) are shown in greater detail, and the surface of the cartilage is evaluated substantially better at 3.0 T than at 1.5 T.

and quantitative MR imaging sequences performed at 3.0 T with five identical scanners from the same manufacturer.[22]

To date, MR imaging at 7.0 T is a research application, and only limited studies have been performed in human participants.[23,24] Currently available sequence protocols have not been shown to be superior to 3.0 T in the assessment of OA. Future research work clearly will need to focus on developing adequate surface coils and optimized sequences for imaging at 7.0 T.

EXTREMITY AND OPEN MR IMAGING

Peripheral extremity magnets have lower installation, maintenance, and management costs than whole-body systems, and these systems are beneficial for patients who have claustrophobia. Moreover, they do not require the amount of shielding necessary for a whole-body system and potentially can be used in private offices, thus making MR imaging widely available. Dedicated extremity scanners operating at higher field strength have been developed to overcome the limitations of 0.2-T MR imaging scanners in visualizing cartilage and other anatomic structures such as ligaments (Fig. 4). Using a dedicated peripheral extremity-only MR imaging system operating at 1.0 T, Roemer and colleagues[25] examined 34 knees using fat-suppressed FSE proton density (PD)-weighted sequences. They found good to excellent interobserver performance in assessing OA-associated abnormalities, including cartilage lesions (Fig. 5). These high-field peripheral scanners may offer a low-cost alternative providing adequate image quality for assessing cartilage pathology. Currently, peripheral extremity

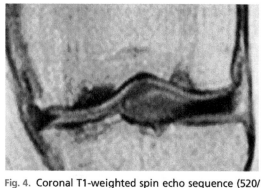

Fig. 4. Coronal T1-weighted spin echo sequence (520/24 milliseconds) of the right knee obtained at 0.2 T with a dedicated extremity scanner in a patient who has subchondral bone infarcts. The limitations of image SNR and spatial resolution that limit visualization of cartilage abnormalities are demonstrated clearly.

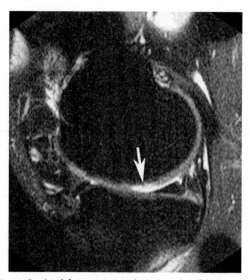

Fig. 5. Sagittal fat-suppressed PD-weighted MR image at 1.0 T depicts a focal cartilage defect (arrow) at the central weight-bearing medial femoral condyle. (Courtesy of Ali Guermazi, MD, Boston University.)

scanners operating at 1.5-T field strength are available also.

Depending on the open MR imaging configuration, patients can be placed in the scanner in either a supine or weight-bearing position. Open MR imaging scanners allow the functional aspects of joint function to be assessed and may therefore be useful in investigating conditions associated with abnormal articulation in certain joint positions that may lead to accelerated OA. For example, femoroacetabular impingement is a condition in which labral and cartilage damage results from an abnormal morphology of the head–neck junction (cam-type impingement) or an abnormally deep acetabulum (pincer-type impingement). This impingement typically occurs with flexion, abduction, and external rotation. Open MR imaging can be used to assess these functional aspects of the hip joint. Yamamura and colleagues[26] demonstrated that, although impingement occurred frequently during daily activities, it was not associated with accelerated OA of the hip in male and female Japanese participants.

Open MR imaging scanners also can be used to assess patella kinematics and patellofemoral contact areas, which may play a role in development of femoropatellar OA. Hinterwimmer and colleagues[27] studied a sample of 15 patients who had genu varum and mild OA and 15 healthy volunteers in an open MR imaging scanner. Three-dimensional (3D) gradient echo sequences of the knee were obtained in 0°, 30°, and 90° with and without activity of the extensor muscles. Contact areas between patella and femur cartilage were defined by intersection of opposing cartilage volumes. These investigators, however, were not able to demonstrate significant differences in patella kinematics and patellofemoral contact areas ($P > .05$) between varus knees with mild OA and healthy knees either at the different flexion angles or under extending muscle activity.

WEIGHT-BEARING MR IMAGING

Weight-bearing MR imaging can be performed using open MR imaging systems that have vertically orientated magnets or with whole-body MR imaging systems that use special loading devices for the knee, such as the one described by Nishii and colleagues.[28] Although the vertical alignment of the magnets in a double-doughnut system allows true weight-bearing MR imaging studies, the field strength and image quality of these scanners are limited, affecting cartilage imaging in particular. Image quality in whole-body systems generally is superior, and loading devices also have been applied successfully in 3.0-T scanners.[28] Static loading conditions usually are obtained by applying an axial compression force of approximately 50% of body weight during imaging.

Anterior cruciate ligament (ACL) tears have been identified as an important factor in the pathogenesis of OA, and it also has been found that patients who have ACL repair experience accelerated OA.[29] Logan and colleagues[30] used a vertical open MR imaging system to study the tibiofemoral kinematics of ACL-deficient weight-bearing in 10 patients. The tibiofemoral motion was assessed through the arc of flexion from 0° to 90° in the ACL-deficient and normal contralateral knees. These investigators found that ACL tears change tibiofemoral kinematics, producing anterior subluxation of the lateral tibial plateau. They hypothesized that altered kinematics may explain, at least in part, the increased incidence of secondary OA in patients who have had an ACL tear. In another study, the same investigators[31] used the same weight-bearing technique in an open MR imaging system to study 10 patients who had isolated reconstruction of the ACL (hamstring autograft) in one knee and a normal contralateral knee. They found that ACL reconstruction reduces sagittal laxity to within normal limits but does not restore normal tibiofemoral kinematics; the abnormal kinematics, again, may explain the relatively high rate of accelerated OA in this patient population.

Currently there has been substantial interest in studying changes in cartilage volume and biochemical matrix in response to load-bearing. It has been suggested that failure to respond to normal load-bearing may be caused by the disorder or degeneration of articular cartilage with collagen disorganization or abnormal water content.[28] Nishii and colleagues[28] used T2 relaxation time measurements to study the biochemical composition of the normal hyaline knee cartilage under loading. Using 3.0-T MR imaging and applying an axial compression force of 50% of body weight during imaging, they obtained sagittal T2 maps of the medial and lateral femorotibial joints of 22 healthy volunteers. They compared the T2 values of the femoral and tibial cartilage at the weight-bearing area in the unloading and loading conditions. These investigators found that under loading conditions, mean cartilage T2 values generally decreased. At the medial joint compartment, a significant decrease in T2 values with loading was observed at the femoral region in direct contact with the opposing tibial cartilage. A significant decrease in T2 values with loading also was observed at the medial and lateral tibia, at regions both covered and not covered by the meniscus.

In addition, the role of the meniscus during weight-bearing is critical in preventing OA. While axial compression forces are applied, MR imaging directly visualizes changes of the meniscus in morphology, deformity, extrusion, and, potentially, biochemistry (Fig. 6). These findings may help elucidate the evolution and pathophysiology of OA, but at present the experience in direct visualization of meniscal abnormalities with weight-bearing MR imaging is limited.

SURFACE COILS

In addition to adequate field strength, dedicated surface coils are important prerequisites to achieve good image quality and visualization of the joint tissues involved in OA. Currently, surface coils for the wrist, shoulder, knee, and ankle are standard; most of these coils are multichannel phased-array coils. For visualization of smaller structures such as the fingers and toes, smaller (so-called "microscopy") coils have been developed. These coils allow imaging with small fields of view and high spatial resolution.

Fig. 7 shows the effect of the coil on the image quality. In panel A, a non-dedicated two-element paddle coil was used; in panel B, a dedicated three-element shoulder coil was applied. The effect on visualization of the cartilage is evident. Even if a high-quality, high-field scanner is used, inadequate coils limit image quality substantially, as shown by Lutterbey and colleagues.[32] These investigators found that using the standard body coil at 3.0 T for imaging of the knee gave a lower

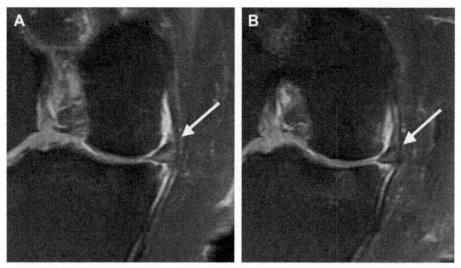

Fig. 6. Coronal MR image of the knee in a patient who has mild knee OA obtained using fat-suppressed PD-weighted FSE sequences (3000/10.3 milliseconds) (*A*) without and (*B*) with loading (50% body weight) in a whole-body 3.0-T MR scanner. Note that the medial meniscal extrusion (*arrow*) is increased under loading conditions and also that the shape of the meniscus is changed slightly.

image performance than achieved using a 1.5-T scanner with a dedicated knee coil.

Multichannel phased-array coils give high SNR and allow parallel imaging, which can provide better image quality with the same acquisition time or can shorten acquisition time by maintaining image quality. With parallel imaging, each of the coil elements/channels provides image information separately; the information then is fused to obtain one image (Fig. 8).

In an in vitro study performed in human cadaver ankles, Bauer and colleagues[33] compared an autocalibrating parallel imaging technique at 3.0 T with standard acquisitions at 3.0 T for small field-of-view imaging of the ankle. Using parallel imaging techniques, these investigators obtained a reduction in scan time of approximately 44%. All images were analyzed for image quality by two radiologists. Macroscopic findings after dissection served as a reference for the pathologic evaluation. This study did not find a significant difference in ligament and cartilage visualization or in image quality between standard and generalized, autocalibrating, partially parallel acquisitions

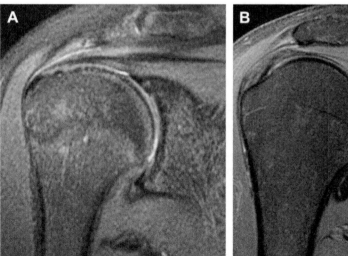
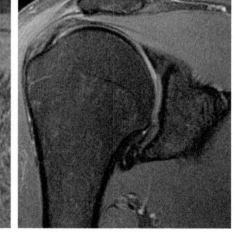

Fig. 7. Coronal MR image of the shoulder obtained at 3.0 T using fat-suppressed IM-weighted FSE sequences (3300/51 milliseconds) with (*A*) a non-dedicated paddle coil and (*B*) a three-element shoulder phased-array coil. Differences in image quality, especially in the visualization of the cartilage and bone marrow, are evident.

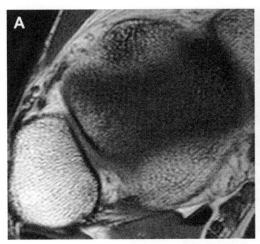 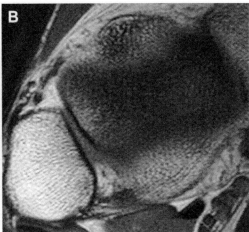

Fig. 8. MR image of a human cadaver ankle joint obtained at 3.0 T using a T1-weighted (675/15.7 milliseconds) FSE sequence (*A*) without and (*B*) with parallel imaging. Images in *B* were obtained with a 44% shorter acquisition time. There is no difference in image quality, particularly in visualizing the ligaments.

reconstructions at 3.0 T. The authors concluded that parallel imaging can provide more flexibility in protocol design by either shortening image acquisition time or improving image quality with the same acquisition time.

Zuo and colleagues[34] evaluated the feasibility and reproducibility of quantitative cartilage imaging with parallel imaging at 3.0 T and determined the impact of the acceleration factor on morphologic and relaxation measurements. They found that morphologic parameters and relaxation time maps from parallel imaging showed results comparable with those obtained by the conventional technique. Intraclass correlation coefficients of the two methods for measuring cartilage volume and mean cartilage thickness were very high both for T1rho, and T2 measurements, and the reproducibility was excellent. In summary, for both quantitative and morphologic OA imaging, multichannel phased-array coils with parallel imaging techniques are recommended.

SEQUENCE PROTOCOLS

Because different tissues are involved in OA and both morphologic and quantitative analyses are required, a number of different sequences have been tailored and developed for "whole-organ" assessment of OA. The workhorse sequences for morphologic imaging of the joints are FSE sequences. In particular fluid-sensitive fat-suppressed sequences have been found useful to assess cartilage, bone marrow, ligaments, menisci, and tendons. Most experience and good results in morphologic imaging of cartilage and subchondral pathology were gathered with (1) two-dimensional

(2D) PD-, IM-, and T2-weighted FSE and (2) 3D SPGR or fast low-angle shot (FLASH) gradient echo sequences. Additional fat suppression in these sequences was found useful to visualize cartilage pathology better and to reduce chemical shift artifacts.

There is some controversy about how exactly to define T2-, IM-, and PD-weighted sequences. In general established terminology, IM-weighted sequences have echo times (TE) in the range of 30 to 60 milliseconds, T2-weighted sequences have TEs of 70 to 80 milliseconds, and PD-weighted sequences have TEs of 10 to 30 milliseconds.[19,35] In the author's experience, fat-suppressed IM-weighted FSE sequences are most useful for imaging joints with OA, because they are fluid sensitive, provide good visualization of cartilage, menisci, and ligaments, and also allow assessment of the bone marrow. These sequences also provide better visualization of anatomic structures than T2-weighted FSE sequences. PD-weighted sequences with lower TE values may be more helpful in assessing the menisci and give additional information concerning tendons and ligaments, but they are less fluid sensitive.

Intermediate- and T2-Weighted Fast Spin-Echo Sequences

The sequence most frequently used for OA assessment in clinical practice is an IM-weighted fat-suppressed FSE sequence, which allows good visualization of cartilage defects, the pattern of bone marrow edema, menisci, and tendons (Fig. 9). The standard parameters used for this sequence are a repetition time (TR) of 3000 to

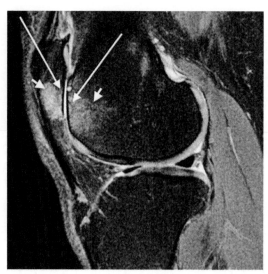

Fig. 9. Sagittal fat-suppressed IM-weighted FSE (3200/30 milliseconds) MR image of the knee obtained in a 48-year-old man who had advanced degenerative disease of the femoropatellar joint. Cartilage lesions (*long arrows*), bone marrow edema pattern (*short arrows*) at the trochlea and patella, osteophytes, tendons, menisci, and ligaments are well visualized with this fluid-sensitive sequence.

4000 milliseconds; a TE of 30 to 60 milliseconds; and an echo train length of 8. This TE range is chosen because it provides higher intrinsic contrast of the cartilage and is less prone to magic angle effects than "true" PD-weighted pulse sequences obtained at shorter TEs. Slice thickness varies between 2 and 4 mm; 3 mm usually is used in a clinical setting. To maintain an acceptable acquisition time and to achieve a good SNR, the matrix size is in the order of 256 × 256 pixels but may be increased if imaging is performed at 3.0 T. Sequence parameters must be adjusted to the joint; the parameter most affected is the field of view. A clinically acceptable acquisition time is in the order of 3 to 6 minutes.

With IM- and T2-weighted FSE sequences, normal hyaline cartilage has intermediate signal intensity, and fluid is bright, allowing good contrast to identify surface abnormalities as well as pathologies of the cartilage matrix. Using 3.0-T MR imaging, Saadat and colleagues[36] analyzed the performance of IM-weighted sequences in relation to histology in patients who had advanced OA before undergoing total knee arthroplasty (Fig. 10). Intraoperatively obtained specimens underwent histologic analysis, and sections were matched with preoperative MR images. Findings on preoperative MR imaging were compared with the corresponding region in histologic sections. Parameters assessed included thinning of cartilage (differentiating < 50%, > 50%, and full-thickness lesions), surface integrity (including fissuring and fraying), and abnormalities in cartilage signal pattern.

Histologic findings related to the pattern of bone marrow edema and cartilage swelling were documented also. The overall sensitivity, specificity, and accuracy of their imaging findings were 72%, 69%, and 70%, respectively, for cartilage thinning, 69%, 74%, and 73%, respectively, for surface irregularities, and 36%, 62%, and 45%, respectively, for intracartilaginous signal abnormalities. The authors concluded that MR imaging using fat-suppressed IM-weighted FSE sequences was useful in assessing cartilage thickness and surface lesions, but changes in cartilage signal were not useful for characterizing the severity of cartilage degeneration. Thus signal abnormalities visualized on IM-weighted FSE sequences of the cartilage matrix may have limited value in characterizing cartilage degeneration and softening. In this study, the areas of bone marrow edema pattern corresponded to fibrovascular tissue ingrowths.

Multiple clinical studies have found IM- and T2-weighted FSE sequences have high sensitivity and specificity in assessing tissue abnormalities that may be related to OA.[14,37–40] The diagnostic performance for cartilage lesions improves when different imaging planes are used. Bredella and colleagues[41] studied how the use of a combination of different imaging planes affects the detection and grading of articular cartilage defects in the knee. They found that the sensitivity of a sagittal T2-weighted FSE sequence was only 40%, and the specificity was 100%. The sensitivity of a combination of axial and coronal fat-suppressed

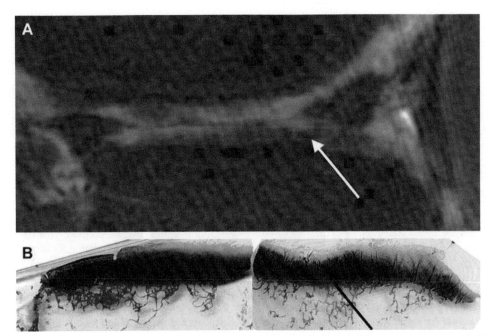

Fig.10. (A) Sagittal MR image of the knee obtained in a patient undergoing total knee replacement at 3.0 T using a fat-suppressed IM-weighted FSE sequence (4300/51 milliseconds) shows focal cartilage thinning and fraying (arrow). The MR image also shows additional abnormal signal of the cartilage. (B) Corresponding histologic slide (hematoxylin and eosin staining) obtained after surgery demonstrates the same focal cartilage thinning and fraying (arrow).

T2-weighted FSE sequences and sagittal T2-weighted FSE sequences was 94%, specificity was 99%, and accuracy was 98%, using arthroscopy as a standard of reference.

Three-Dimensional Spoiled Gradient-Echo and Fast Low-Angle Shot Sequences

3D SPGR and FLASH sequences are well suited for depicting the cartilage volume and, to some extent, the cartilage surface. Sequence parameters used to visualize cartilage are in the range of TR: 20 to 35 milliseconds, TE: 7 to 12 milliseconds, and flip angle: 12° to 30°; parameters need to be optimized according to the field strength. The bright signal of cartilage in the SPGR and FLASH images limits the visualization of internal cartilage pathology to some extent; fissures, for example, may not be as well visualized. These gradient-echo sequences are not suited for visualizing bone marrow pathology and are very limited in assessing menisci, ligaments, and tendons. They have been found useful, however, in segmenting cartilage for quantitative measurement of volume and thickness.[9,21,42]

A number of studies have compared SPGR versus IM- or T2-weighted FSE sequences[18,19,43] and have found that the two sequence types have similar overall diagnostic performance in detecting focal cartilage lesions. 3D SPGR and FLASH sequences provide high spatial resolution but usually require fairly long imaging time, and motion artifacts can degrade image quality. These gradient-echo sequences also are very sensitive to susceptibility artifacts, a consideration after previous surgery and in particular after cartilage repair procedures. In their clinical practice, the author and colleagues have found IM-weighted FSE sequences easier to use and more practically applicable than SPGR or FLASH sequences. More recent studies also suggest that SPGR sequences may be less suited than IM-weighted FSE sequences for visualizing subtle cartilage abnormalities (Fig. 11).[14,15]

Other Sequences

In addition to these sequences, 3D double-echo steady-state sequences (DESS) also have shown good results in detecting cartilage lesions (Fig. 12). This mixed T1/T2*-weighted sequence provides high spatial resolution with the cartilage appearing more intermediate in signal. In an experimental study, Woertler and colleagues[3] found that fat-suppressed 3D FLASH and water-excited 3D DESS sequences performed similarly in detecting cartilage surface lesions. Ruehm and colleagues[44] analyzed patellar cartilage

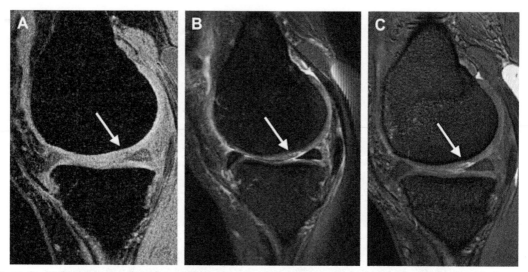

Fig. 11. Sagittal MR images of the knee obtained in a middle-aged runner using (*A*) fat-suppressed SPGR (21/12.5 milliseconds, flip angle: 15°), (*B*) IM-weighted FSE (4300/51 milliseconds), and (*C*) a non–fat-suppressed fluid-sensitive fast imaging employing steady-state acquisition (FIESTA; 5.9/1.9 milliseconds, flip angle: 15°) sequence. Cartilage delamination (*arrow*) is well visualized on the fluid-sensitive sequences (*B* and *C*) but not on the SPGR sequence (*A*) in which the cartilage appears uniformly bright.

abnormalities in 58 consecutive patients using a 3D DESS and a T2-weighted FSE sequence. These authors concluded that the DESS sequence was less accurate in detecting cartilage surface abnormalities but was more accurate in diagnosing cartilage softening. 3D DESS sequences usually are obtained with thin sections, allowing relatively high-quality reconstructions in additional imaging planes.

A number of sequences have been developed to improve morphologic depiction of cartilage. These sequences include driven equilibrium Fourier transform (DEFT) and steady-state free precision (SSFP) imaging. DEFT imaging makes use of a much higher cartilage-to-fluid contrast; the signal of synovial fluid is higher than in SPGR sequences, and the signal of cartilage is higher than in T2-weighted FSE sequences.[45] Yoshioka

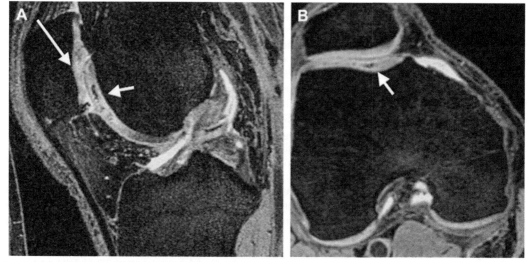

Fig. 12. (*A*) Sagittal 3D DESS MR image (16.3/4.7 milliseconds, flip angle: 25°) of the knee obtained in a 50-year-old man. (*B*) Axial reconstruction from the image dataset. Note femoropatellar cartilage degeneration with surface irregularity (*long arrow*) and signal changes (*short arrow*). Low-intensity signal changes at the trochlea are consistent with chondrocalcinosis.

and colleagues[43] used this sequence in 35 OA knees and correlated imaging findings with arthroscopy. In their study the fat-suppressed 3D DEFT images showed results similar to SPGR and IM-weighted FSE sequences with high sensitivity but relatively low specificity. Gold and colleagues[46] compared 3D DEFT and T2-weighted FSE sequences in 104 consecutive patients who had knee pain and used arthroscopy in 24 patients as a standard of reference. These investigators found that the 3D DEFT sequences provided excellent synovial fluid-to-cartilage contrast while preserving signal from cartilage, giving this method a high cartilage SNR. In addition 3D DEFT showed the full cartilage thickness better than T2-weighted FSE sequences, but T2-weighted FSE sequences had better fat suppression and fewer artifacts than 3D DEFT sequences.

SSFP imaging has been described as an efficient, high-signal method for obtaining 3D images and may be useful for depicting cartilage, because cartilage signal is higher than in conventional sequences.[47] Kornaat and colleagues[48] used this sequence in volunteers at 1.5 and 3 T and found that SSFP-based techniques showed higher SNR and increased contrast-to-noise efficiency at 3.0 T than SPGR sequences. **Fig. 11** shows images of cartilage delamination at the medial femoral condyle of the knee obtained with an SSFP sequence (fast imaging employing steady state acquisition, FIESTA) and SPGR and IM-weighted FSE sequences. Bauer and colleagues[49] compared the performance of SSFP, IM-weighted FSE, and SPGR sequences in assessing cartilage

lesions at cadaver ankles and found the highest ROC values for the IM-weighted FSE sequences at 3.0 T, but IM-weighted FSE and SSFP sequences showed a similar performance at 1.5 T, and both showed better results than the SPGR sequence at 3.0 T and 1.5 T. To the author's knowledge, larger clinical studies have not yet been performed using this sequence. The previously described DESS sequence also is a steady-state sequence and thus has cartilage signal features similar to the SSFP sequences, but the parameters differ in some respects.

Recently 3D FSE sequences have been used for clinical imaging of the knee and ankle.[50,51] These sequences generate isotropic voxels and allow high-quality reformations in any plane. Thus it may be possible to obtain only one sequence dataset and get the additional planes as reformations (**Fig. 13**). This technique potentially would save acquisition time and shorten patient examinations substantially. Ristow and colleagues[50] compared the image quality and diagnostic performance in assessing abnormal findings of the knee of a fat-suppressed IM-weighted 3D FSE sequence and a standard 2D IM-weighted FSE sequence. They found that isotropic 3D IM-weighted FSE imaging enhanced standard knee MR imaging by better visualizing high-contrast lesions; however, 3D FSE image quality was lower, and there were limitations in diagnostic performance compared with standard 2D FSE imaging. Clearly this technique has potential, however, and with further improvements in the sequence design it may replace 2D IM-weighted FSE sequences.

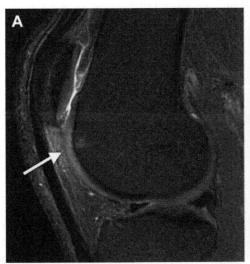 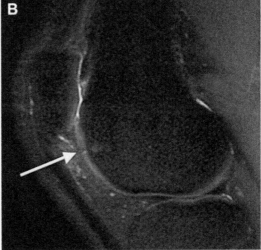

Fig. 13. (A) Sagittal 2D (4200/51 milliseconds) and (B) 3D (2500/38 milliseconds) FSE sequences of the knee show bone marrow edema pattern and a focal cartilage lesion. The cartilage fissure (*arrow*) is well depicted in (B) but is not well visualized in (A).

MR Arthrography

Direct MR arthrography with use of T1-weighted pulse sequences following intra-articular injection of gadolinium chelates has been shown to be a reliable imaging technique for detecting surface lesions of articular cartilage, with sensitivity and specificity ranging from 85% to 100%.[52,53] The injected fluid produces high contrast between joint space, cartilage, and subchondral bone and at the same time distends the joint and thus improves the separation of corresponding joint surfaces. Because of its invasive nature, however, this technique is of limited use for OA imaging.

A simple method for producing artificial arthrographic contrast in a T1-like FSE sequence using a driven equilibrium pulse (DRIVE) has been described recently. In contrast to the 3D DEFT sequence mentioned previously, this 2D technique provides bright signal intensity of joint fluid; signal intensities otherwise are the same as in a normal T1-weighted FSE sequence obtained at high spatial resolution and short scan times.[54] DRIVE also can be used to increase the contrast and/or spatial resolution of IM-weighted FSE images. This new technique and its value for cartilage imaging are still under clinical evaluation, however.

Quantitative Imaging of the Cartilage Matrix

In addition to assessing cartilage pathology, thickness, and volume, recent studies have shown the potential of MR imaging parameters to reflect changes in the biochemical composition of cartilage with early OA. These techniques include T2 quantification,[55] T1rho quantification,[13,56] and dGEMRIC.[57,58] These techniques allow characterization of the cartilage matrix and, potentially, quality before morphologic damage occurs.

T2 quantification

It has been shown that increased T2 relaxation time is proportional to the distribution of cartilage water and is sensitive to small changes in water content.[59] In an early study Dardzinski and colleagues[60] examined the spatial variation of in vivo cartilage T2 in young asymptomatic adults and found a reproducible pattern of increasing T2 that was proportional to the known spatial variation in cartilage water and that was inversely proportional to the distribution of proteoglycans. These authors postulated that the regional T2 differences were secondary to the restricted mobility of cartilage water within an anisotropic solid matrix. Thus measurement of the spatial distribution of the T2 reflecting areas of increased and decreased water content may be used to quantify cartilage degeneration before morphologic changes are appreciated.

In a preliminary study Mosher and colleagues[61] showed that aging is associated with an asymptomatic increase in T2 of the transitional zone of articular cartilage. The results of this study indicated that the diffuse increase in T2 relaxation time in senescent cartilage is different in appearance than the focally increased T2 observed in damaged articular cartilage.[61] Dunn and colleagues[55] analyzed 55 participants who were categorized radiographically as healthy (n = 7), as having mild OA (n = 20), or as having severe OA (n = 28). They found that healthy participants had mean T2 values of 32.1 to 35.0 milliseconds, whereas patients who had mild and severe OA had mean T2 values of 34.4 to 41.0 milliseconds. All cartilage compartments except the lateral tibia showed significant ($P < .05$) differences in T2 relaxation time between healthy and diseased knees. Correlation of T2 values with clinical symptoms and cartilage morphology was found predominantly in the medial compartments.

T1rho quantification

A different parameter that has been proposed for measuring cartilage composition is 3D T1rho relaxation mapping. T1rho describes the spin-lattice relaxation in the rotating frame, and changes in the extracellular matrix of cartilage (eg, the loss of glycosaminoglycans, GAG), may be reflected in measurements of T1rho because of the less restricted motion of water protons. Preliminary results demonstrated the in vivo feasibility of quantifying early biochemical changes in participants who had symptomatic OA using T1rho-weighted MR imaging on a 1.5-T clinical scanner.[13,56] In a study with a limited number of symptomatic participants, T1rho-weighted MR imaging provided a noninvasive marker for quantifying early degenerative changes in cartilage in vivo.[13] Li and colleagues[62] examined 10 healthy volunteers, and 9 patients who had OA at 3.0 T and found a significant difference ($P = .002$) in the average T1rho within patellar and femoral cartilage between controls (45.04 ± 2.59 milliseconds) and patients who had OA (53.06 ± 4.60 milliseconds). A significant correlation was found between T1rho and T2 relaxation measurements; however, the difference in T2 measurements between controls and patients who had OA was not significant. These initial results suggest that T1rho relaxation mapping may be a promising clinical tool for detecting OA and monitoring treatment. Stahl and colleagues[63] analyzed the diagnostic value of T2 and T1rho measurements in identifying asymptomatic physically active subjects with and without focal cartilage pathology. These investigators found that T1rho and T2 composition of cartilage differed in subjects with and without focal cartilage pathology and concluded that T1rho and T2 may be suitable parameters for identifying asymptomatic subjects at higher risk for developing cartilage degeneration (Fig. 14).

Further studies are underway in larger symptomatic populations to correlate T1rho measurements with early OA with arthroscopy as a standard of reference. The advantage of T1rho and T2 measurements is that these techniques are noninvasive and do not require contrast injection.

Delayed gadolinium-enhanced MR imaging of cartilage

Cartilage consists of approximately 70% water, and the remainder is predominantly type II collagen fibers and GAG. The GAG macromolecules contain negative charges that attract sodium ions. One of the most commonly used MR imaging contrast agents, $Gd\text{-}DTPA^{2-}$ has a negative charge and therefore does not penetrate cartilage in areas where GAG concentrations are high. In fact, its distribution is concentrated in areas with lower GAG concentrations and thus pathologic cartilage composition. $Gd\text{-}DTPA^{2-}$ concentrations in cartilage can be quantified, and this technique has been defined as "delayed gadolinium-enhanced MR imaging of cartilage," dGEMRIC.

Initial studies have shown that the dGEMRIC measurement of GAG corresponds to the true GAG concentration as measured with biochemistry and histology.[57,64] This technique has also been used in a number of clinical studies, and variations in this measurement have been shown in patients who have OA, in trials of autologous chondrocyte implants, and in comparisons between participants with a sedentary lifestyle and those who exercise regularly.[11,65–67]

Sequence protocols in relation to joint-specific requirements

MR imaging of OA currently concentrates mostly on the knee joint, but an increasing number of studies have focused on the hip joint.[68–72] There is a limited role for wrist and ankle MR imaging in OA.[73] The shoulder and elbow are rarely affected by OA, and thus MR imaging is not expected to have a significant role in assessing OA in these joints.

An optimal MR imaging protocol for knee OA would include morphologic IM-weighted FSE sequences in a coronal and sagittal orientation as well as quantitative sequences for volumetric and cartilage matrix assessment (SPGR/FLASH sequence as well as T1rho, T2, or dGEMRIC maps). Depending on clinical or research indications, axial IM-weighted sequences may be included for better assessment of the patella. Imaging of the hip would include coronal and

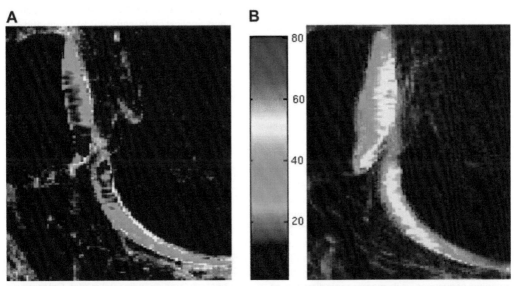

Fig. 14. Sagittal T1rho color maps [ms] of the patellofemoral cartilage. (*A*) An asymptomatic subject without focal cartilage pathology (low T1rho values). (*B*) An asymptomatic subject who has early, diffuse cartilage degeneration (high T1rho values) and focal cartilage defects (not shown). (*From* Stahl R, Luke A, Li X, et al. T1rho, T(2) and focal knee cartilage abnormalities in physically active and sedentary healthy subjects versus early OA patients–a 3.0-Tesla MRI study. Eur Radiol 2009;19:132–43.)

sagittal IM-weighted FSE sequences. Oblique axial images are useful in measuring the alpha angle, which is required for assessment of femoroacetabular impingement and plays a major role in the evolution of accelerated OA.[74] Morphologic evaluation of cartilage and labrum at the hip joint without intra-articular contrast is limited. Initial studies have focused on quantitative MR imaging of the hip,[68,69,72,74] but segmentation of the femoral and acetabular cartilage layers at the hip is challenging, and frequently the two cartilage layers cannot be differentiated.

SUMMARY

To assess all tissues affected by OA, "whole-organ" MR imaging protocols are required. These protocols include morphologic sequences, such as IM-weighted FSE sequences, that are well suited to detect abnormalities of cartilage, menisci, bone marrow, ligaments, and tendons, and quantitative sequences that allow the assessment of cartilage volumes (SPGR, FLASH) and the analysis of cartilage biochemical composition (T2, T1rho, and dGEMRIC techniques). Dedicated surface coils are required for optimal visualization of joints affected by OA, in particular the knee joint, and multichannel phased-array coils with parallel imaging have been shown to improve image quality and/or shorten acquisition time. Image quality also benefits from increased field strength, and 3.0-T MR imaging is used increasingly for assessing joints with OA.

REFERENCES

1. Kladny B, Gluckert K, Swoboda B, et al. Comparison of low-field (0.2 Tesla) and high-field (1.5 Tesla) magnetic resonance imaging of the knee joint. Arch Orthop Trauma Surg 1995;114:281–6.
2. Rand T, Imhof H, Turetschek K, et al. Comparison of low field (0.2T) and high field (1.5T) MR imaging in the differentiation of torn from intact menisci. Eur J Radiol 1999;30:22–7.
3. Woertler K, Strothmann M, Tombach B, et al. Detection of articular cartilage lesions: experimental evaluation of low- and high-field-strength MR imaging at 0.18 and 1.0 T. J Magn Reson Imaging 2000;11:678–85.
4. Ahn JM, Kwak SM, Kang HS, et al. Evaluation of patellar cartilage in cadavers with a low-field-strength extremity-only magnet: comparison of MR imaging sequences, with macroscopic findings as the standard. Radiology 1998;208:57–62.
5. Felson D, Chaisson C, Hill C, et al. The association of bone marrow lesions with pain in knee osteoarthritis. Ann Intern Med 2001;134:541–9.
6. Hunter DJ, Lo GH, Gale D, et al. The reliability of a new scoring system for knee osteoarthritis MRI and the validity of bone marrow lesion assessment: BLOKS (Boston Leeds Osteoarthritis Knee Score). Ann Rheum Dis 2008;67:206–11.
7. Link TM, Steinbach LS, Ghosh S, et al. Osteoarthritis: MR imaging findings in different stages of disease and correlation with clinical findings. Radiology 2003;226:373–81.
8. Phan CM, Link TM, Blumenkrantz G, et al. MR imaging findings in the follow-up of patients with different stages of knee osteoarthritis and the correlation with clinical symptoms. Eur Radiol 2006;16:608–18.
9. Eckstein F, Heudorfer L, Faber SC, et al. Long-term and resegmentation precision of quantitative cartilage MR imaging (qMRI). Osteoarthr Cartil 2002;10:922–8.
10. Peterfy CG, Guermazi A, Zaim S, et al. Whole-Organ Magnetic Resonance Imaging Score (WORMS) of the knee in osteoarthritis. Osteoarthr Cartil 2004;12:177–90.
11. Burstein D, Gray M. New MRI techniques for imaging cartilage. J Bone Joint Surg Am 2003;85(Suppl 2):70–7.
12. Mosher TJ, Dardzinski BJ. Cartilage MRI T2 relaxation time mapping: overview and applications. Semin Musculoskelet Radiol 2004;8:355–68.
13. Regatte RR, Akella SV, Wheaton AJ, et al. 3D-T1rho-relaxation mapping of articular cartilage: in vivo assessment of early degenerative changes in symptomatic osteoarthritic subjects. Acad Radiol 2004;11:741–9.
14. Barr C, Bauer JS, Malfair D, et al. MR imaging of the ankle at 3 Tesla and 1.5 Tesla: protocol optimization and application to cartilage, ligament and tendon pathology in cadaver specimens. Eur Radiol 2007;17:1518–28.
15. Bauer JS, Barr C, Henning TD, et al. Magnetic resonance imaging of the ankle at 3.0 Tesla and 1.5 Tesla in human cadaver specimens with artificially created lesions of cartilage and ligaments. Invest Radiol 2008;43:604–11.
16. Bauer JS, Krause SJ, Ross CJ, et al. Volumetric cartilage measurements of porcine knee at 1.5-T and 3.0-T MR imaging: evaluation of precision and accuracy. Radiology 2006;241:399–406.
17. Kijowski R, Blankenbaker D, Davis K, et al. Comparison of 1.5T and 3T magnetic resonance imaging systems for evaluating the articular cartilage of the knee joint. Chicago: RSNA; 2007. p. 125.
18. Link TM, Sell CA, Masi JN, et al. 3.0 vs 1.5T MRI in the detection of focal cartilage pathology—ROC analysis in an experimental model. Osteoarthr Cartil 2005;14:63–70.
19. Masi JN, Sell CA, Phan C, et al. Cartilage MR imaging at 3.0 versus that at 1.5 T: preliminary results in a porcine model. Radiology 2005;236:140–50.

20. Kijowski R, Blankenbaker DG, Davis KW, et al. Comparison of 1.5- and 3.0-T MR imaging for evaluating the articular cartilage of the knee joint. Radiology 2009.

21. Eckstein F, Charles HC, Buck RJ, et al. Accuracy and precision of quantitative assessment of cartilage morphology by magnetic resonance imaging at 3.0T. Arthritis Rheum 2005;52:3132–6.

22. Peterfy CG, Schneider E, Nevitt M. The osteoarthritis initiative: report on the design rationale for the magnetic resonance imaging protocol for the knee. Osteoarthr Cartil 2008;16:1433–41.

23. Kraff O, Theysohn JM, Maderwald S, et al. MRI of the knee at 7.0 Tesla. Rofo 2007;179:1231–5.

24. Krug R, Carballido-Gamio J, Banerjee S, et al. In vivo bone and cartilage MRI using fully-balanced steady-state free-precession at 7 Tesla. Magn Reson Med 2007;58:1294–8.

25. Roemer FW, Guermazi A, Lynch JA, et al. Short tau inversion recovery and proton density-weighted fat suppressed sequences for the evaluation of osteoarthritis of the knee with a 1.0 T dedicated extremity MRI: development of a time-efficient sequence protocol. Eur Radiol 2005;15:978–87.

26. Yamamura M, Miki H, Nakamura N, et al. Open-configuration MRI study of femoro-acetabular impingement. J Orthop Res 2007;25:1582–8.

27. Hinterwimmer S, von Eisenhart-Rothe R, Siebert M, et al. Patella kinematics and patello-femoral contact areas in patients with genu varum and mild osteoarthritis. Clin Biomech (Bristol, Avon) 2004;19:704–10.

28. Nishii T, Kuroda K, Matsuoka Y, et al. Change in knee cartilage T2 in response to mechanical loading. J Magn Reson Imaging 2008;28:175–80.

29. Amin S, Guermazi A, Lavalley MP, et al. Complete anterior cruciate ligament tear and the risk for cartilage loss and progression of symptoms in men and women with knee osteoarthritis. Osteoarthr Cartil 2008;16:897–902.

30. Logan M, Dunstan E, Robinson J, et al. Tibiofemoral kinematics of the anterior cruciate ligament (ACL)-deficient weightbearing, living knee employing vertical access open "interventional" multiple resonance imaging. Am J Sports Med 2004;32:720–6.

31. Logan MC, Williams A, Lavelle J, et al. Tibiofemoral kinematics following successful anterior cruciate ligament reconstruction using dynamic multiple resonance imaging. Am J Sports Med 2004;32:984–92.

32. Lutterbey G, Behrends K, Falkenhausen MV, et al. Is the body-coil at 3 Tesla feasible for the MRI evaluation of the painful knee? A comparative study. Eur Radiol 2007;17:503–8.

33. Bauer JS, Banerjee S, Henning TD, et al. Fast high-spatial-resolution MRI of the ankle with parallel imaging using GRAPPA at 3 T. AJR Am J Roentgenol 2007;189:240–5.

34. Zuo J, Li X, Banerjee S, et al. Parallel imaging of knee cartilage at 3 Tesla. J Magn Reson Imaging 2007;26:1001–9.

35. Naraghi A, White L. MRI evaluation of the postoperative knee: special considerations and pitfalls. Clin Sports Med 2006;25:703–25.

36. Saadat E, Jobke B, Chu B, et al. Diagnostic performance of in vivo 3T fast spin echo MRI for articular cartilage abnormalities in human osteoarthritic knees using histology as standard of reference. Eur Radiol 2008;18:2292–302.

37. Kawahara Y, Uetani M, Nakahara N, et al. Fast spin-echo MR of the articular cartilage in the osteoarthrotic knee. Correlation of MR and arthroscopic findings. Acta Radiol 1998;39:120–5.

38. Link TM, Sell CA, Masi JN, et al. 3.0 vs 1.5 T MRI in the detection of focal cartilage pathology–ROC analysis in an experimental model. Osteoarthr Cartil 2006;14:63–70.

39. Potter HG, Linklater JM, Allen AA, et al. Magnetic resonance imaging of articular cartilage in the knee. An evaluation with use of fast-spin-echo imaging. J Bone Joint Surg Am 1998;80:1276–84.

40. Ramnath RR, Magee T, Wasudev N, et al. Accuracy of 3-T MRI using fast spin-echo technique to detect meniscal tears of the knee. AJR Am J Roentgenol 2006;187:221–5.

41. Bredella MA, Tirman PF, Peterfy CG, et al. Accuracy of T2-weighted fast spin-echo MR imaging with fat saturation in detecting cartilage defects in the knee: comparison with arthroscopy in 130 patients. AJR Am J Roentgenol 1999;172:1073–80.

42. Eckstein F, Burstein D, Link TM. Quantitative MRI of cartilage and bone: degenerative changes in osteoarthritis. NMR Biomed 2006;19:822–54.

43. Yoshioka H, Stevens K, Hargreaves BA, et al. Magnetic resonance imaging of articular cartilage of the knee: comparison between fat-suppressed three-dimensional SPGR imaging, fat-suppressed FSE imaging, and fat-suppressed three-dimensional DEFT imaging, and correlation with arthroscopy. J Magn Reson Imaging 2004;20:857–64.

44. Ruehm S, Zanetti M, Romero J, et al. MRI of patellar articular cartilage: evaluation of an optimized gradient echo sequence (3D-DESS). J Magn Reson Imaging 1998;8:1246–51.

45. Hargreaves BA, Gold GE, Lang PK, et al. MR imaging of articular cartilage using driven equilibrium. Magn Reson Med 1999;42:695–703.

46. Gold GE, Fuller SE, Hargreaves BA, et al. Driven equilibrium magnetic resonance imaging of articular cartilage: initial clinical experience. J Magn Reson Imaging 2005;21:476–81.

47. Hargreaves BA, Gold GE, Beaulieu CF, et al. Comparison of new sequences for high-resolution cartilage imaging. Magn Reson Med 2003;49:700–9.

48. Kornaat PR, Reeder SB, Koo S, et al. MR imaging of articular cartilage at 1.5T and 3.0T: comparison of SPGR and SSFP sequences. Osteoarthr Cartil 2005;13:338–44.

49. Bauer J, Barr C, Steinbach L, et al. Imaging of the articular cartilage of the ankle at 3.0 and 1.5 Tesla. Eur Radiol 2006;16(Suppl 1):238 [abstract].

50. Ristow O, Steinbach L, Sabo G, et al. Isotropic 3D fast spin-echo imaging versus standard 2D imaging at 3.0 T of the knee-image quality and diagnostic performance. Eur Radiol 2009;19:1263–72.

51. Stevens KJ, Busse RF, Han E, et al. Ankle: isotropic MR imaging with 3D-FSE-cube—initial experience in healthy volunteers. Radiology 2008;249:1026–33.

52. Gagliardi JA, Chung EM, Chandnani VP, et al. Detection and staging of chondromalacia patellae: relative efficacies of conventional MR imaging, MR arthrography, and CT arthrography. AJR Am J Roentgenol 1994;163:629–36.

53. Kramer J, Recht MP, Imhof H, et al. Postcontrast MR arthrography in assessment of cartilage lesions. J Comput Assist Tomogr 1994;18:218–24.

54. Woertler K, Rummeny EJ, Settles M. A fast high-resolution multislice T1-weighted turbo spin-echo (TSE) sequence with a DRIVen equilibrium (DRIVE) pulse for native arthrographic contrast. AJR Am J Roentgenol 2005;185:1468–70.

55. Dunn TC, Lu Y, Jin H, et al. T2 relaxation time of cartilage at MR imaging: comparison with severity of knee osteoarthritis. Radiology 2004;232:592–8.

56. Regatte RR, Akella SV, Borthakur A, et al. In vivo proton MR three-dimensional T1rho mapping of human articular cartilage: initial experience. Radiology 2003;229:269–74.

57. Bashir A, Gray ML, Hartke J, et al. Nondestructive imaging of human cartilage glycosaminoglycan concentration by MRI. Magn Reson Med 1999;41:857–65.

58. Burstein D, Bashir A, Gray ML. MRI techniques in early stages of cartilage disease. Invest Radiol 2000;35:622–38.

59. Liess C, Lusse S, Karger N, et al. Detection of changes in cartilage water content using MRI T2-mapping in vivo. Osteoarthr Cartil 2002;10:907–13.

60. Dardzinski BJ, Mosher TJ, Li S, et al. Spatial variation of T2 in human articular cartilage. Radiology 1997;205:546–50.

61. Mosher TJ, Dardzinski BJ, Smith MB. Human articular cartilage: influence of aging and early symptomatic degeneration on the spatial variation of T2—preliminary findings at 3 T. Radiology 2000;214:259–66.

62. Li X, Han ET, Ma CB, et al. In vivo 3T spiral imaging based multi-slice T(1rho) mapping of knee cartilage in osteoarthritis. Magn Reson Med 2005;54:929–36.

63. Stahl R, Luke A, Li X, et al. T1rho, T(2) and focal knee cartilage abnormalities in physically active and sedentary healthy subjects versus early OA patients—a 3.0-Tesla MRI study. Eur Radiol 2009;19:132–43.

64. Trattnig S, Mlynarik V, Breitenseher M, et al. MRI visualization of proteoglycan depletion in articular cartilage via intravenous administration of Gd-DTPA. Magn Reson Imaging 1999;17:577–83.

65. Gillis A, Bashir A, McKeon B, et al. Magnetic resonance imaging of relative glycosaminoglycan distribution in patients with autologous chondrocyte transplants. Invest Radiol 2001;36:743–8.

66. Williams A, Gillis A, McKenzie C, et al. Glycosaminoglycan distribution in cartilage as determined by delayed gadolinium-enhanced MRI of cartilage (dGEMRIC): potential clinical applications. AJR Am J Roentgenol 2004;182:167–72.

67. Williams A, Sharma L, McKenzie CA, et al. Delayed gadolinium-enhanced magnetic resonance imaging of cartilage in knee osteoarthritis: findings at different radiographic stages of disease and relationship to malalignment. Arthritis Rheum 2005;52:3528–35.

68. Carballido-Gamio J, Link TM, Li X, et al. Feasibility and reproducibility of relaxometry, morphometric, and geometrical measurements of the hip joint with magnetic resonance imaging at 3T. J Magn Reson Imaging 2008;28:227–35.

69. Cheng Y, Wang S, Yamazaki T, et al. Hip cartilage thickness measurement accuracy improvement. Comput Med Imaging Graph 2007;31:643–55.

70. Kim YJ, Bixby S, Mamisch TC, et al. Imaging structural abnormalities in the hip joint: instability and impingement as a cause of osteoarthritis. Semin Musculoskelet Radiol 2008;12:334–45.

71. Taljanovic MS, Graham AR, Benjamin JB, et al. Bone marrow edema pattern in advanced hip osteoarthritis: quantitative assessment with magnetic resonance imaging and correlation with clinical examination, radiographic findings, and histopathology. Skeletal Radiol 2008;37:423–31.

72. Tiderius CJ, Jessel R, Kim YJ, et al. Hip dGEMRIC in asymptomatic volunteers and patients with early osteoarthritis: the influence of timing after contrast injection. Magn Reson Med 2007;57:803–5.

73. Eckstein F, Siedek V, Glaser C, et al. Correlation and sex differences between ankle and knee cartilage morphology determined by quantitative magnetic resonance imaging. Ann Rheum Dis 2004;63:1490–5.

74. Pfirrmann CW, Mengiardi B, Dora C, et al. Cam and pincer femoroacetabular impingement: characteristic MR arthrographic findings in 50 patients. Radiology 2006;240:778–85.

MR Imaging-Based Semiquantitative Assessment in Osteoarthritis

Frank W. Roemer, MD[a,b,c],*, Ali Guermazi, MD[a,c]

KEYWORDS

- MR Imaging • Osteoarthritis • Knee
- Semiquantitative scoring
- Whole-Organ Magnetic Resonance Imaging Score (WORMS)
- Boston Leeds Osteoarthritis Knee Score (BLOKS)
- Knee Osteoarthritis Scoring System (KOSS)
- Cross-sectional and longitudinal assessment

Over the past 2 decades MR imaging has established itself as the most important imaging modality in assessing joint pathology in the clinical and research environments. Its tomographic viewing perspective obviates morphologic distortion, magnification, and superimposition. MR imaging is uniquely able to depict all tissues of the joint directly. This allows the joint to be evaluated as a whole organ and provides a much more detailed picture of the changes associated with osteoarthritis (OA) than is possible with other techniques.

In relation to knee OA, MR imaging studies initially focused on the assessment of articular cartilage as the main outcome measure in clinical and epidemiologic studies (Fig. 1).[1–7] Several methodologies have been introduced and validated to assess many properties of articular cartilage using MR imaging, including compositional and biochemical analysis,[8–11] cartilage thickness and volume measurements,[12–16] and semiquantitative (SQ) analysis of surface damage, which allows cross-sectional and longitudinal evaluation (Fig. 2).[17–20] In addition, the great potential of MR imaging for the assessment of other joint structures that are involved in the OA process was soon recognized.[21–25] Subsequently, validated tools for

whole-organ (or, synonymously, whole-joint) assessment of the OA joint were introduced, which help in discriminating different patterns of intra-articular involvement in OA.[18,26–28] Furthermore, MR imaging detects pathologic changes of pre-radiographic OA at a much earlier stage of the disease than conventional radiography is able to detect.[29]

Although MR imaging has enormous potential, methods of standardized whole-organ analysis of joints are still in their infancy. SQ whole-organ scoring was originally introduced by Peterfy and colleagues[28] in 1999 and has since been applied to a multitude of OA studies. The analyses based on SQ scoring have deeply added to the understanding of the pathophysiology and natural history of OA and the clinical implications of structural changes assessed.[20,30–38] SQ scoring of MR imaging is a valuable method for performing multifeature assessment of the knee, using conventional MR imaging acquisition techniques that are commonly applied in a clinical environment. Such approaches score, in a SQ manner, a variety of features that are currently believed to be relevant to the functional integrity of the knee, are potentially involved in the

[a] Quantitative Imaging Center, Department of Radiology, Boston University School of Medicine, 820 Harrison Avenue, FGH Building, 3rd Floor, Boston, MA 02118, USA
[b] Department of Radiology, Klinikum Augsburg, Stenglinstr 2, 86156 Augsburg, Germany
[c] Boston Imaging Core Lab (BICL), LLC, 580 Harrison Avenue, 4th Floor, Boston, MA 02118, USA
* Corresponding author. Department of Radiology, Boston University School of Medicine, 820 Harrison Avenue, FGH Building, 3rd Floor, Boston, MA 02118.
E-mail address: froemer@bu.edu (F.W. Roemer).

Radiol Clin N Am 47 (2009) 633–654
doi:10.1016/j.rcl.2009.03.005
0033-8389/09/$ – see front matter © 2009 Elsevier Inc. All rights reserved.

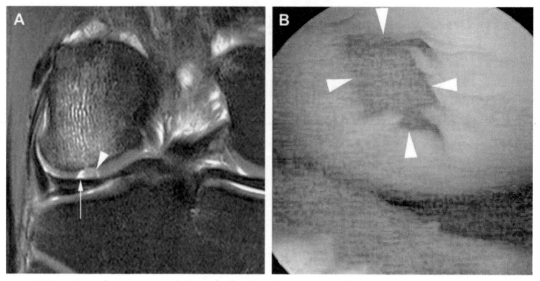

Fig. 1. MR imaging-arthroscopic correlation of a focal cartilage defect. (*A*) Coronal proton density fat-suppressed image. A full-thickness focal cartilage defect is depicted in the weight-bearing region of the lateral femoral condyle. The cartilage fragment is only partially detached (*arrow*). A portion of the fragment is still visualized in situ (*arrowhead*). Note also the extensive bone marrow lesion (BML) in the adjacent subchondral bone, visualized as an ill-defined area of signal hyperintensity (*no arrows*). (*B*) Arthroscopic documentation of same defect. After debridement of the in situ fragment, the full extent of the defect is visualized by arthroscopy (*arrowheads*). (*Courtesy of* W. Fischer, MD, Hessinpark Clinic, Augsburg, Germany.)

pathophysiology of OA, or both. These articular features include articular cartilage integrity, subarticular bone marrow abnormalities, subchondral cysts, subarticular bone attrition, marginal and central osteophytes (Fig. 3), medial and lateral meniscal integrity, anterior and posterior cruciate ligament integrity, medial and lateral collateral ligament integrity, synovitis and effusion,

intra-articular loose bodies, and periarticular cysts (Fig. 4) and bursitis.

The aim of this article is to review the different SQ approaches for MR imaging-based whole-organ assessment of knee OA and also to discuss practical aspects of whole-joint assessment. Alternative SQ scoring approaches are presented in addition. Thoughts on pulse sequence protocol

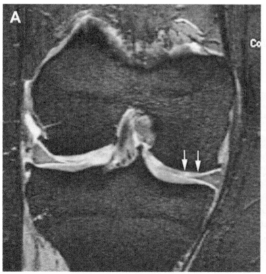
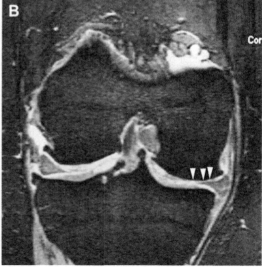

Fig. 2. Progressive cartilage loss in a 6-month interval. (*A*) Baseline reformatted coronal double-echo steady-state sequence shows diffuse thinning of cartilage in the central medial femur (*arrows*). (*B*) Follow-up image depicts subtle but definite progression of cartilage damage (*arrowheads*).

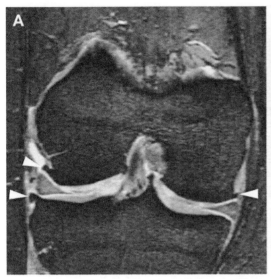
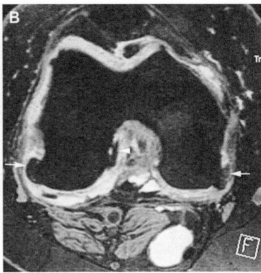

Fig. 3. Osteophytes. (A) Coronal reformatted double-echo steady-state image shows marginal osteophytes (*arrowheads*). (B) Axial image shows additional posterior osteophytes (*arrows*) and a notch osteophyte (*small arrowhead*).

selection and image quality required for SQ scoring are incorporated, although the more technical aspects are covered in the article on hardware and sequences by Link and colleagues elsewhere in this issue. The clinical relevance of the different noncartilaginous tissues assessed with SQ scoring is discussed in the article on MR imaging of intra- and periarticular soft tissues and subchondral bone in knee osteoarthritis by Crema and colleagues in this issue and in the article on the role of the meniscus by Englund and Lohmander in this issue and are not focus of this article.

WHOLE-JOINT ASSESSMENT ON MR IMAGING OF THE KNEE

Whole-organ assessment of scoring different joint structures on MR imaging has shown adequate reliability, specificity, and sensitivity, in addition to an ability to detect lesion progression.[18,26,32,39,40] To date, three SQ scoring systems for whole-organ assessment of knee OA have been published and have been applied in epidemiologic studies or clinical trials: the whole-organ MR imaging score (WORMS),[18] the knee osteoarthritis scoring system (KOSS),[26] and the Boston-Leeds osteoarthritis knee score (BLOKS).[27] Additional scoring tools have been introduced covering joint pathology that may not be adequately assessed by the previously mentioned systems or offer alternative approaches. Examples are the assessment of synovitis on contrast-enhanced MR imaging or detailed evaluation of the intercondylar tibial region.[41,42] To date, no study has been performed

that directly compares the established scoring systems concerning longitudinal sensitivity to change and correlates the different systems to clinical outcomes. Because a reference standard, such as histology, is not available, the true superiority of one system over the other probably cannot be proved. The three different scoring systems are summarized in Table 1.

When deciding which scoring system should be applied for the assessment of a given study, many aspects have to be considered. The most

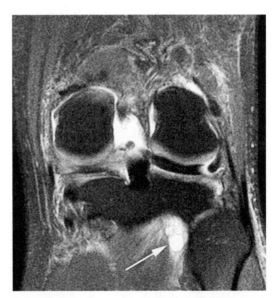

Fig. 4. Periarticular cysts. A tibiofibular joint cyst is depicted on coronal proton density fat-suppressed image (*arrow*).

Table 1
Comparison of three different semiquantitative scoring systems of knee osteoarthritis

	BLOKS	KOSS	WORMS
Number of knees scored in original publication	10 knees (71 knees for validity exercise of BML scoring)	25 knees	19 knees
MR imaging protocol of original publication (all publications used 1.5-T systems)	For reliability exercise (10 knees): sag/cor T2w FS, sag T1w SE, axial/cor 3D FLASH; For validity of BML assessment: sag PDw/T2w; Cor/axial PDw/T2w FS	Cor/sag T2w and PDw, sag 3D SPGR, axial PDw and axial T2w FS	Axial T1w SE, cor T1w SE, sag T1w SE, sag T2w FS, sag 3D SPGR
Subregional division of knee	9 subregions: medial/lateral patella, medial/lateral trochlea, medial, lateral weight bearing femur, medial/lateral weight bearing tibia, subspinous tibia	9 subregions: medial patella, patellar crest, lateral patella, medial/lateral trochlea, medial/lateral femoral condyle, medial/lateral tibial plateau	15 subregions: medial/lateral patella, medial/lateral femur (anterior/central/posterior), medial/lateral tibia (anterior/central/posterior), subspinous tibia
Interreader reliability	Performed on 10 knees; w-kappa between 0.51 (meniscal extrusion) and 0.79 (meniscal tear)	Performed on 25 knees; w-kappa between 0.57 (osteochondral defects) and 0.88 (bone marrow edema)	Performed on 19 knees; ICC between 0.74 (bone marrow abnormalities and synovitis/effusion) and 0.99 (cartilage)
Intrareader reliability	Not presented	Performed on 25 knees; w-kappa between 0.56 (intrasubstance meniscal degeneration) and 0.91 (bone marrow edema and Baker's cyst)	Not presented
Scored MR imaging features			
Cartilage	Two different scores; Score 1: subregional approach; A. Percentage of any cartilage loss in subregion; B. Percentage of full-thickness cartilage loss in subregion; Score 2: site-specific approach. Scoring of cartilage thickness at 11 specific locations (not subregions) from 0 (none) to 2 (full thickness loss)	Subregional approach: focal and diffuse defects are differentiated. Depth of lesions is scored from 0 to 3. Diameter of lesion is scored from 0 to 3. Osteochondral defects are scored separately	Subregional approach: scored from 0 to 6 depending on depth and extent of cartilage loss. Intrachondral cartilage signal additionally scored as present or absent

Bone marrow lesions	Scoring of individual lesions 3 different aspects of BMLs are scored: A. Size of BML scored from 0 to 3 concerning percentage of subregional bone volume B. Percentage of surface area adjacent to subchondral plate C. Percentage of BML that is noncystic	Scoring of individual lesions from 0 to 3 concerning maximum diameter of lesion	Summed BML size/volume for subregion from 0 to 3 in regard to percentage of subregional bone volume
Subchondral cysts	Scored together with BMLs	Scoring of individual lesions from 0 to 3 concerning maximum diameter of lesion	Summed cyst size/volume for subregion from 0 to 3 in regard to percentage of subregional bone volume
Osteophytes	Scored at 12 sites from 0 to 3	Scored from 0 to 3 Marginal intercondylar and central osteophytes are differentiated Locations/sites of osteophyte scoring not forwarded	Scored at 16 sites from 0 to 7
Bone attrition	Not scored	Not scored	Scored in 14 subregions from 0 to 3
Effusion	Scored from 0 to 3	Scored from 0 to 3	Scored from 0 to 3
Synovitis	A. Scoring of size of signal changes in Hoffa's fat pad B. Five additional sites scored as present or absent (details of scoring not described)	Synovial thickening scored as present or absent on sagittal T1w SPGR sequence (location not described)	Combined effusion/synovitis score.
Meniscal status	Anterior horn, body, posterior horn scored separately in medial/lateral meniscus Presence/absence scored: • Intrameniscal signal • Vertical tear • Horizontal tear • Complex tear • Root tear • Macerated • Meniscal cyst	No subregional division of meniscus described. Presence or absence of following tears: • Horizontal tear • Vertical tear • Radial tear • Complex tear • Bucket-handle tear • Meniscal intrasubstance degeneration scored from 0 to 3	Anterior horn, body, posterior horn scored separately in medial/lateral meniscus from 0 to 4: 1: Minor radial or parrot beak tear 2: Nondisplaced tear or prior surgical repair 3: Displaced tear or partial resection 4: Complete maceration or destruction or complete resection

(continued on next page)

Table 1
(continued)

	BLOKS	KOSS	WORMS
Meniscal extrusion	Scored as medial and lateral extrusion on coronal image and anterior extrusion for medial or lateral meniscus on sagittal image from 0 to 3	Scored on coronal image from 0 to 3	Not scored
Ligaments	Cruciate ligaments scored as normal or complete tear Associated insertional BMLs are scored in tibia and in femur collateral ligaments not scored	Not scored	Cruciate ligaments and collateral ligaments scored as intact or torn
Periarticular features	The following features are scored as present or absent: • Patella tendon signal • Pes anserine bursitis • Iliotibial band signal • Popliteal cyst • Infrapatellar bursa • Prepatellar bursa • Ganglion cysts of the TFJ, meniscus, ACL, PCL, semimembranosus, semitendinosus, other	Only popliteal cysts scored from 0 to 3	Popliteal cysts, anserine bursitis, semimembranosus bursa meniscal cyst, infrapatellar bursitis, prepatellar bursitis, tibiofibular cyst scored from 0 to 3
Loose bodies	Scored as absent or present	Not scored	Scored from 0 to 3 depending on number of loose bodies

Abbreviations: ACL, anterior cruciate ligament; BLOKS, Boston Leeds Osteoarthritis Knee Score; BML, bone marrow lesion; cor, coronal; ICC, intraclass correlation coefficient; KOSS, Knee Osteoarthritis Scoring System; PCL, posterior cruciate ligament; PDw, proton density weighted; sag, sagittal; T2w FS, T2-weighted fat-suppressed sequence; T1 SE, T1-weighted spin echo sequence; w-kappa, weighted kappa; TFJ, tibio-fibular joint; WORMS, whole-organ MR imaging score; 3D FLASH, three-dimensional fast low-angle shot sequence; 3D SPGR, three-dimensional spoiled gradient echo sequence.

important factors are certainly the outcome measures that are relevant to the study. Second, resources have to be taken into account, because assessment using a complete whole-organ score differs from scoring only certain selected features. Finally, the available image data set plays an important role, because not all features are scorable on all sequences or with any given sequence protocol. For example, none of the scoring systems incorporates contrast-enhanced MR imaging.

When estimating the time involved to apply any of these SQ systems and, consequently, projecting the resources needed for assessment of a given study, the imaging protocol (especially the number of sequences and individual images), the quality of images, and the degree of joint abnormalities attributable to OA have to be taken into account. Time needed for scoring cross-sectionally differs from longitudinal scoring, and the number of time points to be assessed needs to be considered. Finally, the method of documenting the scores (manually or electronically) is a crucial factor when estimating effort and resources required for the specific research endeavor.

To date, no data are available if several consecutive MR imaging examinations from the same subject are evaluated semiquantitatively in known chronologic order or if the images are presented with the reader blinded to the sequence in which they were acquired (ie, the order of films is not revealed). Studies evaluating blinded versus non-blinded reading to date have only been performed concerning radiographic SQ assessment of spinal fractures and in rheumatoid arthritis (RA).[43–46] The primary rationale behind blinding to sequence is to reduce reader bias toward finding change in the expected direction. As long as readers are blinded to treatment assignment in a clinical trial, however, it is not necessary to blind them to the chronologic sequence of the image data, because possible bias cannot influence the trial results. If the research aim is not treatment but rather the natural history and the question is how often progression or other change occurs, blinding might be of advantage. If films are read with known chronology in these studies, a reader could have the inclination to overread progression, although the experience from RA has shown otherwise.[47]

WHOLE-ORGAN MR IMAGING SCORE

Peterfy and colleagues[18] published WORMS in 2004. Many epidemiologic studies and clinical trials have used WORMS to assess several OA features of the knee semiquantitatively.[20,48–50] WORMS uses a complex subregional division of the different knee compartments: the patella is divided into the medial facet and lateral facet. The medial femur and lateral femur and tibial plateau, respectively, are subdivided into anterior, central, and posterior

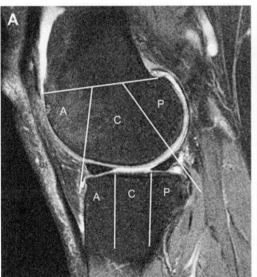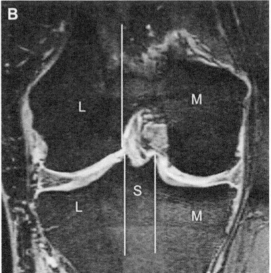

Fig. 5. Subregional division of the knee joint in WORMS. (A) Sagittal intermediate-weighted fat-suppressed image. The tibial plateau is subdivided into anterior (A), central (C), and posterior (P) subregions defined by meniscal coverage. The femur is subdivided into anterior (A), central (C), and posterior (P) portions defined by the anterior and posterior margins of the meniscus. (B) Coronal reformatted double-echo steady-state image. In the coronal plane, the tibia is divided into the medial (M) and lateral (L) tibial plateaus and the subspinous region (S) that is not covered by articular cartilage. The femur is divided into lateral (L) and medial (M) facets, whereas the femoral notch is considered a part of the medial femur.

subregions (Fig. 5). Finally, the subspinous tibial region not covered by cartilage is defined as an additional distinct subregion. The following features are covered by the WORMS system: cartilage, subchondral bone marrow lesions (BMLs), subchondral cysts, osteophytes, bone attrition, meniscal status, a combined effusion/synovitis score, and collateral and cruciate ligaments. In addition, several periarticular features are evaluated, such as meniscal and popliteal cysts, periarticular bursitis, and loose bodies (Fig. 6).

Cartilage is scored on a scale from 0 to 6 considering the extent of cartilage damage that is superficial or full thickness in each of the articular subregions (Fig. 7). Subchondral BMLs are defined as ill-delineated areas of hyperintensity adjacent to the subchondral plate on T2-weighted or proton density (PD)-weighted fat-suppressed fast spin echo (FSE) images (Fig. 8). Several differential diagnoses and possible artifacts need to be considered and ruled out when assessing subchondral BMLs (Fig. 9). Subchondral cysts, which

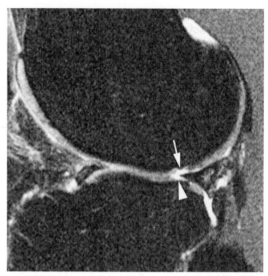

Fig. 7. Focal cartilage defects. Sagittal intermediate-weighted fat-suppressed sequence. The arrow depicts a small partial-thickness cartilage lesion in the central femoral condyle. In addition, a small full-thickness lesion is visualized in the posterior tibia (*arrowhead*).

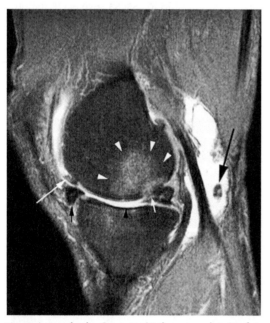

Fig. 6. Loose body. On a sagittal proton-density fat-suppressed image, a loose body within a popliteal (Baker's) cyst is visualized (*large black arrow*). Other typical MR imaging features of advanced knee OA are depicted in addition: a large subchondral bone marrow lesion in the weight-bearing region of the medial femur (*white arrowheads*), an anterior osteophyte of the medial femur (*large white arrow*), diffuse full-thickness cartilage loss of the central medial tibia (*black arrowhead*), anterior extrusion of the anterior horn of the medial meniscus (*short black arrow*), and a horizontal tear of the posterior horn of the medial meniscus (*small white arrow*).

represent well-defined lesions of fluid-equivalent signal intensity, are scored as separate entities. BMLs and cysts are scored from 0 to 3 depending on the percentage amount of subregion. Thus, a lesion that is partially cystic and partially noncystic is assigned two separate scores (Fig. 10). When compared with the other systems, WORMS uses a strict subregional rather than lesion-oriented approach to scoring, especially of cartilage, BMLs, and subchondral cysts. This has the possible advantage of summing several lesions per subregion and may facilitate reading and subsequent analyses. Using a lesional approach,[24,26,27] definition of the exact number of individual lesions is sometimes difficult, because lesions may be directly adjacent to each other or may be merging or splitting in longitudinal assessments. WORMS is the only SQ scoring system that assesses subchondral bone attrition, which is defined as flattening or depression of the articular surface not related to trauma and is scored from 0 to 3 (Fig. 11).

KNEE OSTEOARTHRITIS SCORING SYSTEM

KOSS, introduced by Kornaat and colleagues,[26] covers similar MR imaging-detected OA features as WORMS, but the following differences have to be mentioned. Cartilage status, subchondral BMLs, and cysts are scored individually for each subregion, and each score is differentiated by the size of the lesion. Osteophytes are

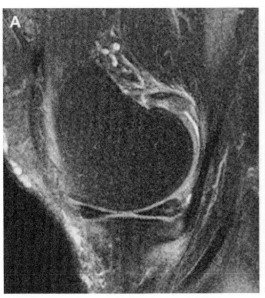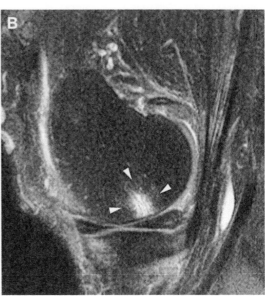

Fig. 8. Incident BML. (*A*) Sagittal intermediate-weighted fat-suppressed sequence. No BML is present at baseline. (*B*) At 24 months of follow-up, an incident non-cystic BML (*arrowheads*) is observed.

differentiated into marginal, intercondylar, and central. Although KOSS uses a more complex meniscal score concerning tear morphology than WORMS, it does not describe regional subdivision or partial or total meniscal maceration or resection. Meniscal subluxation is scored in addition to meniscal morphology (Fig. 12). Effusion is scored in

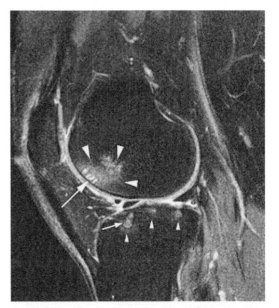

Fig. 10. Example of BML scoring. Sagittal intermediate-weighted fat-suppressed sequence. A large BML in the lateral femoral trochlea is shown. The BML consists of cystic (*large arrow*) and noncystic (*large arrowheads*) parts. In the BLOKS system, this is considered one entity, whereas in the WORMS and KOSS systems, this lesion is scored as two separate entities. The tibial plateau exhibits three separate lesions of ill-defined delineation (*small arrowheads*). The most anterior BML also consists of a cystic portion (*small arrow*).

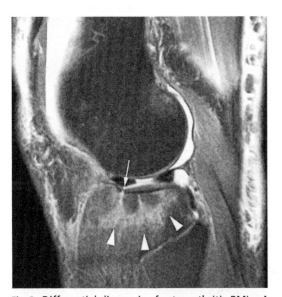

Fig. 9. Differential diagnosis of osteoarthritic BMLs. A sagittal PD fat-suppressed image shows acute traumatic osteochondral depression of the lateral tibial plateau. Note disruption of the articular cartilage (*arrow*) and the large associated traumatic bone contusion (*arrowheads*).

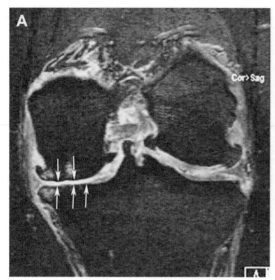
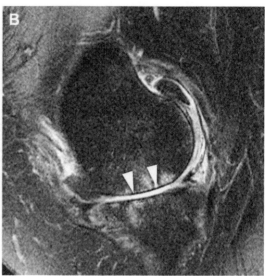

Fig. 11. Attrition. (*A*) Coronal reformatted double-echo steady-state image. Flattening of the central medial femoral condyle and tibial plateau is depicted (*arrows*). (*B*) Sagittal intermediate-weighted fat-suppressed image. Flattening of the central medial condyle is shown (*arrowheads*).

a similar fashion as in WORMS (Fig. 13). In addition, synovitis scoring is described for sagittal T1-weighted gradient-recalled echo images as present or absent. Concerning periarticular features, only popliteal cysts are assessed. KOSS uses a different subregional division than WORMS and differentiates the patellar crest (crista patellae), the medial patellar facet and lateral patellar facet, the medial trochlear articular facet and lateral trochlear articular facet, the medial femoral condyle and lateral femoral condyle (excluding the trochlear groove), and the medial tibial plateau and lateral tibial plateau.

BOSTON-LEEDS OSTEOARTHRITIS KNEE SCORE

The BLOKS system was published by Hunter and colleagues[27] in 2008. Concerning the subregional division of the articular surfaces, BLOKS uses a similar approach to KOSS, focusing on the

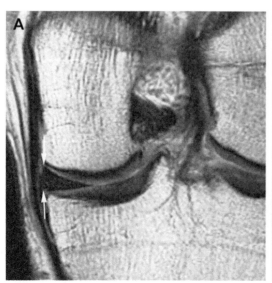
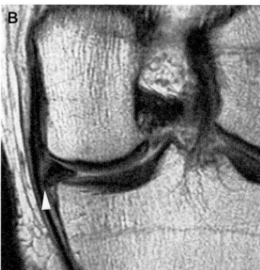

Fig. 12. Meniscal extrusion. (*A*) Coronal intermediate-weighted fast spin echo image. Regular position of the meniscus is observed at baseline (*arrows*). (*B*) Incident meniscal extrusion is observed at 12 months of follow-up (*arrowhead*).

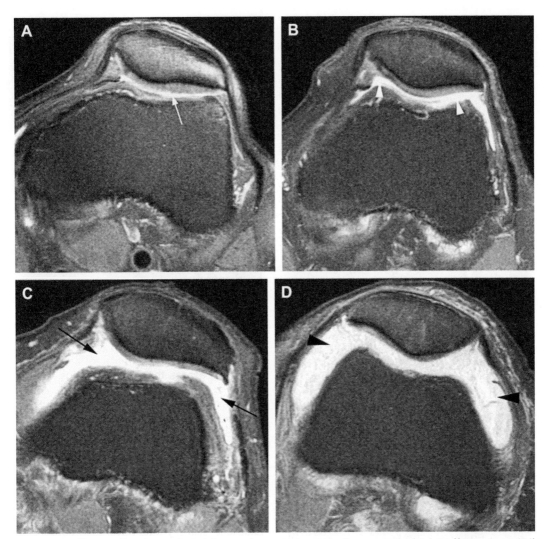

Fig. 13. Joint effusion. The three whole-joint scoring systems assess the amount of joint effusion in a similar fashion according to the degree of joint capsule distention. (*A*) Axial proton-density (PD) fat-suppressed (fs) image shows a physiologic amount of effusion (*white arrow*). (*B*) Axial PD fs image depicts grade 1 joint effusion (*white arrowheads*). (*C*) Grade 2 effusion is visualized (*black arrows*). (*D*) Axial PD fs image shows an extensive grade 3 joint effusion with marked distention of the joint capsule (*black arrowheads*).

weight-bearing components versus the patellofemoral joint (**Fig. 14**). As in WORMS, the patella is subdivided into the medial and lateral facets (**Fig. 15**). BMLs and cysts are scored in a complex manner, taking into account the size of the BML, percentage of involved subchondral surface area of the BML, and percentage of the BML that is cystic. Thus, subchondral cysts are defined as cystic portions of the BML and are not assessed separately as in the other two scoring systems (**Fig. 16**). The lesional approach for BMLs allows for superior longitudinal analysis of individual lesions, especially concerning the percentage of the lesion that is cystic or noncystic. Conversely,

the definition of each lesion is time-consuming, and the ill-delineated nature of these lesions makes differentiation among individual lesions difficult in certain instances. In addition, the BLOKS assesses the amount of the BML that is adjacent to the subchondral plate and allows for differentiation of depth of BMLs in regard to the subchondral plate.

Cartilage scoring is performed reporting two scores. The first score describes the percentage of any cartilage loss in the subregion and percentage of cartilage damage that represents full-thickness loss. The second cartilage score describes the cartilage status at defined locations

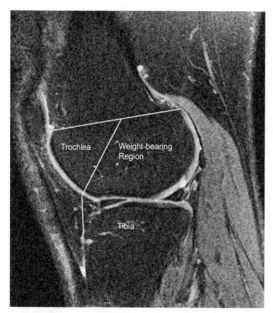

Fig. 14. Subregional division in BLOKS and KOSS. Sagittal intermediate-weighted fat-suppressed image. The femur is subdivided into the femoral trochlea and the weight-bearing region. The medial and lateral tibial plateaus are defined as one subregion, respectively.

on specific landmark-defined image sections in the coronal plane and differentiates partial- and full-thickness cartilage loss. Signal changes in Hoffa's fat pad are scored as a surrogate for synovitis.[51] BLOKS uses a complex scoring

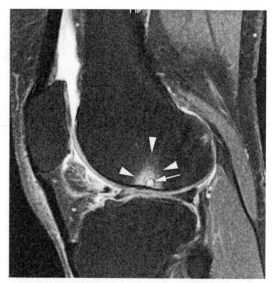

Fig. 16. BML. Sagittal intermediate-weighted fat-suppressed image shows a BML with cystic (*arrow*) and noncystic (*arrowheads*) portions in the central part of the lateral femoral condyle.

system to assess the meniscal status, including tears (Fig. 17), signal changes (Fig. 18), and meniscal extrusion. The original BLOKS publication included a comparison between WORMS and BLOKS concerning the validity of BML scoring. Slight superiority was reported for the BLOKS system.

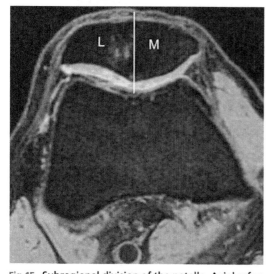

Fig. 15. Subregional division of the patella. Axial reformatted DESS image in WORMS and BLOKS, the patella is divided into the medial (M) and lateral (L) facets, whereas the patellar crest is defined as medial. In KOSS, the patella crest is a separate entity; thus, the patella has three subregions.

RELIABILITY

Excellent reliability data have been published for all three whole-organ SQ scoring systems. A comparative overview of the reliability exercises is presented in Table 2. The usual range of these exercises represents good to excellent agreement between two independent radiologists after an intensive training and validation exercise. It has to be kept in mind, however, that these numbers are highly dependent on the MR imaging protocol and on the experience of the individual expert readers. The numbers presented in Table 2 reflect only the data on published features (eg, the cruciate ligaments are scored with BLOKS and the Baker's cysts are assessed with WORMS, but these features were not included in the reliability exercises). Intraobserver data have only been published for the KOSS system and showed comparable results as interobserver reliability. Additional reliability exercises were performed for aspects of the WORMS system in the Multicenter Osteoarthritis (MOST) study and have been published.[32,34,36,37]

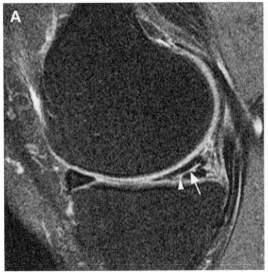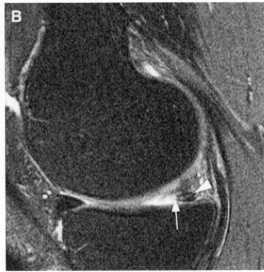

Fig. 17. Meniscal damage. (*A*) Sagittal intermediate-weighted fat-suppressed image. A horizontal tear (*small arrow*) extending to the inferior meniscal surface (*small arrowhead*) is shown. (*B*) Meniscal maceration. Missing central portion of meniscus (*large arrow*). In addition, a horizontal tear is depicted (*large arrowhead*).

ADDITIONAL SEMIQUANTITATIVE SCORING SYSTEMS

Additional methods to score different tissue pathologies on MR imaging in knee OA have been suggested. Examples are presented in this section to illustrate these alternative approaches.

Several SQ grading schemes for the evaluation of articular cartilage have been proposed, with most of them being derived from the surgery-based scoring method suggested by Outerbridge[52] in 1961. Arthroscopic scoring systems usually assess cartilage macroscopically on a scale from 0 to 4 based on visual evaluation and direct probing.[53] MR imaging-adapted modifications of these systems grade the depth of articular cartilage damage and differentiate between surface defects of less or more than 50% of cartilage thickness but rarely incorporate the involved area of superficial or full-thickness defects.[54–57] Biswal and colleagues[19] suggested a scoring system similar to WORMS, grading cartilage on a six-point scale and also incorporating lesion size.

Synovitis is frequently present in OA and may predict other structural changes in OA and correlate with pain and other clinical outcomes.[25,58] Quantitative MR imaging markers of synovitis include the volume of synovial tissue and fluid and synovial enhancement after intravenous injection of contrast material. Because the published whole-organ scoring systems are based on non-enhanced MR imaging, only indirect surrogate imaging features may be used to estimate the degree of synovitis. One of these is joint effusion

as a reflection of inflammatory synovial activation of the joint.[37] Synovitis has been scored semiquantitatively in the absence of gadopentetate dimeglumine[25,58] as signal alterations in the infrapatellar fat pad on noncontrast MR imaging correlated with mild chronic synovitis on histologic analysis, however.[51] This surrogate assessment seems to be nonspecific, albeit sensitive.[59] Other differential diagnoses, such as nonspecific edema

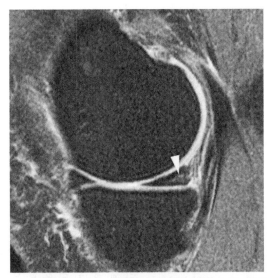

Fig. 18. Mucoid intrameniscal degeneration. Sagittal intermediate-weighted fat-suppressed image shows intrameniscal signal change in the posterior horn of the medial meniscus (*arrowhead*).

Table 2
Published inter- and intraobserver reliability results for reading of MR imaging features using different whole-joint scoring systems

Joint Feature	WORMS Interreader Agreement (ICC)	KOSS Interreader (ICC [95% CI]/w kappa)	KOSS Intrareader (ICC [95% CI]/w kappa)	BLOKS Interreader (w kappa [95% CI])
BML size	0.74	0.91 [0.88–0.93]/0.88	0.93 [0.91–0.94]/0.91	0.72 [0.58–0.87]
BML % area (BLOKS only)	N/A	N/A	N/A	0.69 [0.55–0.82]
% of lesion BML (BLOKS only)	N/A	N/A	N/A	0.72 [0.58–0.87]
Osteophytes	0.97	0.71 [0.67–0.76]/0.67	0.76 [0.72–0.80]/0.79	0.65 [0.52–0.77]
Cartilage morphology	0.99	0.64 [0.58–0.69]/0.57	0.78 [0.74–0.81]/0.67	0.72 [0.59–0.85]
Cartilage 2 (BLOKS only)	N/A	N/A	N/A	0.73 [0.60–0.85]
Osteochondral defects (KOSS only)	N/A	0.63 [0.55–0.70]/0.66	0.87 [0.83–0.90]/0.87	N/A
Synovitis	0.74	0.74 [0.58–0.85]	0.81 [0.69–0.89]/0.77	0.62 [0.05–1.00]
Effusion	See synovitis; scores combined	See synovitis; scores combined	See synovitis; scores combined	0.61 [0.05–0.85]
Meniscal extrusion/subluxation	N/A	0.67 [0.57–0.75]/0.65	0.82 [0.75–0.86]/0.82	0.51 [0.24–0.78]
Meniscal signal/Intrasubstance degeneration	N/A	0.78 [0.68–0.85]/0.66	0.76 [0.66–0.83]/0.56	0.68 [0.44–0.93]
Meniscal tear	0.87	0.70 [0.61–0.77]/0.70	0.78 [0.70–0.83]/0.78	0.79 [0.40–1.00]
Ligaments	1.0	N/A	N/A	N/A
Subchondral cysts	0.94	0.87 [0.83–0.89]/0.83	0.90 [0.87–0.92]/0.87	Part of %BML score
Baker's cysts	N/A	0.89 [0.76–0.95]/0.80	0.96 [0.90–0.98]/0.91	N/A

Abbreviations: BLOKS, Boston Leeds Osteoarthritis Knee Score; BML, bone marrow lesion; ICC, intraclass correlation coefficient; KOSS, Knee Osteoarthritis Scoring System; N/A, not applicable; w kappa, weighted kappa; WORMS, whole-organ MR imaging score; 95% CI, 95% confidence interval.

or chronic fibrotic changes, might present with a similar aspect on MR imaging.[60] Another scoring system assessing synovitis on non-enhanced images has been introduced recently.[61] The researchers suggest scoring synovial thickening at four different locations in the peripatellar region on a T1-weighted gradient echo type sequence and showed good intra- and interreader reliability. Validation data comparing the system with an established reference standard, such as histology or contrast-enhanced MR imaging, was not provided.[62] A detailed whole-joint synovitis scoring system measuring synovial thickness on T1-weighted, fat-suppressed, contrast-enhanced images was presented recently. Synovitis is assessed at 11 defined joint locations and is scored semiquantitatively from 0 to 3 (Fig. 19). Good reliability and a correlation with pain could be shown.[42] In a recent publication considering microscopic analysis as a "gold standard," only the MR imaging total synovitis score performed on injected images correlated with synovial membrane inflammation, with histology as the reference standard.[63]

There are few MR imaging scoring systems published for evaluating ligaments in OA of the knee joint. One report scored the medial collateral ligament for no, weak, and high signal intensity on coronal and axial sections.[22] Another study used a classification system based on ligamentous injury grading of 0 to 3, ranging from edema on one side of the ligament fibers to edema on both sides and edema with ligamentous disruption.[64]

It has to be kept in mind, however, that this classification assesses traumatic injury and is not necessarily applicable to osteoarthritic joints.

Concerning BML assessment, Felson and colleagues[24,31] introduced a lesional approach to be graded from 0 to 3. Expanding this scoring method and incorporating the number of slices that depict a specific lesion were suggested by other research groups.[57,65] Recently, one publication assessed BMLs using software cursors applied to the greatest diameter of each lesion.[66] A drawback seems to be that large diameters do not necessarily reflect BML volume.

SEQUENCE PROTOCOLS FOR SEMIQUANTITATIVE WHOLE-ORGAN ASSESSMENT

When designing any imaging protocol for whole-organ assessment, it has to be considered which articular tissues are to be included in the assessment and which measurement methods are to be applied to assess the individual tissue or feature. Full anatomic coverage has to be supported by the MR imaging system. Other quality parameters, such as signal homogeneity, correct image orientation, sufficient signal-to-noise ratio, and spatial resolution, in addition to the minimization of technical artifacts, have to be taken into account. Length of the protocol based on the number of sequences applied, the number of acquisitions per sequence, spatial resolution, and type of sequence needs to be determined to find

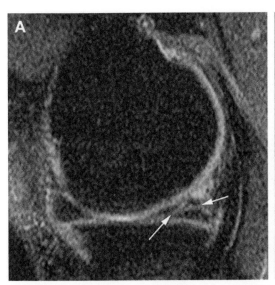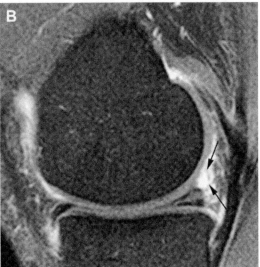

Fig. 19. Localized synovitis. (A) Sagittal PD fat-suppressed (fs) image shows a horizontal meniscal tear extending to the inferior surface and posterior aspect of the posterior horn of the medial meniscus (arrows). (B) T1-weighted fs image after intravenous contrast administration shows marked perimeniscal enhancement reflecting synovitic thickening (arrows) not depicted on the nonenhanced sequence.

a compromise between patient comfort and tolerance, costs, and image quality.

Suggestions for MR imaging protocols focusing on whole-organ assessment have been described in detail in an Osteoarthritis Research Society International (OARSI)/Outcome Measures in Rheumatoid Arthritis Clinical Trials (OMERACT) consensus review by Peterfy and colleagues.[67] A minimalist protocol still allowing for assessment of most articular features that are included in whole-organ scoring would consist of PD-weighted or T2-weighted fat-suppressed sequences in three orthogonal planes.[68] Additional sequences add information for the assessment of certain tissues, such as cartilage-dedicated gradient echo type sequences or T1-weighted spin echo sequences for assessment of sclerosis or superior visualization of loose bodies. Individualized angulation of sequences helps in delineating specific structures and should be considered if the focus of a study is not assessment of multiple features but only of a few features. An example is the paracoronal T2-weighted sequence depicting the anterior cruciate ligament (ACL) in its full extent, which helps in differentiating partial from complete ACL disruption (Fig. 20). It has to be kept in mind that additional sequences increase imaging time and, consequently, participant comfort, however. Also, image preparation before scoring becomes more time-consuming. A detailed description of the rationales for choosing the protocol for the Osteoarthritis Initiative (OAI) has been reported recently.[69] Concerning whole-organ assessment,

a drawback of the OAI protocol seems to be the availability of only one water-sensitive, fat-suppressed, FSE sequence acquired in one plane (in the OAI, the sagittal intermediate-weighted turbo spin echo sequence with fat suppression [IW TSE FS]) that allows for detailed BML assessment. The sagittal IW TSE FS sequence depicts cartilage defects superiorly and should be considered for cartilage assessment in addition to the also available cartilage-dedicated double-echo steady-state (DESS) sequence or fast low-angle shot sequence (for one knee) when performing SQ assessment in the OAI (Fig. 21).[70] The DESS sequence, conversely, is extremely sensitive to magnetic susceptibility and allows for detection of discrete meniscal or intrachondral calcification, which is not possible with conventional FSE sequences (Fig. 22).

IMAGE QUALITY

Sufficient image quality is crucial for SQ whole-organ assessment. MR imaging needs to be acquired in a standardized fashion adhering to protocol requirements.[67] An example of how to acquire optimal image data, what kind of problems are likely to be encountered, and how to deal with such problems is presented in the publicly available OAI MR imaging operations manual.[71] Despite sufficient anatomic coverage, field homogeneity, absence of motion artifacts, and sufficient fat suppression in fat-saturated sequences are paramount for reliable SQ scoring of osteoarthritic

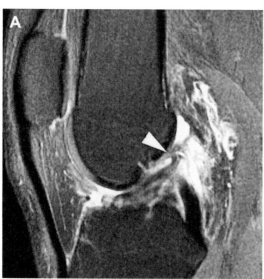
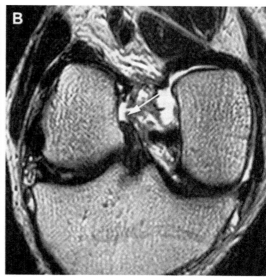

Fig. 20. Proximal ACL disruption. (*A*) Sagittal PD fat-suppressed image shows damage of the femoral ACL attachment (*arrowhead*). The sagittal image does not allow differentiation between a partial and full-thickness tear. (*B*) Paracoronal T2-weighted image shows discontinuation of the ligament, reflecting a complete proximal intraligamentous tear (*arrow*).

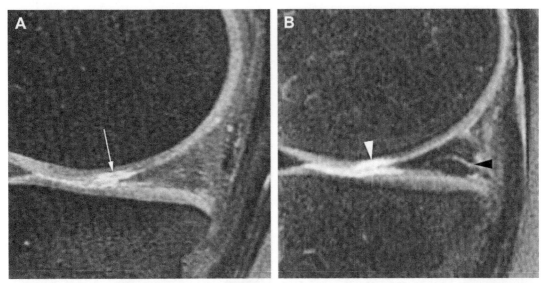

Fig. 21. Assessment of focal cartilage lesions. (*A*) Sagittal DESS image shows superficial thinning of cartilage in the weight-bearing region of the medial femur (*arrow*). (*B*) Sagittal IW fat-suppressed (fs) image superiorly depicts the defect because of better contrast between the intra-articular joint fluid and cartilage surface (*white arrowhead*). Note also the horizontal tear of the posterior horn of the medial meniscus only visualized on IW fs image (*black arrowhead*).

joints. Knowledge of additional possible artifacts, such as susceptibility (including metallic artifacts), vascular pulsation, and aliasing, is crucial.[67] Examples of possible artifacts and commonly encountered image quality impairment are presented in Fig. 23.

SEMIQUANTITATIVE SCORING OF OTHER JOINTS

Currently, most research teams using MR imaging-based SQ assessment of OA focus on the knee joint. Reasons for this are the size of the joint, with relatively thick articular cartilage in comparison to other diarthrodial joints; high prevalence of knee OA; and joint anatomy that allows

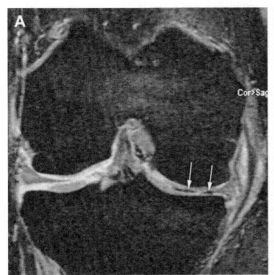
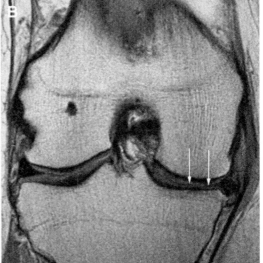

Fig. 22. Susceptibility artifact. (*A*) Reformatted coronal DESS sequence. Discrete calcification of chondral surface in the weight-bearing region of the medial tibiofemoral compartment is depicted (*short arrows*). (*B*) On a coronal IW sequence, calcification may not be appreciated and can only be delineated in the knowledge of the findings on the DESS image (*long arrows*).

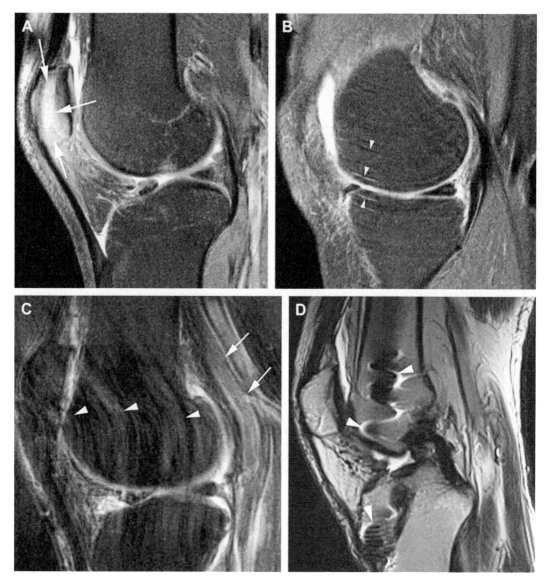

Fig. 23. Artifacts. (*A*) Insufficient fat suppression. Sagittal PD fat-suppressed (fs) image shows hyperintense bone marrow within the patella that is consistent with bone marrow edema (*arrows*). The association of high signal extending across adjacent tissue compartments (prepatellar soft tissues and Hoffa's fat pad) suggests failed fat suppression as an alternative cause, however. This artifact reduces the diagnostic accuracy of this scan for assessment of patellar BMLs. (*B*) Motion artifact. Sagittal PD fs image of the medial tibiofemoral compartment. Repetitive band-like high- and low-intensity signal changes are observed in the anterior femur and tibia (*arrowheads*). These are a result of motion during the sequence acquisition and impair assessment of the subchondral bone marrow in these subregions. (*C*) Pulsation artifact. Midsagittal PD fs image shows marked pulsation artifacts from the popliteal artery (*arrows*) in the phase-encoding direction (anterior-posterior), obscuring the articular anatomy of the knee. Band-like repetition artifacts of the vessel impair bone marrow assessment in the adjacent femur and tibia (*arrowheads*). (*D*) Susceptibility artifacts after reconstructive surgery. A sagittal T2-weighted FSE image shows severe metallic artifacts in the femur and tibia associated with surgical ACL repair and an intraosseous marrow implant after diaphyseal femoral fracture (*arrowheads*).

convenient assessment of most structures in two orthogonal planes. SQ assessment of facet joint OA on multidetector CT scans has been introduced.[72] Recently, a SQ system to assess early hip OA was presented.[73] To the authors' knowledge, additional MR imaging- or CT-based SQ assessment of OA of other joints has not been performed to date (**Fig. 24**).

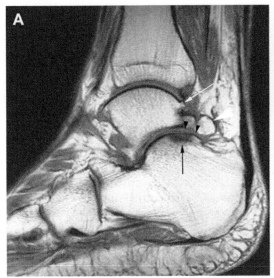 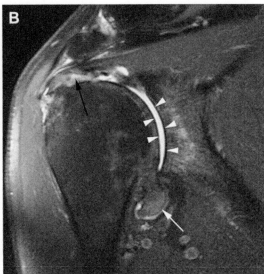

Fig. 24. OA of other joints. (*A*) Sagittal T1-weighted image shows severe OA of the subtalar joint. Note cartilage loss (*black arrowheads*) and subchondral calcaneal BML (*black arrow*). In addition, osteophytes at the posterior tibiotalar (*white arrow*) and subtalar (*white arrowhead*) joints are depicted. (*B*) Coronal PD fat-suppressed image of shoulder OA. Diffuse humeral and glenoidal cartilage loss is depicted (*arrowheads*). In addition, an articular-sided partial tear of the supraspinatus tendon is shown (*black arrow*). Note the huge osteophyte at the caudal humeral head (*white arrow*).

SUMMARY

With several large currently ongoing epidemiologic studies, huge amounts of image data are being acquired and, in the case of the OAI, made publicly available. This should allow the research community ample opportunity for SQ, quantitative, and compositional MR imaging assessment to deepen their knowledge of risk factors for disease development and progression. In addition, novel analytic approaches have to be developed to define those subcohorts that are likely to be of relevance for answering the specific research question and, specifically, increasing knowledge on disease progression. Because resources are limited, complete assessment of the MR imaging data sets is not likely to become feasible (especially in the OAI) in the near future. Interdisciplinary collaboration is likely to be crucial in determining which imaging biomarkers may superiorly predict clinical outcomes. Several reliable SQ scoring approaches have been introduced that offer the possibility of whole-joint assessment or assessment of only certain features pertinent to the research focus of a given study. MR imaging-based SQ assessment of knee OA has proved to be a powerful and applicable methodology that has profoundly contributed to the understanding of disease characterization and its natural history.

REFERENCES

1. Eckstein F, Schnier M, Haubner M, et al. Accuracy of cartilage volume and thickness measurements with magnetic resonance imaging. Clin Orthop Relat Res 1998;352:137–48.
2. Burgkart R, Glaser C, Hyhlik-Durr A, et al. Magnetic resonance imaging-based assessment of cartilage loss in severe osteoarthritis: accuracy, precision, and diagnostic value. Arthritis Rheum 2001;44:2072–7.
3. Cicuttini F, Forbes A, Asbeutah A, et al. Comparison and reproducibility of fast and conventional spoiled gradient-echo magnetic resonance sequences in the determination of knee cartilage volume. J Orthop Res 2000;18:580–4.
4. Gahunia HK, Babyn P, Lemaire C, et al. Osteoarthritis staging: comparison between magnetic resonance imaging, gross pathology and histopathology in the rhesus macaque. Osteoarthritis Cartilage 1995;3:169–80.
5. Broderick LS, Turner DA, Renfrew DL, et al. Severity of articular cartilage abnormality in patients with osteoarthritis: evaluation with fast spin-echo MR vs arthroscopy. AJR Am J Roentgenol 1994;162:99–103.
6. Chan WP, Lang P, Stevens MP, et al. Osteoarthritis of the knee: comparison of radiography, CT, and MR imaging to assess extent and severity. AJR Am J Roentgenol 1991;157:799–806.
7. Blackburn WD Jr, Bernreuter WK, Rominger M, et al. Arthroscopic evaluation of knee articular cartilage: a

comparison with plain radiographs and magnetic resonance imaging. J Rheumatol 1994;21:675–9.

8. Burstein D, Bashir A, Gray ML. MRI techniques in early stages of cartilage disease. Invest Radiol 2000;35:622–38.

9. Burstein D, Velyvis J, Scott KT, et al. Protocol issues for delayed Gd(DTPA)(2-)-enhanced MRI (dGEMRIC) for clinical evaluation of articular cartilage. Magn Reson Med 2001;45:36–41.

10. Gray ML, Burstein D, Lesperance LM, et al. Magnetization transfer in cartilage and its constituent macromolecules. Magn Reson Med 1995;34: 319–25.

11. Kimelman T, Vu A, Storey P, et al. Three-dimensional T1 mapping for dGEMRIC at 3.0 T using the Look Locker method. Invest Radiol 2006;41:198–203.

12. Eckstein F, Glaser C. Measuring cartilage morphology with quantitative magnetic resonance imaging. Semin Musculoskelet Radiol 2004;8:329–53.

13. Eckstein F, Burstein D, Link TM. Quantitative MRI of cartilage and bone: degenerative changes in osteoarthritis. NMR Biomed 2006;19:822–54.

14. Eckstein F, Westhoff J, Sittek H, et al. In vivo reproducibility of three-dimensional cartilage volume and thickness measurements with MR imaging. AJR Am J Roentgenol 1998;170:593–7.

15. Gandy SJ, Dieppe PA, Keen MC, et al. No loss of cartilage volume over three years in patients with knee osteoarthritis as assessed by magnetic resonance imaging. Osteoarthritis Cartilage 2002;10: 929–37.

16. Inglis D, Pui M, Ioannidis G, et al. Accuracy and test-retest precision of quantitative cartilage morphology on a 1.0 T peripheral magnetic resonance imaging system. Osteoarthritis Cartilage 2007;15:110–5.

17. Sowers MF, Hayes C, Jamadar D, et al. Magnetic resonance-detected subchondral bone marrow and cartilage defect characteristics associated with pain and X-ray-defined knee osteoarthritis. Osteoarthritis Cartilage 2003;11:387–93.

18. Peterfy CG, Guermazi A, Zaim S, et al. Whole-Organ Magnetic Resonance Imaging Score (WORMS) of the knee in osteoarthritis. Osteoarthritis Cartilage 2004;12:177–90.

19. Biswal S, Hastie T, Andriacchi TP, et al. Risk factors for progressive cartilage loss in the knee: a longitudinal magnetic resonance imaging study in forty-three patients. Arthritis Rheum 2002;46: 2884–92.

20. Hunter DJ, Zhang Y, Niu JB, et al. The association of meniscal pathologic changes with cartilage loss in symptomatic knee osteoarthritis. Arthritis Rheum 2006;54:795–801.

21. Zanetti M, Bruder E, Romero J, et al. Bone marrow edema pattern in osteoarthritic knees: correlation between MR imaging and histologic findings. Radiology 2000;215:835–40.

22. Pham XV, Monteiro I, Judet O, et al. Magnetic resonance imaging changes in periarticular soft tissues during flares of medial compartment knee osteoarthritis. Preliminary study in 10 patients. Rev Rhum Engl Ed 1999;66:398–403.

23. Gale DR, Chaisson CE, Totterman SM, et al. Meniscal subluxation: association with osteoarthritis and joint space narrowing. Osteoarthritis Cartilage 1999;7:526–32.

24. Felson DT, Chaisson CE, Hill CL, et al. The association of bone marrow lesions with pain in knee osteoarthritis. Ann Intern Med 2001;134:541–9.

25. Hill CL, Gale DG, Chaisson CE, et al. Knee effusions, popliteal cysts, and synovial thickening: association with knee pain in osteoarthritis. J Rheumatol 2001; 28:1330–7.

26. Kornaat PR, Ceulemans RY, Kroon HM, et al. MRI assessment of knee osteoarthritis: Knee Osteoarthritis Scoring System (KOSS)—inter-observer and intra-observer reproducibility of a compartment-based scoring system. Skeletal Radiol 2005;34:95–102.

27. Hunter DJ, Lo GH, Gale D, et al. The reliability of a new scoring system for knee osteoarthritis MRI and the validity of bone marrow lesion assessment: BLOKS (Boston Leeds Osteoarthritis Knee Score). Ann Rheum Dis 2008;67:206–11.

28. Peterfy CG, White D, Tirman P, et al. Whole-organ evaluation of the knee in osteoarthritis using MRI. Ann Rheum Dis 1999;38:342 [abstract].

29. Guermazi A, Hunter DJ, Roemer FW, et al. Magnetic resonance imaging prevalence of different features of knee osteoarthritis in persons with normal knee x-rays. Arthritis Rheum 2007; 56(Suppl):S128.

30. Hernandez-Molina G, Neogi T, Hunter DJ, et al. The association of bone attrition with knee pain and other MRI features of osteoarthritis. Ann Rheum Dis 2008; 67:43–7.

31. Felson DT, McLaughlin S, Goggins J, et al. Bone marrow edema and its relation to progression of knee osteoarthritis. Ann Intern Med 2003;139: 330–6.

32. Felson DT, Niu J, Guermazi A, et al. The development of knee pain correlates with enlarging bone marrow edema lesions on MRI. Arthritis Rheum 2007;56:2986–92.

33. Englund M, Guemazi A, Gale D, et al. Incidental meniscal findings on knee MRI in middle-aged and elderly persons. N Engl J Med 2008;359: 1108–15.

34. Englund M, Guermazi A, Roemer FW, et al. Meniscal tear in knee without surgery and the development of radiographic osteoarthritis among middle-aged and elderly persons: the multicenter osteoarthritis study. Arthritis Rheum 2009;60:831–9.

35. Hunter DJ, Zhang Y, Tu X, et al. Change in joint space width: hyaline articular cartilage loss or

alteration in meniscus? Arthritis Rheum 2006;54: 2488–95.

36. Roemer FW, Guermazi A, Javaid MK, et al. Change in MRI-detected subchondral bone marrow lesions is associated with cartilage loss—the MOST study. A longitudinal multicenter study of knee osteoarthritis. Ann Rheum Dis 2008; [Epub ahead of print].

37. Roemer FW, Guermazi A, Hunter DJ, et al. The association of meniscal damage with joint effusion in persons without radiographic osteoarthritis: the Framingham and MOST osteoarthritis studies. Osteoarthritis Cartilage 2008;[Epub ahead of print].

38. Reichenbach S. Does cartilage volume or thickness distinguish knees with and without mild radiographic osteoarthritis? The Framingham study. Ann Rheum Dis 2009;[Epub ahead of print].

39. Hunter DJ, Gerstenfeld L, Bishop G, et al. Bone marrow lesions from osteoarthritis knees are characterized by sclerotic bone that is less well mineralized. Arthritis Res Ther 2009;11:R11.

40. Englund M, Niu J, Guermazi A, et al. Effect of meniscal damage on the development of frequent knee pain, aching, or stiffness. Arthritis Rheum 2007;56: 4048–54.

41. Hernandez-Molina G, Guermazi A, Niu J, et al. Central bone marrow lesions in symptomatic knee osteoarthritis and their relationship to anterior cruciate ligament tears and cartilage loss. Arthritis Rheum 2008;58:130–6.

42. Guermazi A, Roemer FW, Crema MD, et al. Assessment of synovitis in knee osteoarthritis on contrast-enhanced MRI using a novel comprehensive semiquantitative scoring system. Arthritis Rheum 2008;58(Suppl):S696–7.

43. van Der Heijde D, Boonen A, Boers M, et al. Reading radiographs in chronological order, in pairs or as single films, has important implications for the discriminative power of rheumatoid arthritis clinical trials. Rheumatology (Oxford) 1999;38: 1213–20.

44. Salaffi F, Carotti M. Interobserver variation in quantitative analysis of hand radiographs in rheumatoid arthritis: comparison of 3 different reading procedures. J Rheumatol 1997;24:2055–6.

45. Ross PD, Huang C, Karpf D, et al. Blinded reading of radiographs increases the frequency of errors in vertebral fracture detection. J Bone Miner Res 1996;11:1793–800.

46. Bruynesteyn K, Van Der Heijde D, Boers M, et al. Detecting radiological changes in rheumatoid arthritis that are considered important by clinical experts: influence of reading with or without known sequence. J Rheumatol 2002;29: 2306–12.

47. Felson DT, Nevitt MC. Blinding images to sequence in osteoarthritis: evidence from other diseases. Osteoarthritis Cartilage 2009;17:281–3.

48. Amin S, Guermazi A, Lavalley MP, et al. Complete anterior cruciate ligament tear and the risk for cartilage loss and progression of symptoms in men and women with knee osteoarthritis. Osteoarthritis Cartilage 2008;16:897–902.

49. Reichenbach S, Guermazi A, Niu J, et al. Prevalence of bone attrition on knee radiographs and MRI in a community based cohort. Osteoarthritis Cartilage 2008;16:1005–10.

50. Hunter DJ, Zhang Y, Niu J, et al. Increase in bone marrow lesions associated with cartilage loss: a longitudinal magnetic resonance imaging study of knee osteoarthritis. Arthritis Rheum 2006;54: 1529–35.

51. Fernandez-Madrid F, Karvonen RL, Teitge RA, et al. Synovial thickening detected by MR imaging in osteoarthritis of the knee confirmed by biopsy as synovitis. Magn Reson Imaging 1995;13:177–83.

52. Outerbridge RE. The etiology of chondromalacia patellae. J Bone Joint Surg Br 1961;43-B:752–7.

53. Noyes FR, Stabler CL. A system for grading articular cartilage lesions at arthroscopy. Am J Sports Med 1989;17:505–13.

54. Sonin AH, Pensy RA, Mulligan ME, et al. Grading articular cartilage of the knee using fast spin-echo proton density-weighted MR imaging without fat suppression. AJR Am J Roentgenol 2002;179:1159–66.

55. Disler DG, McCauley TR, Wirth CR, et al. Detection of knee hyaline cartilage defects using fat-suppressed three-dimensional spoiled gradient-echo MR imaging: comparison with standard MR imaging and correlation with arthroscopy. AJR Am J Roentgenol 1995;165:377–82.

56. Duc SR, Koch P, Schmid MR, et al. Diagnosis of articular cartilage abnormalities of the knee: prospective clinical evaluation of a 3D water-excitation true FISP sequence. Radiology 2007;243:475–82.

57. Ding C, Garnero P, Cicuttini F, et al. Knee cartilage defects: association with early radiographic osteoarthritis, decreased cartilage volume, increased joint surface area and type II collagen breakdown. Osteoarthritis Cartilage 2005;13:198–205.

58. Hill CL, Hunter DJ, Niu J, et al. Synovitis detected on magnetic resonance imaging and its relation to pain and cartilage loss in knee osteoarthritis. Ann Rheum Dis 2007;66:1599–603.

59. Roemer FW, Guermazi A, Zhang Y, et al. Evaluation of Hoffa's fat pad findings on non-contrast enhanced MR imaging as a measure of patello-femoral knee synovitis in osteoarthritis. AJR Am J Roentgenol, in press.

60. Saddik D, McNally EG, Richardson M. MRI of Hoffa's fat pad. Skeletal Radiol 2004;33:433–44.

61. Pelletier JP, Raynauld JP, Abram F, et al. A new noninvasive method to assess synovitis severity in relation to symptoms and cartilage volume loss in knee osteoarthritis patients using MRI. Osteoarthritis Cartilage 2008;3(Suppl 16):S8–13.

62. Roemer FW, Hunter DJ, Guermazi A. Semiquantitative assessment of synovitis in osteoarthritis on non contrast-enhanced MRI. Osteoarthritis Cartilage 2008;[Epub ahead of print].

63. Loeuille D, Rat AC, Goebel JC, et al. Magnetic resonance imaging in osteoarthritis: which method best reflects synovial membrane inflammation? Correlations with clinical, macroscopic and microscopic features. Osteoarthritis Cartilage 2009;[Epub ahead of print].

64. Bergin D, Keogh C, O'Connell M, et al. Atraumatic medial collateral ligament oedema in medial compartment knee osteoarthritis. Skeletal Radiol 2002;31:14–8.

65. Davies-Tuck ML, Wluka AE, Wang Y, et al. The natural history of cartilage defects in people with knee osteoarthritis. Osteoarthritis Cartilage 2008;16:337–42.

66. Raynauld JP, Martel-Pelletier J, Berthiaume MJ, et al. Correlation between bone lesion changes and cartilage volume loss in patients with osteoarthritis of the knee as assessed by quantitative magnetic resonance imaging over a 24-month period. Ann Rheum Dis 2008;67:683–8.

67. Peterfy CG, Gold G, Eckstein F, et al. MRI protocols for whole-organ assessment of the knee in osteoarthritis. Osteoarthritis Cartilage 2006;14(Suppl A):A95–111.

68. Roemer FW, Guermazi A, Lynch JA, et al. Short tau inversion recovery and proton density-weighted fat suppressed sequences for the evaluation of osteoarthritis of the knee with a 1.0 T dedicated extremity MRI: development of a time-efficient sequence protocol. Eur Radiol 2005;15:978–87.

69. Peterfy CG, Schneider E, Nevitt M. The Osteoarthritis Initiative: report on the design rationale for the magnetic resonance imaging protocol for the knee. Osteoarthritis Cartilage 2008;16:1433–41.

70. Roemer FW, Kwoh CK, Hannon MJ, et al. Semiquantitative assessment of focal cartilage lesions of the knee: a comparison of fat-suppressed intermediate weighted fast spin echo and double echo steady state sequences at 3.0T MRI. Eur Radiol 2009; 19(Suppl):S246–7.

71. Available at: http://www.oai.ucsf.edu/datarelease/OperationsManuals.asp. Accessed February 11, 2009.

72. Kalichman L, Li L, Kim DH, et al. Facet joint osteoarthritis and low back pain in the community-based population. Spine 2008;33:2560–5.

73. Kress I, Mamisch TC, Werlen S, et al. MRI-based morphologic grading system for early hip osteoarthritis. Osteoarthritis Cartilage 2008;16(Suppl 4): S173.

Quantitative MR Imaging of Cartilage and Trabecular Bone in Osteoarthritis

Felix Eckstein, MD[a,b],*, Ali Guermazi, MD[c,d],
Frank W. Roemer, MD[c,e]

KEYWORDS

- Osteoarthritis • MR imaging • Cartilage • Trabecular bone
- Knee • Progression • Risk factors • Subregional

Quantitative measurement of cartilage morphology exploits the three-dimensional (3D) nature of MR imaging data sets to assess tissue dimensions (eg, volume, thickness) or signal as continuous variables (Fig. 1). The strengths of quantitative measurements of cartilage or other articular tissues in osteoarthritis (OA) are that they are less observer dependent and more objective than scoring methods and that relatively small changes in cartilage thickness and cartilage volume (VC) over time (that occur relatively homogeneously over larger areas) may be detected, which are not apparent to the naked eye. A recent study, for instance, found that quantitative measures of cartilage morphometry[1] were more powerful in revealing significant relations between local risk factors (meniscal damage and malalignment) and knee cartilage loss than a semi-quantitative (SQ) approach using ordinal data (whole-organ magnetic resonance imaging score [WORMS]).[2] The disadvantage of quantitative measurement, however, is that it requires specialized software and is time-intensive, because tissue boundaries need to be tracked through series of slices (segmentation) using trained technical personnel. Moreover, quantitative measurement is less sensitive to small focal changes within larger structures (eg, focal cartilage lesions), which may be more readily picked up by an expert reader, particularly if the location within the larger structure is variable from person to person. A recent study showed, for instance, that MR imaging-based SQ assessment of cartilage status differed substantially (and significantly) between participants with and without radiographic OA in a large community-based cohort, whereas quantitative measures of cartilage morphology displayed no or little difference between these groups.[3] Whether SQ or quantitative cartilage assessment is better suited as an outcome measure for

Felix Eckstein is co-owner and Chief Executive Officer of Chondrometrics GmbH, a company that provides image analysis service for academic researchers and the pharmaceutics industry. Felix Eckstein provides consulting services to Pfizer, Inc.; Merck Serono, Inc.; Wyeth, Inc.; and Novo Nordisk Inc. Ali Guermazi is co-owner and President of Boston Imaging Core Laboratory, LLC. He is a shareholder at Synarc, Inc. Frank Roemer is co-owner of Boston Imaging Core Laboratory, LLC.
[a] Institute of Anatomy and Musculoskeletal Research, Paracelsus Medical University, Strubergasse 21, A5020 Salzburg, Austria
[b] Chondrometrics GmbH, Ainring, Germany
[c] Department of Radiology, Quantitative Imaging Center, Boston University School of Medicine, Boston, MA, USA
[d] Boston Imaging Core Laboratory, LLC, Boston, MA, USA
[e] Department of Radiology, Klinikum Augsburg, Augsburg, Germany
* Corresponding author. Institute of Anatomy and Musculoskeletal Research, Paracelsus Medical University, Strubergasse 21, A5020 Salzburg, Austria.
E-mail address: felix.eckstein@pmu.ac.at (F. Eckstein).

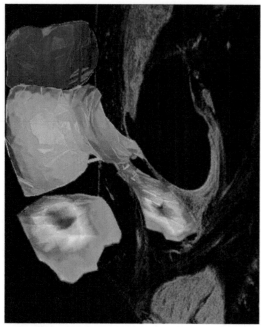

Fig. 1. 3D reconstruction and visualization of quantitative cartilage measurements in the human knee obtained from a sagittal MR imaging data set; oblique view from anterior and medial. The segmented patellar cartilage is shown in magenta, and the segmented trochlea femoris is shown in turquoise. The cartilage thickness in the medial and lateral tibia is displayed in colors, with red areas corresponding to areas with the greatest cartilage thickness and dark blue areas corresponding to areas with the lowest cartilage thickness.

a particular study therefore needs to be carefully considered in the context of the particular question of interest. Generally speaking, when minute changes occur homogeneously throughout larger areas or at highly predictable locations within larger areas, quantitative measures seem to be more powerful than SQ scoring, whereas SQ scoring of cartilage may be more powerful when local changes (in tissue dimensions or signal intensity) occur at unpredictable locations within the structure of interest and involve only small parts of this structure. Ideally, therefore, both approaches should be used in a complimentary rather than competing fashion in studies assessing the status and the progression of OA.

The progression of structural changes in OA has generally been shown to be slow, whether applying radiography[4,5] (see the article by Hellio Le Graverand and colleagues in this issue) or MR imaging.[6] The tissue that has been the primary target for quantitative measurement in OA using MR imaging is the articular cartilage because it provides the weight-bearing surface of the joint and its loss is commonly (albeit not strongly) associated with functional impairment and symptoms. This article focuses on quantitative studies on cartilage morphology in OA and also includes a short review of quantitative measurements of trabecular bone architecture. Also in this issue, SQ assessment of cartilage and other tissues is reviewed by Roemer and colleagues, quantitative measurements of cartilage composition are reviewed by Burstein and colleagues, and quantitative measurements of the meniscus are reviewed by Englund and colleagues. The current article focuses exclusively on knee OA in humans, because this is where most of the work has been performed to date.

MEASUREMENT PROCESS AND OUTCOME MEASURES OF CARTILAGE MORPHOLOGY IN OSTEOARTHRITIS

To obtain a quantitative measurement of the cartilage, all or some cartilage plates of a joint are segmented by a trained user, with or without assistance from segmentation software,[7–15] with the choice of several input devices, such as a regular computer mouse, graphics table, or touch-sensitive screens.[16] These can be used to trace the bone-cartilage interface and the surface of the cartilage, respectively. Because there are various sources of artifacts on MR imaging, and because signal intensity and contrast may vary substantially between baseline and follow-up acquisitions, there is consensus that expert quality control is key to the analysis, with the time required for segmentation or the correction of computer-generated segmentation taking several hours per joint. When all slices of interest have been segmented, image analysis software can be used to compute a variety of morphologic parameters of total cartilage plates, such as the size of the total area of subchondral bone (tAB), the area of the cartilage surface (AC), the denuded (dAB) and cartilage covered (cAB) subchondral bone area, the cartilage thickness over the tAB (ThCtAB) or cAB (ThCcAB) (see **Fig. 1**), the VC, the cartilage volume normalized to the tAB (VCtAB), cartilage signal intensity,[17–19] and others. A system of consensus-based nomenclature and definition for these outcome measures, for features of cartilage composition, and for regions of interest in the knee (**Fig. 2**) was proposed by a group of experts[20] and is used throughout this review.

Most investigations dealing quantitatively with cartilage morphology in OA have focused on VC, but this outcome measure has several limitations. The ability to discriminate between subjects who have OA and healthy subjects is limited, because people with larger bones display larger VC,[21,22]

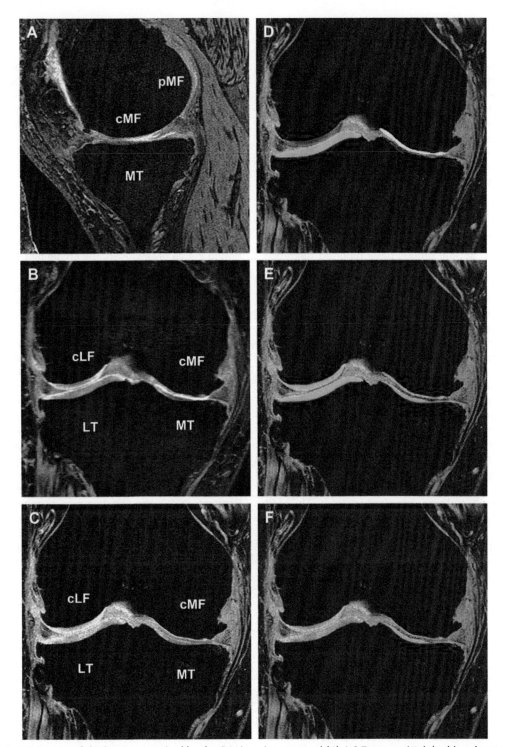

Fig. 2. MR images of the knee as acquired by the OAI imaging protocol (*A*) A 0.7-mm sagittal double-echo steady-state (DESS) sequence with water excitation. cMF, central (weight-bearing) femoral cartilage; MT, medial tibia; pMF, posterior femoral cartilage. (*B*) A 1.5-mm double-oblique coronal multiplanar reconstruction (MPR) of the sagittal DESS sequence. cLF, central weight-bearing lateral femoral cartilage; LT, lateral tibia. (*C*) A 1.5-mm double-oblique, coronal, fast low-angle shot (FLASH) sequence with water excitation. (*D*) Same image as in *C* with the MT (*blue*), cMF (*yellow*), LT (*green*), and cLF (*red*) segmented. (*E*) Same image as in *C* with the areas of the cartilage surface (AC, magenta) and the total area of the subchondral bone (tAB, *green*) segmented in MT, cMF, LT, and cLT. (*F*) Same image as in *C* with only the area of the cartilage surface (AC) and tAB of the MT segmented. Please note that there is a denuded area of subchondral bone (dAB) wherein the AC does not cover the tAB. (*From* NIAMS/NIH OAI Study. Available at: http://www.niams.nih.gov/Funding/Funded_Research/Osteoarthritis_Initiative/default.asp.)

thus creating wide overlap between the groups. Men have larger joint surfaces than women (and hence larger VCs), even after adjustment for body height and weight,[23] and VC is thus difficult to compare between genders. In longitudinal studies, the subchondral bone area has been shown to increase with aging in healthy reference subjects and in patients who have OA.[24–26] Such effects may mask a reduction in cartilage thickness in OA because of the expansion of the bone and cartilage layer. Therefore, alternative outcomes have been suggested, such as VCtAB or ThCtAB.[21,27] In the context of cross-sectional studies, several groups have reported reference values of cartilage morphology in healthy volunteers[21,28–30] or templates or atlases for comparison of cartilage thickness distribution patterns between healthy reference subjects and patients who have OA.[27,31]

Some studies showed that the sensitivity to change (standardized response mean [SRM] = mean change/SD of change) for ThCtAB or VCtAB was higher than for VC,[32,33] whereas others found comparable SRMs for VC, VCtAB, or ThCtAB.[34,35] A recent article[33] reported that when cartilage loss is relatively rapid, attributable to high mechanical challenge, "horizontal" cartilage loss (increase in dAB) made a stronger contribution to the total cartilage loss (reduction in ThCtAB), whereas when cartilage loss was relatively slow, the "vertical" cartilage loss (reduction in ThCcAB) made a stronger contribution. This finding needs to be confirmed, however, in other cohorts and pathophysiologic conditions.

Quantitative measures of surface curvature and joint incongruity have been determined[36] and were reported to discriminate among subjects with various radiographic OA grades cross sectionally at 0.2 T.[37,38] Curvature estimates at different scales (at 0.2 T) were also reported to predict cartilage loss longitudinally.[39] Also, at 0.2 T, cartilage homogeneity (quantified by measuring entropy from the distribution of signal intensities in tibial cartilage) was reported to discriminate between subjects without and with early radiographic OA[19] and was proposed to be particularly sensitive in peripheral regions, wherein the cartilage is covered by the meniscus.[40] These results are surprising, because other MR imaging techniques that have been validated for targeting relatively specific macromolecules of the cartilage, such as collagen, proteoglycans, or water (eg, T2 mapping, T1rho, delayed gadolinium enhanced MRI [dGEMRIC]) have not commonly been successful in discriminating between healthy volunteers and subjects who have early OA (see the review by Burstein and colleagues in this issue).

Recently, several researchers have proposed the measurement of certain anatomically defined subregions (Fig. 3) within cartilage plates to determine the spatial pattern of cartilage loss.[41–43] Results of these studies are discussed later in this article.

IMAGING PROTOCOLS FOR MEASUREMENT OF CARTILAGE MORPHOLOGY AND VALIDATION

Quantitative work performed on cartilage with MR imaging between 1994 and 2006 has been thoroughly summarized previously[44–51] and is not reiterated in this review. Also, the article by Link and colleagues elsewhere in this issue covers hardware and imaging sequences for OA imaging in detail. Briefly, for quantifying cartilage morphology, water-excitation (or fat-suppressed) T1-weighted spoiled gradient recalled echo acquisition in the steady state (SPGR) or fast low-angle shot (FLASH) sequences at 1.5 or 3 T represent the current "gold standard."[46,49,52] Double-echo steady-state (DESS) imaging with water excitation has recently gained interest because of the faster acquisition time and lower slice thickness that can be achieved (see Fig. 2).[53–56] SPGR/FLASH sequences are readily available on virtually all MR imaging scanners and do not require specific hardware or software, whereas DESS imaging is currently only available from one vendor.[54] Because DESS imaging acquires two separate images with different echo times simultaneously, this provides an opportunity to estimate T2 and to obtain morphologic and compositional information about the cartilage from a single high-resolution data set.[57] This approach, however, is still undergoing validation.

The Osteoarthritis Initiative (OAI)[58] is a large research endeavor jointly sponsored by the National Institutes of Health (NIH), the National Institute of Arthritis and Musculoskeletal and Skin Diseases (NIAMS), and the pharmaceutics industry. In a cohort of almost 5000 participants, this study is currently focusing on identifying imaging (and other) biomarkers for predicting and monitoring the onset and progression of symptomatic knee OA applying 3 T MR imaging over a 4-year period. The OAI relies on a nearly isotropic sagittal DESS sequence with water excitation in both knees for quantifying cartilage morphology and on a coronal FLASH sequence with water excitation in one knee of all participants (see Fig. 2).[59] Sagittal images have the advantage that all cartilage plates of the knee (including the femoropatellar and femorotibial compartments) are visualized but have the disadvantage of partial volume effects in the internal and external

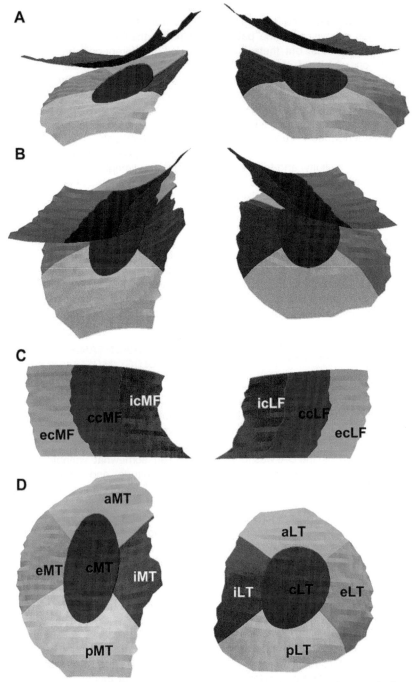

Fig. 3. Figure displays commonly used anatomic subregions in the weight-bearing femorotibial joint, as outlined in Tables 1 and 2. (*A*) Posterior view onto the weight-bearing femorotibial joint shows the medial and lateral tibia (*bottom*) and the medial and lateral weight-bearing part of the femoral condyle (*top*). (*B*) Superior view onto the weight-bearing femorotibial joint shows the medial and lateral tibia (*background*) and the medial and lateral weight-bearing part of the femoral condyle (*foreground*). (*C*) Inferior view onto the central medial (cMF) and lateral (cLF) (weight-bearing) part of the femoral condyle. c, central subregions (*red*); e, external subregions (*green*); i, internal subregions (*blue*). (*D*) Superior view onto the medial (MT) and lateral (LT) tibia. a, anterior subregion (turquoise); c, central subregions (*red*); e, external subregions (*green*); i, internal subregions (*blue*); p, posterior subregion (*yellow*).

subregions of the knee cartilage plates. Coronal images, in contrast, can delineate the femorotibial joint, and axial images can visualize the patella with few partial volume effects, but there is no current consensus on which of these is the preferred orientation. Because of the isotropic character of sagittal DESS imaging, multiplanar reconstruction (MPR) in the coronal and axial planes is feasible, and segmentation of the articular cartilage can be performed in reconstructed images.[54–56]

The technical accuracy (validity) and test-retest precision (reproducibility) of quantitative cartilage measurements at 1.5 T have been summarized in previous reviews.[46,47] Analyses based on images acquired with a dedicated 1.0-T extremity scanner were found to be consistent with 1.5-T imaging, albeit less precise (reproducible).[60] Use of peripheral MR imaging scanners at lower fields potentially permits more widespread distribution of this technology, especially when access to high-field MR imaging is limited. Also, quantitative cartilage measurement at 0.2 T has been proposed[14,15,19,37–39] but has not been validated versus external standards or measurement at higher field strength.

Cartilage imaging at 3 T has been cross-calibrated with that at 1.5 T, and lower precision errors than for 1.5-T imaging were reported when acquiring thinner (coronal) slices of 1.0 mm on a 3 T system.[61] Morphometric analysis from DESS images acquired at 3 T in the OAI was found to be consistent with that from FLASH images and to display similar test-retest precision errors as FLASH images in the femorotibial joint, using unpaired[54] and paired reading approaches.[55,56] In terms of sensitivity to change, a small comparative analysis in the OAI pilot study[56] and a comparison of two studies performed on the first release of baseline and year 1 follow-up data in the OAI progression subcohort by two groups (one analyzing signal knees using sagittal DESS imaging[34] and one analyzing right knees using coronal FLASH imaging[32]) found similar rates of change, sensitivity to change, and patterns of cartilage loss in the femorotibial joint.

Generally, results from different vendors for cartilage morphometry were shown to be comparable at 1.5 T[62] and at 3 T,[63] although one study reported slight offsets between different scanners and protocols from the same vendor.[64] At 3 T, precision errors of cartilage morphometry were observed to be similar for different vendors and scanners in a multicenter trial, and measurements were relatively stable over a 3-month observation period.[25] The stability of geometric measurements over longer periods on phantoms was found to be satisfactory and comparable among several scanners from the same manufacturer over a 3-year period in the OAI.[65]

Use of different coils has been evaluated at 3 T. Although the test-retest precision was similar between a phased array and quadrature coil, certain offsets in cartilage morphology outcomes were observed between these,[55] prohibiting changes of the coil between baseline and follow-up measurements. Cartilage morphometry on images acquired 2 hours after intravenous gadopentetate dimeglumine (Gd-DTPA) injection (for the purpose of simultaneous dGEMRIC imaging; see the review by Burstein and colleagues in this issue) was reported to be highly correlated (r = 0.85–0.95) with that on images obtained before the injection of the contrast agent at baseline.[66] A recent 2-year longitudinal analysis in participants who had OA found the sensitivity to change of post–Gd-DTPA cartilage imaging to be substantially less than acquisition acquired before intravenous Gd-DTPA injection, however.[67]

LONGITUDINAL MEASUREMENT OF CARTILAGE MORPHOLOGY IN OSTEOARTHRITIS
Rate of Change and Sensitivity to Change in Osteoarthritis

Several reports on longitudinal changes of cartilage morphology in subjects with OA have been published.[32–34,42,46,47,68–77] These studies have revealed somewhat variable results in terms of the magnitude and SRM of annual cartilage loss[46,47,78]: Two studies reported almost no loss in VC over 1-year[75] and 3-year[68] periods, whereas other studies reported up to a 7% annual loss in the femorotibial joint.[70] Reasons for this may include variability in imaging and image analysis technology, differences in risk factor profiles among cohorts, differences in study duration, experience and blinding of the readers, and others. Recent analyses of a first release of 160 participants of the OAI progression cohort (baseline and year 1 follow-up data) displayed substantially higher rates of progression in the weight-bearing medial femur than in the medial tibia,[32,34,77] but this was not a consistent finding across cohorts, particularly not when focusing on the SRM (Table 1). Several studies have thus taken the approach of additionally reporting the aggregate thickness in the tibia and weight-bearing femur.[32,33,55,76,79] One study suggested that longitudinal changes in VC in the tibia and in the weight-bearing femur are highly correlated[70] and that measurement of only tibial cartilage is therefore sufficient. Given the fact that at least some cohorts display larger changes and higher

SRMs in the weight-bearing femur than in the tibia, however,[32,34,77] this approach has limitations.

Lateral and medial femorotibial cartilage loss and patellar cartilage loss were found not to be significantly associated with each other.[80] The ratio of medial versus lateral cartilage loss was reported to be 1.4:1 in knees with neutral biomechanical alignment, consistent with higher medial loads in neutral knees.[33] In varus knees, the ratio was 3.7:1, and in valgus knees, it was 1:6.0, confirming that knee alignment is an important determinant of medial versus lateral cartilage loss.[33]

After anterior cruciate ligament rupture,[81] a reduction of VC and cartilage thickness was observed in the femoral trochlea, whereas an increase was found in the weight-bearing medial femur. The latter observation may be consistent with cartilage swelling or hypertrophy observed as a sign of early OA in various animal models.[82–86]

MR Imaging-based Cartilage Morphology Versus Radiography in Osteoarthritis

Several studies found only weak correlations between MR imaging-detected cartilage loss and OA progression in radiography,[71,75,87] but a recent publication reported a higher correlation when the longitudinal reduction in joint space width (JSW) in radiographs was compared with cartilage loss in the central aspect of the femorotibial joint.[42] Whereas some studies found a higher rate and sensitivity to change of cartilage morphology compared with radiography,[71,73,88] a recent 2-year study reported a somewhat higher SRM (−0.62) for Lyon Schuss radiography versus cartilage thickness of the medial tibia as measured with MR imaging (−0.59)[76] but a lower SRM for fixed flexion radiography (SRM = −0.20), as used in the OAI,[89–93] in the same study.[76] It was discussed that the relatively high SRM of the minimal JSW measured with Lyon Schuss radiography may be attributable to fluoroscopic guidance providing optimal alignment of the anterior and posterior tibial rim and to radiography being performed under weight-bearing conditions, whereas MR imaging is performed in a supine non–weight-bearing position. On weight bearing, slightly swollen cartilage may be compressed mechanically. Also, it must be kept in mind that radiographic assessment of JSW also depends on meniscal extrusion and not only on cartilage thickness.[94–96]

Spatial Patterns of Cartilage Loss as Derived from Subregional Cartilage Analysis

Pelletier and colleagues[42] recently reported that the rate of change in cartilage morphology in the central aspects of the femorotibial joint exceeded that in total cartilage plates but found that the SRM was not improved because of the higher variability (SD) of the regional changes.[35] Wirth and colleagues[77] found the sensitivity to change (SRM) in the central tibia to be slightly higher than for the total medial tibial cartilage, but this was not the case in the weigh-bearing medial femur. Minimal thickness in a central subregion displayed the greatest rate of change, but lower SRMs than mean regional thickness, because of the high SD.[77]

Table 1 summarizes the rate of change of cartilage thickness in subregions (shown in Fig. 3) of the femorotibial joint. Results are displayed as percentage per annum, independent of the study duration, for the following:

1. A 2-year multicenter study at 3 T (Pfizer A 9001140), with results being shown for the 24-month time point. This study involved 99 healthy participants (data not shown), 30 with Kellgren Lawrence grade (KLG) 2 and 28 with KLG 3.[76] Because the participants with KLG 2 did not show significant changes in cartilage morphology over the study period, results are shown for KLG 3 participants only.

2. A first release of baseline and year 1 follow-up data from the OAI progression subcohort.[77] Only right knees were analyzed, because the coronal FLASH sequence was only available for the right knee, and not all knees analyzed had radiographic or symptomatic OA. For this reason, the results are also given for a subcohort with a high risk for progression, including only subjects with obesity (body mass index [BMI] >30) and definite radiographic OA (KLG ≥2).

3. The Mechanical Factors in Arthritis of the Knee Study (MAK) study, an epidemiologic study investigating the effect of local factors (eg, alignment, joint laxity, meniscal status) on OA progression.[1,33] Data are given for a subcohort of 74 participants with neutral knee alignment (mechanical knee axis from −2° to +2°) and for subjects with malalignment. The subregional progression in the medial compartment is given for 57 participants with varus malalignment (because little to no progression was observed in the lateral compartment), and progression in the lateral compartment is given for 43 participants with valgus malalignment (because little change was observed in the medial compartment).

To synthesize findings regarding the pattern of cartilage loss, the eight medial and eight lateral femorotibial subregions (see Fig. 3) were ranked, with the subregion encountering the greatest

Table 1
Mean changes of cartilage thickness in percent per annum: summary of longitudinal studies involving subregional analysis of the weight-bearing femorotibial joint

	A 9001140 KLG 3 (n = 28)		OAI (n = 156)		OAI High Risk (n = 54)		MAK Neutral (n = 74)		MAK Varus/Valgus (n = 57/43)				Versus Plate[c]
	MC (%)	Rank[b]	MC (%)	Rank[b]	MC (%)	Rank[b]	MC (%)	Rank[b]	MC (%)	Rank[b]	Sum	Rank[b]	
MFTC	−1.6	—	−1.2	—	−2.5	—	−1.4	—	−2.6	—	—	—	—
cMFTC	−2.2	—	−1.7	—	−3.5	—	—	—	—	—	—	—	+++
MT	−1.4	—	−0.5	—	−1.0	—	−1.1	—	−2.6	—	—	—	—
cMT[a]	−2.0	4	−0.9	4	−1.6	4	−1.5	3	−3.1	3	18	4	+++++
eMT[a]	−3.4	1	−0.8	5	−1.4	5	−1.7	2	−5.1	2	14	2	+++++
iMT[a]	−0.6	6	−0.6	6	−0.9	6	−0.1	8	−1.5	8	34	7	−+−−−
aMT[a]	−1.2	5	−0.2	7	−0.2	8	−1.4	5	−2.5	5	30	6	−−−+−
pMT[a]	0.0	8	−0.2	7	−0.7	7	−0.7	7	−1.8	7	36	8	−−−−−
cMF	−1.9	—	−1.9	—	−4.1	—	−1.7	—	−2.6	—	—	—	—
ccMF[a]	−2.4	3	−2.8	1	−5.8	1	−2.2	1	−3.3	1	8	1	+++++
ecMF[a]	−3.0	2	−1.6	2	−3.8	2	−1.2	6	−2.9	4	16	3	+−−−+
icMF[a]	−0.5	7	−1.4	3	−2.8	3	−1.5	3	−1.9	6	22	5	−−−−−
LFTC	0.1	—	−0.3	—	−0.5	—	−1.0	—	−2.4	—	—	—	—
cLFTC	−0.3	—	−0.5	—	−0.8	—	—	—	—	—	—	—	+++
LT	−0.5	—	−0.7	—	−1.1	—	−0.9	—	−3.0	—	—	—	—
cLT[a]	−0.8	2	−0.9	1	−1.6	2	−1.1	3	−4.7	1	9	1	+++++
eLT[a]	−0.4	3	−0.9	1	−1.0	4	0.0	4	−2.4	4	20	4	−+−−+

iLT[a]	−0.3	4	−0.8	4	−1.2	3	−1.8	1	−4.2	2	14	2	−++++
aLT[a]	0.2	6	0.2	7	0.3	7	−1.1	3	−1.2	8	31	7	−−+−
pLT[a]	−1.0	1	−0.9	1	−1.9	1	−0.3	7	−2.0	5	15	3	+++−−
cLF	0.8	—	0.1	—	0.1	—	−1.0	—	−1.9	—	—	—	—
ccLF[a]	0.4	7	0.1	6	0.3	7	−0.9	6	−1.7	6	32	8	na
ecLF[a]	1.9	8	0.0	5	0.1	6	−1.2	2	−2.9	3	24	5	na
icLF[a]	0.1	5	0.3	8	0.0	5	−1.0	5	−1.3	7	30	6	na

A9001140, Osteoarthritis Initiative (OAI), and MAK: longitudinal studies involving quantitative measurement of cartilage morphology in patients who have OA.

Abbreviations: cLF, central weight-bearing lateral femoral condyle; cLFTC, central lateral femorotibial compartment (cLT + ccLF); cMF, central weight-bearing medial femoral condyle; cMFTC, central medial femorotibial compartment (cMT + ccMF); KLG, Kellgren Lawrence grade; LFTC, lateral femorotibial compartment; LT, lateral tibia; MMC, mean change; MC%, mean change of cartilage thickness in percent per year; MFTC, medial femorotibial compartment; MT, medial tibia; n, number of participants in (sub)study; na, not applicable; sum, sum of the ranks in the studies of the five subregions listed below; ThCtAB, cartilage thickness over total area of subchondral bone.

[a] Subregions in MT, cMF, LT, and cLF are as follows: c, central; e, external; i, internal; a, anterior; p, posterior.

[b] Rank (1–8): subregions in the medial and lateral femorotibial compartment are ranked according to the rate of cartilage loss (rank 1 = subregion with the greatest cartilage loss; rank 8 = subregion with the least cartilage loss or with the greatest cartilage increase).

[c] Versus plate, information on whether a subregion displayed a higher rate of change than the total plate (+), the same rate (=), or a lower rate (−) in the five (sub)studies listed previously.

cartilage loss being assigned to rank 1 and the subregion with the smallest loss (or greatest increase in cartilage thickness) assigned to rank 8, respectively. In Table 1, the ranks were then added to determine which subregion(s) displayed the greatest change across these studies. Additionally, it was determined how often across the five populations the subregional change exceeded that in the total cartilage plate.

- Rate of change, medial femorotibial compartment (see Table 1): The central part of the weight-bearing femoral condyle (ccMF sum = 8), the external aspect of the medial tibia (eMT, sum = 14), the external aspect of the femoral condyle (ecMF, sum = 16), and the central tibia (cMT, sum = 18) displayed the relatively greatest change across subregions. The ccMF, eMT, and cMT also consistently displayed greater changes than the total cartilage plate across the studies (see Table 1, last column).
- Rate of change, lateral femorotibial compartment (see Table 1): The central lateral tibia (cLT, sum = 9), the internal lateral tibia (iLT, sum = 14), and the posterior lateral tibia (pLT, sum = 15) displayed the relatively greatest changes, and only small changes were observed in the lateral femoral condyle across the studies. Rates of change in the cLT and iLT were consistently greater than for the total cartilage plates.
- Sensitivity to change, medial and lateral femorotibial compartment (Table 2): Ranks for the SRM were similar to those for the rates of change but not identical (compare with Table 1). In line with other observations,[35] the sensitivity to change in the subregions was not consistently higher than in the total plates across studies. Only analysis of the central compartment (cMFTC = cMT + ccMF, and cLFTC = cLT + ccLF) revealed consistently greater SRMs than analysis of the entire medial (MFTC = MT + cMF) or lateral femorotibial (LFTC = LT + cLF) compartment.

Correlation of Cartilage Loss With Long-term Structural Change, Clinical Outcome, and Treatment Response in Osteoarthritis

Estimates of tibial cartilage loss over 2 years were found to be correlated with those over 4.5 years. This suggests that changes in VC measured over 2 years predict long-term cartilage loss.[74] More importantly, the rate of change in VC over 2 years was found to be significantly associated with total

knee arthroplasty (TKA) at year 4.[97] For every 1% increase in the rate of cartilage loss, there was a 20% increased risk for undergoing TKA. Participants in the highest tertile of tibial cartilage loss had 7.1 higher odds of TKA than those in the lowest tertile. In contrast, radiographic scores of OA did not predict TKA in this study. This is an important finding because it links cartilage morphology, as a potential surrogate measure of disease progression, to a clinical outcome, that is, how a patient feels or functions or how long the knee "survives" (TKA). Raynauld and colleagues[88] recently reported that licofelone significantly reduced cartilage loss over time and that MR imaging was superior to radiographs in demonstrating a structure-modifying effect in this multicenter trial. No structure-modifying osteoarthritis drug (SMOAD) or disease-modifying osteoarthritis drug (DMOAD) has yet been approved by regulatory agencies, however.

RISK FACTORS FOR CARTILAGE LOSS AS IDENTIFIED BY QUANTITATIVE CARTILAGE MORPHOMETRY

Great interest is directed at identifying risk factors (predictors) for subsequent cartilage loss so as to understand the pathophysiology of the disease and to be able to identify so-called "fast progressors" for inclusion in pharmacologic intervention studies that attempt to show protection from structural change over relatively short periods. This section focuses exclusively on studies that have reported correlations between risk factors for progression and quantitative measures of cartilage morphology but not on those that have relied on SQ or quantitative assessment of JSW or increases in SQ MR imaging scores. The list of (potential) risk factors for cartilage loss is not comprehensive but encompasses important examples derived from cross-sectional and longitudinal studies. Risk factors associated with higher rates of progression were as follows:

- High BMI[32,42,71,73,77,80,98]: This relation was also suggested to exist in the patella in subjects without OA.[99]
- Meniscal extrusion and tears or damage[42,72,73]: Sharma and colleagues[1] found a significant relation of cartilage loss with meniscal tears but not with meniscal extrusion. Raynauld and colleagues[100] recently reported that selecting a subcohort of participants with meniscal tears or extrusion did not improve the ability to identify treatment effects of a potentially SMOAD because of the larger SD of the change in

the participants who had meniscal pathologic findings. Meniscal tears were frequently observed in asymptomatic subjects[101,102] and were found to be associated with greater tibial plateau bone area but not with reduced tibial VC in a 2-year longitudinal study.[102]

- Knee malalignment[1,22,33,103]: Teichtahl and colleagues[104] showed increasing varus malalignment between baseline and follow-up to be associated with an increase in the rate of medial tibial cartilage loss, whereas it did not significantly affect the rate of loss of the lateral tibia. The investigators concluded that these findings suggest that methods to reduce progression of varus alignment may also delay the progression of medial tibiofemoral OA. Frontal plane knee valgus malalignment also seemed to be correlated with patellar cartilage loss.[105] In a largely nonarthritic cohort, in contrast, no correlation between cartilage loss and malalignment was identified.[106]
- Advanced radiographic OA, as evidenced by higher KLGs,[107] decreased JSW, or increased joint space narrowing[32,42,76,77]: In contrast, one study found increased cartilage loss with higher baseline VC,[69] stating that cartilage loss was greater in the early phase of OA.
- Bone marrow alterations[42,73]: Raynauld and colleagues[100] reported that although bone marrow lesions and cysts did not increase significantly in size over 24 months in an OA cohort, there was a significant correlation between size change of bone marrow lesions and cysts with the loss of VC in the medial femorotibial compartment. A relation between extremely large bone marrow lesions and lateral tibial cartilage loss was also reported in asymptomatic persons.[108,109]
- Focal cartilage lesions or defects, as graded by visual scoring[110,111]: Cartilage defects at baseline seemed to be associated with longitudinal measurement of quantitative cartilage loss in the same compartment in OA subjects, although one study[111] only found a significant relation in the femoropatellar but not in the femorotibial joint. Other studies reported that the presence of cartilage defects also predicted knee cartilage loss in asymptomatic individuals without radiographic knee OA.[112,113]
- Smoking.[113,114]
- Medial-lateral joint laxity, measured with a device applying a fixed varus and valgus

load, was found to have inconsistent effects and was not a significant predictor of cartilage loss in models fully adjusted for alignment and meniscal damage.[1]
- Other factors, such as age, gender, pain, function, physical activity levels, synovitis (effusion), sex hormone levels, and serum or urine biomarkers, were not consistently found to be associated with cartilage loss as measured quantitatively with MR imaging, and studies have produced partially contradictory results.

It was recently hypothesized that tibial subchondral bone area expansion may lead to the development of knee cartilage defects, which, in turn, are associated with future cartilage loss, and is predictive of the need for knee joint replacement in subjects who have knee OA, independent of radiographic change.[115] Hunter and colleagues[116] studied whether thin cartilage (in the contralateral knee) was a predisposing factor for radiographic OA. They observed no difference in the mean cartilage thickness between premorbid knees (no radiographic change but radiographic OA in the contralateral knee) versus knees of a non-OA subsample, but they did find higher numbers of denuded areas, suggesting that the initial pathologic change in OA may be focal cartilage loss and adjacent swelling. This is consistent with observations by Reichenbach and colleagues[3] that focal cartilage lesions (WORMS scores) discriminate better between normal subjects and those who have early radiographic OA than quantitative measures of total plate or subregional cartilage thickness.

QUANTITATIVE TRABECULAR BONE CHANGES IN OSTEOARTHRITIS

Beuf and colleagues[117] were the first to use in vivo MR imaging to investigate the role of trabecular bone quantitatively, using an axial 3D high spatial resolution fast gradient-echo sequence at 1.5 T. In a cross-sectional study, they studied the trabecular bone structure of the distal femur and proximal tibia in normal volunteers and patients who had varying degrees of knee OA and showed that differences in quantitative measures of trabecular bone structure between the tibia and the femur decreased with increasing degree of OA. Apparent bone volume fraction (BV/TV), trabecular number (Tb.N), and trabecular spacing (Tb.Sp) in the femoral condyles seemed to differentiate healthy individuals or patients who had mild OA from patients who had severe OA ($P<.05$). Apparent BV/TV was lower in patients

Table 2

Standardized response mean (mean/SD of change) of cartilage thickness in percent per annum: summary of longitudinal studies involving subregional analysis of the weight-bearing femorotibial joint

	A 9001140 KLG3 (n = 28)		OAI (n = 156)		OAI High Risk (n = 54)		MAK Neutral (n = 74)		MAK Varus/Valgus (n = 57/43)				
	MC (%)	Rank[b]	MC (%)	Rank[b]	MC (%)	Rank[b]	MC (%)	Rank[b]	MC (%)	Rank[b]	Sum	Rank[b]	Versus Plate[c]
MFTC	−0.44	—	−0.31	—	−0.47	—	−0.50	—	−0.62	—	—	—	
cMFTC	−0.48	—	−0.33	—	−0.48	—	—	—	—	—	—	—	+++
MT	−0.59	—	−0.16	—	−0.24	—	−0.50	—	—	—	—	—	–
cMT[a]	−0.53	2	−0.20	4	−0.29	4	−0.49	1	−0.50	1	13	1	–++–
eMT[a]	−0.57	1	−0.13	6	−0.17	7	−0.41	3	−0.43	3	20	4	–––
iMT[a]	−0.29	6	−0.18	5	−0.23	5	−0.06	8	−0.31	8	32	7	–+––
aMT[a]	−0.32	5	−0.05	8	−0.03	8	−0.41	3	−0.37	4	28	6	–––––
pMT[a]	−0.02	8	−0.06	7	−0.18	6	−0.15	7	−0.34	6	34	8	–––––
cMF	−0.34	—	−0.30	—	−0.49	—	−0.37	—	−0.49	—	—	—	
ccMF[a]	−0.35	3	−0.31	3	−0.47	1	−0.34	5	−0.37	4	14	2	++––
ecMF[a]	−0.34	4	−0.22	4	−0.43	2	−0.21	6	−0.32	7	22	5	––––
icMF[a]	−0.18	7	−0.25	7	−0.42	3	−0.42	2	−0.55	1	15	3	–––++
LFTC	0.06	—	−0.11	—	−0.17	—	−0.42	—	−0.61	—	—	—	
cLFTC	−0.15	—	−0.14	—	−0.20	—	—	—	—	—	—	—	+++
LT	−0.35	—	−0.23	—	−0.39	—	−0.32	—	−0.71	—	—	—	–

										n	Rankb	Versus platec
cLTa	−0.29	2	−0.21	1	−0.38	1	−0.25	6	−0.81	11	1	− − − − +
eLTa	−0.19	3	−0.21	1	−0.23	4	−0.01	8	−0.28	23	4	− − − − −
iLTa	−0.16	4	−0.20	3	−0.25	3	−0.55	1	−0.76	13	2	− − − − −
aLTa	0.08	6	0.04	7	0.06	8	−0.36	2	−0.19	31	8	− − − + −
pLTa	−0.31	1	−0.16	4	−0.34	2	−0.05	7	−0.42	18	3	− − − − −
cLF	0.32	—	0.02	—	0.03	—	−0.36	—	−0.42	—	—	
ccLFa	0.16	7	0.01	6	0.05	7	−0.27	3	−0.31	28	7	na
ecLFa	0.56	8	0.00	5	0.02	6	−0.26	5	−0.50	27	5	na
icLFa	0.05	5	0.06	8	0.00	5	−0.27	3	−0.30	27	5	na

A9001140, Osteoarthritis Initiative (OAI), and MAK: longitudinal studies involving quantitative measurement of cartilage morphology in patients who have OA.

Abbreviations: cLF, central weight-bearing lateral femoral condyle; cLFTC, central lateral femorotibial compartment (cLT + ccLF); cMF, central weight-bearing medial femoral condyle; cMFTC, central medial femorotibial compartment (cMT + ccMF); cMFTC, medial femorotibial compartment; LT, lateral tibia; MAK, Mechanical Factors in Arthritis of the Knee Study; MC, mean change; MC%, mean change of cartilage thickness in percent per year; MFTC, medial femorotibial compartment; MT, medial tibia; n, number of participants in (sub)study; na, not applicable; sum, sum of the ranks in the studies of the five subregions listed below; ThCtAB, cartilage thickness over total area of subchondral bone.

a Subregions in MT, cMF, LT, and cLF are as follows: c, central; e, external; i, internal; a, anterior; p, posterior.

b Rank (1–8): subregions in the medial and lateral femorotibial compartment are ranked according to the rate of cartilage loss (rank 1 = subregion with the greatest cartilage loss; rank 8 = subregion with the least cartilage loss or with the greatest cartilage increase).

c Versus plate, information on whether a subregion displayed a higher rate of change than the total plate (+), the same rate (=), or a lower rate (−) in the five (sub)studies listed previously.

who had OA compared with normal controls; Tb.N was lower in patients who had OA and decreased with the degree of OA. Patients who had a mild degree of OA had a lower trabecular thickness than those who had higher degrees of OA. In addition, the structural variation of the lateral and medial femoral condyle among individuals was indicative of the extent of the disease. In another cross-sectional study using the same protocol, Lindsey and colleagues[118] analyzed the relation between VC and trabecular bone structure in the knees of 21 healthy volunteers and 53 patients who had varying degrees of OA. They reported that cartilage thinning was associated with loss of bone structure in the opposite femoral condyle ($P<.05$). In varus OA, a high correlation between cartilage loss in the MT and cMF and loss of bone structure in the LT and cLF was observed. In addition, a significant correlation existed between the compartmental differences (lateral versus medial) of cartilage thickness and bone structure. These researchers concluded that degradation of articular cartilage within a compartment correlated with loss of bone structure in the opposite compartment. Malalignment seemed to be associated with bone formation in the diseased condyle and bone resorption in the opposite compartment. Under ex vivo conditions, Lammentausta and colleagues[119] found that bone structural measures of subchondral bone were different between human patellar samples with no OA and with advanced OA and that mechanical properties of trabecular bone discerned those with no OA from OA samples. More recently, Lancianese and colleagues[120] were able to show ex vivo that MR imaging-derived properties of trabecular bone from whole-joint images of the proximal tibia were significantly correlated with mechanical parameters of the subchondral bone, such as Young's modulus, yield stress, and ultimate stress ($r^2 = 58\%–73\%$). These correlations were similar to those between µCT and the mechanical properties of the subchondral bone in the same specimens.

Blumenkrantz and colleagues[121] were the first to investigate knee trabecular bone structure (and cartilage properties) longitudinally in OA over a 2-year period. They observed a large variation in bone and cartilage parameters among individuals across groups of healthy participants and participants who had OA, with group-specific means showing decreasing trends in bone and cartilage parameters in the participants who had OA. A positive relation was established between cartilage changes and localized bone changes closest to the joint line, whereas a negative correlation was established between cartilage changes and global

bone changes further away from the joint line. These investigators hypothesized that osteoarthritic knees encounter subchondral plate sclerosis, which could cause osteopenia in the subarticular bone attributable to a "stress shielding" effect.

Using 3 T MR imaging, Bolbos and colleagues[122] evaluated knee trabecular bone structure and cartilage morphology using parallel imaging. They showed good reproducibility ranging from 1.8% for apparent Tb.N to 5.5% for apparent Tb.Sp. Significant differences were identified between controls and OA participants for apparent BV/TV and apparent Tb.Sp. T1rho of the cartilage (a measure of glycosaminoglycan content) was negatively correlated with apparent BV/TV, Tb.N, and Tb.Sp at the medial femoral condyle and lateral tibia. Significant correlations were also reported between trabecular bone parameters and cartilage thickness at the lateral tibia and femur, indicating that loss of mineralized bone and alterations in its structure may be associated with early phases of cartilage degeneration.

FUTURE DIRECTIONS

Baseline and year 1 follow-up MR imaging data have been made publicly available for the first half (2678 cases) of the OAI cohort,[58] and further releases of radiographic and MR imaging data are planned in the future. This and the results of other large epidemiologic studies should provide ample opportunity for collaborative research and should allow the research community to make rapid progress in understanding the risk factors involved in quantitative cartilage loss and bone changes in OA. Most importantly, it should make it possible to determine which imaging biomarkers best predict clinical outcomes, such as real or virtual TKA. This is an important step in validating novel cartilage imaging biomarkers and approaches as surrogate measures of disease progression, particularly in therapeutic intervention trials. Once the clinical importance of these imaging biomarkers are established, further improvements in imaging hardware, coils, sequences, and image analysis algorithms may foster a more automated analysis of cartilage morphology, composition, and other articular tissues than is currently possible. This is likely to be of particular importance once SMOADs or DMOADs become available, because of the required monitoring of the treatment response in large sets of patients who have OA. Currently, quantitative MR imaging of articular tissues represents a potent research tool in experimental, epidemiologic, and pharmacologic intervention studies. It is only with the availability of such drugs (SMOADs or DMOADs) that quantitative MR imaging of the cartilage will also play a relevant and important role in clinical decision making and clinical practice.

ACKNOWLEDGMENTS

The authors thank Julio Carballido-Gamio (Department of Radiology, University of California, San Francisco, California) for help with the review of the literature of quantitative assessment of trabecular bone.

REFERENCES

1. Sharma L, Eckstein F, Song J, et al. Relationship of meniscal damage, meniscal extrusion, malalignment, and joint laxity to subsequent cartilage loss in osteoarthritic knees. Arthritis Rheum 2008; 58(6):1716–26.
2. Peterfy CG, Guermazi A, Zaim S, et al. Whole-Organ Magnetic Resonance Imaging Score (WORMS) of the knee in osteoarthritis. Osteoarthr Cartil 2004;12(3):177–90.
3. Reichenbach S, Yang M, Eckstein F, et al. Does cartilage volume or thickness distinguish knees with and without mild radiographic osteoarthritis? The Framingham study. Ann Rheum Dis 2009 Feb 4 [Epub ahead of print].
4. Le Graverand MP, Mazzuca S, Lassere M, et al. Assessment of the radioanatomic positioning of the osteoarthritic knee in serial radiographs: comparison of three acquisition techniques. Osteoarthr Cartil 2006;14(Suppl A):A37–43.
5. Cline GA, Meyer JM, Stevens R, et al. Comparison of fixed flexion, fluoroscopic semi-flexed and MTP radiographic methods for obtaining the minimum medial joint space width of the knee in longitudinal osteoarthritis trials. Osteoarthr Cartil 2006; 14(Suppl A):A32–6.
6. Hunter DJ, Conaghan PG, Peterfy CG, et al. Responsiveness, effect size, and smallest detectable difference of Magnetic Resonance Imaging in knee osteoarthritis. Osteoarthr Cartil 2006; 14(Suppl 1):112–5.
7. Solloway S, Hutchinson CE, Waterton JC, et al. The use of active shape models for making thickness measurements of articular cartilage from MR images. Magn Reson Med 1997;37(6):943–52.
8. Stammberger T, Eckstein F, Michaelis M, et al. Inter-observer reproducibility of quantitative cartilage measurements: comparison of B-spline snakes and manual segmentation. Magn Reson Imaging 1999;17(7):1033–42.
9. Cohen ZA, McCarthy DM, Kwak SD, et al. Knee cartilage topography, thickness, and contact areas

from MRI: in-vitro calibration and in-vivo measurements. Osteoarthr Cartil 1999;7(1):95–109.
10. Lynch JA, Zaim S, Zhao J, et al. Cartilage segmentation of 3D MRI scans of the osteoarthritic knee combining user knowledge and active contours. Proc Soc Photo Opt Instrum Eng 2000;3979: 925–35.
11. Cashman PM, Kitney RI, Gariba MA, et al. Automated techniques for visualization and mapping of articular cartilage in MR images of the osteoarthritic knee: a base technique for the assessment of microdamage and submicrodamage. IEEE Trans Nanobioscience 2002;1(1):42–51.
12. Kauffmann C, Gravel P, Godbout B, et al. Computer-aided method for quantification of cartilage thickness and volume changes using MRI: validation study using a synthetic model. IEEE Trans Biomed Eng 2003;50(8):978–88.
13. Pathak SD, Ng L, Wyman B, et al. Quantitative image analysis: software systems in drug development trials. Drug Discov Today 2003;8(10):451–8.
14. Folkesson J, Dam E, Olsen OF, et al. Automatic segmentation of the articular cartilage in knee MRI using a hierarchical multi-class classification scheme. Med Image Comput Comput Assist Interv Int Conf Med Image Comput Comput Assist Interv 2005;8(Pt 1):327–34.
15. Folkesson J, Dam EB, Olsen OF, et al. Segmenting articular cartilage automatically using a voxel classification approach. IEEE Trans Med Imaging 2007; 26(1):106–15.
16. McWalter EJ, Wirth W, Siebert M, et al. Use of novel interactive input devices for segmentation of articular cartilage from magnetic resonance images. Osteoarthr Cartil 2005;13(1):48–53.
17. Hohe J, Faber S, Stammberger T, et al. A technique for 3D in vivo quantification of proton density and magnetization transfer coefficients of knee joint cartilage. Osteoarthr Cartil 2000;8(6):426–33.
18. Hohe J, Faber S, Muehlbauer R, et al. Three-dimensional analysis and visualization of regional MR signal intensity distribution of articular cartilage. Med Eng Phys 2002;24(3):219–27.
19. Qazi AA, Folkesson J, Pettersen PC, et al. Separation of healthy and early osteoarthritis by automatic quantification of cartilage homogeneity. Osteoarthr Cartil 2007;15(10):1199–206.
20. Eckstein F, Ateshian G, Burgkart R, et al. Proposal for a nomenclature for magnetic resonance imaging based measures of articular cartilage in osteoarthritis. Osteoarthr Cartil 2006;14(10): 974–83.
21. Burgkart R, Glaser C, Hinterwimmer S, et al. Feasibility of T and Z scores from magnetic resonance imaging data for quantification of cartilage loss in osteoarthritis. Arthritis Rheum 2003;48(10): 2829–35.

22. Eisenhart-Rothe R, Graichen H, Hudelmaier M, et al. Femorotibial and patellar cartilage loss in patients prior to total knee arthroplasty, heterogeneity, and correlation with alignment of the knee. Ann Rheum Dis 2006;65(1):69–73.

23. Otterness IG, Eckstein F. Women have thinner cartilage and smaller joint surfaces than men after adjustment for body height and weight. Osteoarthr Cartil 2007;15(6):666–72.

24. Wang Y, Ding C, Wluka AE, et al. Factors affecting progression of knee cartilage defects in normal subjects over 2 years. Rheumatology (Oxford) 2006;45(1):79–84.

25. Eckstein F, Buck RJ, Burstein D, et al. Precision of 3.0 Tesla quantitative magnetic resonance imaging of cartilage morphology in a multicentre clinical trial. Ann Rheum Dis 2008;67(12):1683–8.

26. Eckstein F, Hudelmaier M, Cahue S, et al. Medial-to-lateral ratio of tibiofemoral subchondral bone area is adapted to alignment and mechanical load. Calcif Tissue Int 2009;84(3):186–94.

27. Cohen ZA, Mow VC, Henry JH, et al. Templates of the cartilage layers of the patellofemoral joint and their use in the assessment of osteoarthritic cartilage damage. Osteoarthr Cartil 2003;11(8):569–79.

28. Hudelmaier M, Glaser C, Hohe J, et al. Age-related changes in the morphology and deformational behavior of knee joint cartilage. Arthritis Rheum 2001;44(11):2556–61.

29. Eckstein F, Reiser M, Englmeier KH, et al. In vivo morphometry and functional analysis of human articular cartilage with quantitative magnetic resonance imaging—from image to data, from data to theory. Anat Embryol (Berl) 2001;203(3):147–73.

30. Beattie KA, Duryea J, Pui M, et al. Minimum joint space width and tibial cartilage morphology in the knees of healthy individuals: a cross-sectional study. BMC Musculoskelet Disord 2008;9:119.

31. Tameem HZ, Selva LE, Sinha US. Morphological atlases of knee cartilage: shape indices to analyze cartilage degradation in osteoarthritic and non-osteoarthritic population. Conf Proc IEEE Eng Med Biol Soc 2007;2007:1310–3.

32. Eckstein F, Maschek S, Wirth W, et al. One year change of knee cartilage morphology in the first release of participants from the Osteoarthritis Initiative progression subcohort—association with sex, body mass index, symptoms, and radiographic OA status. Ann Rheum Dis 2009;68(5):674–9.

33. Eckstein F, Wirth W, Hudelmaier M, et al. Patterns of femorotibial cartilage loss in knees with neutral, varus, and valgus alignment. Arthritis Rheum 2008;59(11):1563–70.

34. Hunter DJ, Niu J, Zhang Y, et al. Change in cartilage morphometry: a sample of the progression cohort of the Osteoarthritis Initiative. Ann Rheum Dis 2009;68(3):349–56.

35. Raynauld JP, Martel-Pelletier J, Abram F, et al. Analysis of the precision and sensitivity to change of different approaches to assess cartilage loss by quantitative MRI in a longitudinal multicentre clinical trial in patients with knee osteoarthritis. Arthritis Res Ther 2008;10(6):R129.

36. Hohe J, Ateshian G, Reiser M, et al. Surface size, curvature analysis, and assessment of knee joint incongruity with MRI in vivo. Magn Reson Med 2002;47(3):554–61.

37. Dam EB, Folkesson J, Pettersen PC, et al. Automatic morphometric cartilage quantification in the medial tibial plateau from MRI for osteoarthritis grading. Osteoarthr Cartil 2007;15(7):808–18.

38. Folkesson J, Dam EB, Olsen OF, et al. Accuracy evaluation of automatic quantification of the articular cartilage surface curvature from MRI. Acad Radiol 2007;14(10):1221–8.

39. Folkesson J, Dam EB, Olsen OF, et al. Automatic quantification of local and global articular cartilage surface curvature: biomarkers for osteoarthritis? Magn Reson Med 2008;59(6):1340–6.

40. Qazi AA, Dam EB, Nielsen M, et al. Osteoarthritic cartilage is more homogeneous than healthy cartilage: identification of a superior region of interest colocalized with a major risk factor for osteoarthritis. Acad Radiol 2007;14(10):1209–20.

41. Koo S, Gold GE, Andriacchi TP. Considerations in measuring cartilage thickness using MRI: factors influencing reproducibility and accuracy. Osteoarthr Cartil 2005;13(9):782–9.

42. Pelletier JP, Raynauld JP, Berthiaume MJ, et al. Risk factors associated with the loss of cartilage volume on weight-bearing areas in knee osteoarthritis patients assessed by quantitative magnetic resonance imaging: a longitudinal study. Arthritis Res Ther 2007;9(4):R74.

43. Wirth W, Eckstein F. A technique for regional analysis of femorotibial cartilage thickness based on quantitative magnetic resonance imaging. IEEE Trans Med Imaging 2008;27(6):737–44.

44. Gray ML, Eckstein F, Peterfy C, et al. Toward imaging biomarkers for osteoarthritis. Clin Orthop 2004;(Suppl 427):S175–81.

45. Mosher TJ, Dardzinski BJ. Cartilage MRI T2 relaxation time mapping: overview and applications. Semin Musculoskelet Radiol 2004;8(4):355–68.

46. Eckstein F, Cicuttini F, Raynauld JP, et al. Magnetic resonance imaging (MRI) of articular cartilage in knee osteoarthritis (OA): morphological assessment. Osteoarthr Cartil 2006;14(Suppl 1):46–75.

47. Eckstein F, Burstein D, Link TM. Quantitative MRI of cartilage and bone: degenerative changes in osteoarthritis. NMR Biomed 2006;19(7):822–54.

48. Eckstein F, Hudelmaier M, Putz R. The effects of exercise on human articular cartilage. J Anat 2006;208(4):491–512.

49. Gold GE, Burstein D, Dardzinski B, et al. MRI of articular cartilage in OA: novel pulse sequences and compositional/functional markers. Osteoarthr Cartil 2006;14(Suppl 1):76–86.

50. Mosher TJ. Musculoskeletal imaging at 3T: current techniques and future applications. Magn Reson Imaging Clin N Am 2006;14(1):63–76.

51. Burstein D. MRI for development of disease-modifying osteoarthritis drugs. NMR Biomed 2006; 19(6):669–80.

52. Peterfy CG, Gold G, Eckstein F, et al. MRI protocols for whole-organ assessment of the knee in osteoarthritis. Osteoarthr Cartil 2006;14(Suppl 1):95–111.

53. Hardy PA, Recht MP, Piraino D, et al. Optimization of a dual echo in the steady state (DESS) free-precession sequence for imaging cartilage. J Magn Reson Imaging 1996;6(2):329–35.

54. Eckstein F, Hudelmaier M, Wirth W, et al. Double echo steady state magnetic resonance imaging of knee articular cartilage at 3 Tesla: a pilot study for the Osteoarthritis Initiative. Ann Rheum Dis 2006; 65(4):433–41.

55. Eckstein F, Kunz M, Hudelmaier M, et al. Impact of coil design on the contrast-to-noise ratio, precision, and consistency of quantitative cartilage morphometry at 3 Tesla: a pilot study for the osteoarthritis initiative. Magn Reson Med 2007;57(2):448–54.

56. Eckstein F, Kunz M, Schutzer M, et al. Two year longitudinal change and test-retest-precision of knee cartilage morphology in a pilot study for the osteoarthritis initiative. Osteoarthr Cartil 2007; 15(11):1326–32.

57. Welsch GH, Mamisch TC, Hughes T, et al. Advanced morphological and biochemical magnetic resonance imaging of cartilage repair procedures in the knee joint at 3 Tesla. Semin Musculoskelet Radiol 2008;12(3):196–211.

58. National Institute of Arthritis and Musculoskeletal and Skin Diseases. National Institute of Health, Department of Health and Human Services. Available at: http://www.niams.nih.gov/ne/oi/.

59. Peterfy CG, Schneider E, Nevitt M. The osteoarthritis initiative: report on the design rationale for the magnetic resonance imaging protocol for the knee. Osteoarthr Cartil 2008;16(12):1433–41.

60. Inglis D, Pui M, Ioannidis G, et al. Accuracy and test-retest precision of quantitative cartilage morphology on a 1.0 T peripheral magnetic resonance imaging system. Osteoarthr Cartil 2007; 15(1):110–5.

61. Eckstein F, Charles HC, Buck RJ, et al. Accuracy and precision of quantitative assessment of cartilage morphology by magnetic resonance imaging at 3.0T. Arthritis Rheum 2005;52(10):3132–6.

62. Morgan SR, Waterton JC, Maciewicz RA, et al. Magnetic resonance imaging measurement of knee cartilage volume in a multicentre study. Rheumatology (Oxford) 2004;43(1):19–21.

63. Kornaat PR, Koo S, Andriacchi TP, et al. Comparison of quantitative cartilage measurements acquired on two 3.0T MRI systems from different manufacturers. J Magn Reson Imaging 2006; 23(5):770–3.

64. Hudelmaier M, Horger W, Pfau C, et al. Cross-calibration of magnetic resonance sequences and scanners for quantifying articular cartilage morphology. Osteoarthr Cartil 2003;11(Suppl A): S72 [abstract].

65. Schneider E, NessAiver M, White D, et al. The Osteoarthritis Initiative (OAI) magnetic resonance imaging quality assurance methods and results. Osteoarthr Cartil 2008;16(9):994–1004.

66. Eckstein F, Buck RJ, Wyman BT, et al. Quantitative imaging of cartilage morphology at 3.0 Tesla in the presence of gadopentetate dimeglumine (Gd-DTPA). Magn Reson Med 2007;58(2):402–6.

67. Eckstein F, Wyman BT, Buck RJ, et al. Longitudinal quantitative MR imaging of cartilage morphology in the presence of gadopentetate dimeglumine (Gd-DTPA). Magn Reson Med 2009;61(4):975–80.

68. Gandy SJ, Dieppe PA, Keen MC, et al. No loss of cartilage volume over three years in patients with knee osteoarthritis as assessed by magnetic resonance imaging. Osteoarthr Cartil 2002;10(12): 929–37.

69. Wluka AE, Stuckey S, Snaddon J, et al. The determinants of change in tibial cartilage volume in osteoarthritic knees. Arthritis Rheum 2002;46(8): 2065–72.

70. Cicuttini FM, Wluka AE, Wang Y, et al. Longitudinal study of changes in tibial and femoral cartilage in knee osteoarthritis. Arthritis Rheum 2004;50(1): 94–7.

71. Raynauld JP, Martel-Pelletier J, Berthiaume MJ, et al. Quantitative magnetic resonance imaging evaluation of knee osteoarthritis progression over two years and correlation with clinical symptoms and radiologic changes. Arthritis Rheum 2004; 50(2):476–87.

72. Berthiaume MJ, Raynauld JP, Martel-Pelletier J, et al. Meniscal tear and extrusion are strongly associated with progression of symptomatic knee osteoarthritis as assessed by quantitative magnetic resonance imaging. Ann Rheum Dis 2005;64(4): 556–63.

73. Raynauld JP, Martel-Pelletier J, Berthiaume MJ, et al. Long term evaluation of disease progression through the quantitative magnetic resonance imaging of symptomatic knee osteoarthritis patients: correlation with clinical symptoms and radiographic changes. Arthritis Res Ther 2006;8(1):R21.

74. Wluka AE, Forbes A, Wang Y, et al. Knee cartilage loss in symptomatic knee osteoarthritis over 4.5 years. Arthritis Res Ther 2006;8(4):R90.

75. Bruyere O, Genant H, Kothari M, et al. Longitudinal study of magnetic resonance imaging and standard X-rays to assess disease progression in osteoarthritis. Osteoarthr Cartil 2007;15(1):98–103.

76. Hellio Le Graverand MP, Buck RJ, Wyman BT, et al. Change in regional cartilage morphology and joint space width in osteoarthritis participants versus healthy controls—a multicenter study using 3.0 Tesla MRI and Lyon Schuss radiography. Ann Rheum Dis 2008 Dec 22 [Epub ahead of print].

77. Wirth W, Hellio Le Graverand MP, Wyman BT, et al. Regional analysis of femorotibial cartilage loss in a subsample from the Osteoarthritis Initiative progression subcohort. Osteoarthr Cartil 2009; 17(3):291–7.

78. Guermazi A, Burstein D, Conaghan P, et al. Imaging in osteoarthritis. Rheum Dis Clin North Am 2008;34(3):645–87.

79. Raynauld JP, Kauffmann C, Beaudoin G, et al. Reliability of a quantification imaging system using magnetic resonance images to measure cartilage thickness and volume in human normal and osteoarthritic knees. Osteoarthr Cartil 2003;11(5): 351–60.

80. Cicuttini F, Wluka A, Wang Y, et al. The determinants of change in patella cartilage volume in osteoarthritic knees. J Rheumatol 2002;29(12):2615–9.

81. Frobell RB, Le Graverand MP, Buck R, et al. The acutely ACL injured knee assessed by MRI: changes in joint fluid, bone marrow lesions, and cartilage during the first year. Osteoarthr Cartil 2009;17(2):161–7.

82. Watson PJ, Carpenter TA, Hall LD, et al. Cartilage swelling and loss in a spontaneous model of osteoarthritis visualized by magnetic resonance imaging. Osteoarthr Cartil 1996;4(3):197–207.

83. Calvo E, Palacios I, Delgado E, et al. High-resolution MRI detects cartilage swelling at the early stages of experimental osteoarthritis. Osteoarthr Cartil 2001;9(5):463–72.

84. Calvo E, Palacios I, Delgado E, et al. Histopathological correlation of cartilage swelling detected by magnetic resonance imaging in early experimental osteoarthritis. Osteoarthr Cartil 2004; 12(11):878–86.

85. Vignon E, Arlot M, Hartmann D, et al. Hypertrophic repair of articular cartilage in experimental osteoarthrosis. Ann Rheum Dis 1983;42(1):82–8.

86. Adams ME, Brandt KD. Hypertrophic repair of canine articular cartilage in osteoarthritis after anterior cruciate ligament transection. J Rheumatol 1991;18(3):428–35.

87. Cicuttini F, Hankin J, Jones G, et al. Comparison of conventional standing knee radiographs and magnetic resonance imaging in assessing progression of tibiofemoral joint osteoarthritis. Osteoarthr Cartil 2005;13(8):722–7.

88. Raynauld JP, Martel-Pelletier J, Bias P, et al. Protective effects of licofelone, a 5-lipoxygenase and cyclooxygenase inhibitor, versus naproxen on cartilage loss in knee osteoarthritis: a first multi-centre clinical trial using quantitative MRI. Ann Rheum Dis 2008 Jul 23 [Epub ahead of print].

89. Peterfy C, Li J, Zaim S, et al. Comparison of fixed-flexion positioning with fluoroscopic semi-flexed positioning for quantifying radiographic joint-space width in the knee: test-retest reproducibility. Skeletal Radiol 2003;32(3):128–32.

90. Botha-Scheepers S, Kloppenburg M, Kroon HM, et al. Fixed-flexion knee radiography: the sensitivity to detect knee joint space narrowing in osteoarthritis. Osteoarthr Cartil 2007;15(3):350–3.

91. Charles HC, Kraus VB, Ainslie M, et al. Optimization of the fixed-flexion knee radiograph. Osteoarthr Cartil 2007;15(11):1221–4.

92. Nevitt MC, Peterfy C, Guermazi A, et al. Longitudinal performance evaluation and validation of fixed-flexion radiography of the knee for detection of joint space loss. Arthritis Rheum 2007;56(5): 1512–20.

93. Le Graverand MP, Vignon EP, Brandt KD, et al. Head-to-head comparison of the Lyon Schuss and fixed flexion radiographic techniques. Long-term reproducibility in normal knees and sensitivity to change in osteoarthritic knees. Ann Rheum Dis 2008;67(11):1562–6.

94. Adams JG, McAlindon T, Dimasi M, et al. Contribution of meniscal extrusion and cartilage loss to joint space narrowing in osteoarthritis. Clin Radiol 1999; 54(8):502–6.

95. Gale DR, Chaisson CE, Totterman SM, et al. Meniscal subluxation: association with osteoarthritis and joint space narrowing. Osteoarthr Cartil 1999;7(6): 526–32.

96. Hunter DJ, Zhang YQ, Tu X, et al. Change in joint space width: hyaline articular cartilage loss or alteration in meniscus? Arthritis Rheum 2006;54(8): 2488–95.

97. Cicuttini FM, Jones G, Forbes A, et al. Rate of cartilage loss at two years predicts subsequent total knee arthroplasty: a prospective study. Ann Rheum Dis 2004;63(9):1124–7.

98. Cicuttini FM, Wluka A, Bailey M, et al. Factors affecting knee cartilage volume in healthy men. Rheumatology (Oxford) 2003;42(2):258–62.

99. Teichtahl AJ, Wluka AE, Wang Y, et al. Obesity and adiposity are associated with the rate of patella cartilage volume loss over two years in adults without knee osteoarthritis. Ann Rheum Dis 2008 Jul 16 [Epub ahead of print].

100. Raynauld JP, Martel-Pelletier J, Berthiaume MJ, et al. Correlation between bone lesion changes and cartilage volume loss in patients with osteoarthritis of the knee as assessed by quantitative magnetic resonance imaging over a 24-month period. Ann Rheum Dis 2008;67(5):683–8.

101. Englund M, Guermazi A, Gale D, et al. Incidental meniscal findings on knee MRI in middle-aged and elderly persons. N Engl J Med 2008;359(11): 1108–15.

102. Davies-Tuck ML, Martel-Pelletier J, Wluka AE, et al. Meniscal tear and increased tibial plateau bone area in healthy post-menopausal women. Osteoarthr Cartil 2008;16(2):268–71.

103. Cicuttini F, Wluka A, Hankin J, et al. Longitudinal study of the relationship between knee angle and tibiofemoral cartilage volume in subjects with knee osteoarthritis. Rheumatology (Oxford) 2004; 43(3):321–4.

104. Teichtahl AJ, Davies-Tuck ML, Wluka AE, et al. Change in knee angle influences the rate of medial tibial cartilage volume loss in knee osteoarthritis. Osteoarthr Cartil 2009;17(1):8–11.

105. Teichtahl AJ, Wluka AE, Cicuttini FM. Frontal plane knee alignment is associated with a longitudinal reduction in patella cartilage volume in people with knee osteoarthritis. Osteoarthr Cartil 2008; 16(7):851–4.

106. Zhai G, Ding C, Cicuttini F, et al. A longitudinal study of the association between knee alignment and change in cartilage volume and chondral defects in a largely non-osteoarthritic population. J Rheumatol 2007;34(1):181–6.

107. Kellgren JH, Lawrence JS. Radiological assessment of osteo-arthrosis. Ann Rheum Dis 1957; 16(4):494–502.

108. Wluka AE, Hanna FS, Davies-Tuck M, et al. Bone marrow lesions predict increase in knee cartilage defects and loss of cartilage volume in middle-aged women without knee pain over 2 years. Ann Rheum Dis 2008 Jul 14 [Epub ahead of print].

109. Wluka AE, Wang Y, Davies-Tuck M, et al. Bone marrow lesions predict progression of cartilage defects and loss of cartilage volume in healthy middle-aged adults without knee pain over 2 yrs. Rheumatology (Oxford) 2008;47(9):1392–6.

110. Ding C, Cicuttini F, Scott F, et al. Association of prevalent and incident knee cartilage defects with loss of tibial and patellar cartilage: a longitudinal study. Arthritis Rheum 2005;52(12):3918–27.

111. Wluka AE, Ding C, Jones G, et al. The clinical correlates of articular cartilage defects in symptomatic knee osteoarthritis: a prospective study. Rheumatology (Oxford) 2005;44(10): 1311–6.

112. Cicuttini F, Ding C, Wluka A, et al. Association of cartilage defects with loss of knee cartilage in healthy, middle-age adults: a prospective study. Arthritis Rheum 2005;52(7):2033–9.

113. Ding C, Martel-Pelletier J, Pelletier JP, et al. Two-year prospective longitudinal study exploring the factors associated with change in femoral cartilage volume in a cohort largely without knee radiographic osteoarthritis. Osteoarthr Cartil 2008; 16(4):443–9.

114. Ding C, Cicuttini F, Blizzard L, et al. Smoking interacts with family history with regard to change in knee cartilage volume and cartilage defect development. Arthritis Rheum 2007;56(5):1521–8.

115. Ding C, Cicuttini F, Jones G. Tibial subchondral bone size and knee cartilage defects: relevance to knee osteoarthritis. Osteoarthr Cartil 2007; 15(5):479–86.

116. Hunter DJ, Niu JB, Zhang Y, et al. Premorbid knee osteoarthritis is not characterised by diffuse thinness: the Framingham Osteoarthritis Study. Ann Rheum Dis 2008;67(11):1545–9.

117. Beuf O, Ghosh S, Newitt DC, et al. Magnetic resonance imaging of normal and osteoarthritic trabecular bone structure in the human knee. Arthritis Rheum 2002;46(2):385–93.

118. Lindsey CT, Narasimhan A, Adolfo JM, et al. Magnetic resonance evaluation of the interrelationship between articular cartilage and trabecular bone of the osteoarthritic knee. Osteoarthr Cartil 2004;12(2):86–96.

119. Lammentausta E, Kiviranta P, Toyras J, et al. Quantitative MRI of parallel changes of articular cartilage and underlying trabecular bone in degeneration. Osteoarthr Cartil 2007;15(10):1149–57.

120. Lancianese SL, Kwok E, Beck CA, et al. Predicting regional variations in trabecular bone mechanical properties within the human proximal tibia using MR imaging. Bone 2008;43(6):1039–46.

121. Blumenkrantz G, Lindsey CT, Dunn TC, et al. A pilot, two-year longitudinal study of the interrelationship between trabecular bone and articular cartilage in the osteoarthritic knee. Osteoarthr Cartil 2004;12(12):997–1005.

122. Bolbos RI, Zuo J, Banerjee S, et al. Relationship between trabecular bone structure and articular cartilage morphology and relaxation times in early OA of the knee joint using parallel MRI at 3 T. Osteoarthr Cartil 2008;16(10):1150–9.

Measures of Molecular Composition and Structure in Osteoarthritis

Deborah Burstein, PhD[a],*, Martha Gray, PhD[b], Tim Mosher, MD[c], Bernard Dardzinski, PhD[d]

KEYWORDS
- dGEMRIC • T1rho • Sodium imaging • T2 mapping
- MR imaging • Osteoarthritis

Osteoarthritis (OA) is increasingly recognized as a disease that involves ongoing degradative and healing processes occurring at the molecular level in multiple tissues in the joint in response to a number of biochemical and mechanical factors. Understanding these dynamic processes before they affect the structural aspects of the joint motivates the need for metrics to better visualize the compositional and structural molecular aspects of the tissues in vivo. Most of the work to date in this regard has been focused on cartilage; this article reviews cartilage magnetic resonance (MR) imaging methods designed to interrogate these molecular features with examples of insights gained.

MOLECULAR COMPOSITION OF CARTILAGE

Cartilage can be thought of as a fluid-filled macromolecular network, one that functions to support mechanical loading. Chondrocytes, a sparse population of cells within the network, are presumed to be responsible for any homeostatic and repair processes that modulate the composition of the network. During normal joint loading, the electrolyte-containing interstitial fluid (about 75% of cartilage by weight) becomes pressurized to the extent that its movement is restricted by the macromolecular network. As such, the pressurized fluid serves to distribute and support the mechanical load.

The macromolecular network itself consists mainly of collagen and proteoglycans. Collagen, a fibrillar macromolecule, is by far the most abundant macromolecule, accounting for about 20% of cartilage volume by weight (approximately 70%–80% of the dry weight). Normally, the collagen network is highly organized and serves as the tissue's structural framework and its principal source of tensile and shear strength. Although the collagen network becomes disrupted in OA and there is a net loss in total collagen content, its concentration is not appreciably affected in disease states.[1–3]

Aggrecan is the second most abundant macromolecule of the extracellular matrix network of cartilage. Aggrecan is a large aggregating proteoglycan, with a bottle-brush appearance on electron microscopy,[4] wherein the "wire" of the brush is a protein core to which the "bristles"—glycosaminoglycan (GAG) molecules—are covalently attached. The GAGs are repeating disaccharides with carboxyl and sulfate groups that are charged under physiologic conditions. Consequently, the

[a] Department of Radiology, Beth Israel Deaconess Medical Center, Harvard Medical School, 330 Brookline Avenue, Boston, MA 02115, USA
[b] Department of Health Sciences and Technology, Department of Electrical Engineering and Computer Science, Massachusetts Institute of Technology, Cambridge, MA 02139, USA
[c] Department of Radiology, Pennsylvania State College of Medicine, The Milton S. Hershey Medical Center, Hershey, PA 17033, USA
[d] Merck Research Laboratories, Merck, Inc., West Point, PA 19486, USA
* Corresponding author.
E-mail address: dburstei@bidmc.harvard.edu (D. Burstein).

Radiol Clin N Am 47 (2009) 675–686
doi:10.1016/j.rcl.2009.04.003

GAG molecules possess considerable net negative charge, and confer to the cartilage considerable compressive strength.[5,6]

Because of the well-documented importance of collagen and aggrecan-associated GAG to the functional and structural integrity of cartilage, efforts toward developing MR imaging methods to interrogate cartilage macromolecules have focused on collagen and GAG.

THE METRICS
T2 Mapping

T2 of cartilage has been the subject of numerous studies since 1989, when the variation of T2 across cartilage was demonstrated.[7] T2 is an MR relaxation time reflecting interactions between water molecules and between water and surrounding macromolecules; increased interaction results in decreased T2. Not surprisingly, T2 is affected by many physiologic and pathophysiologic processes that relate to the state of cartilage.

T2 is sensitive to changes in hydration (or, nearly equivalently, collagen concentration),[8] and orientation of the highly organized anisotropic arrangement of collagen fibrils in the extracellular cartilage matrix.[9] As illustrated in **Fig. 1**, the signal intensity of normal cartilage varies with depth from the

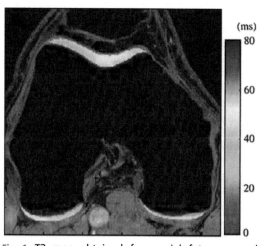

Fig. 1. T2 map obtained from axial fat-suppressed SPGR T1-weighted MR imaging shows the signal intensity in T2 or proton density–weighted images of normal cartilage varies with location in the joint and with depth from the articular surface. This variation, due to the structural and compositional molecular architecture of cartilage, needs to be taken into account when interpreting images of osteoarthritis. (*Reproduced from* Li X, Benjamin Ma C, Link TM, et al. In vivo T(1rho) and T(2) mapping of articular cartilage in osteoarthritis of the knee using 3T MRI. Osteoarthr Cartil 2007;15(7):789–97; with permission.)

articular surface. Regional and zonal differences in density and structural organization of the type II collagen matrix are primarily responsible for this variation in cartilage T2. Near the bone cartilage interface, densely packed collagen fibrils are preferentially aligned perpendicular to the subchondral cortex. In this region, termed the radial zone, the high density and anisotropic orientation of collagen fibrils provides efficient T2 relaxation, leading to low signal intensity on proton density–(PD) or T2-weighted images. Closer to the articular surface, less fibril anisotropy and oblique orientation of the collagen matrix in the transitional zone lead to a gradual increase in T2 relaxation time and thus a relative increase in signal intensity on T2-weighted images. At the articular surface collagen fibers are oriented parallel to the articular surface. The superficial tangential layer and the lamina splendens is approximately 20 μm thick and can be identified on MR microscopy images of excised cartilage specimens as a thin hypointense layer; however, it is too thin to resolve on routine clinical MR imaging.

In addition to variation in signal intensity with respect to depth from the articular surface, there are differences with respect to location in the joint and relative orientation of cartilage to the applied magnetic field. Goodwin and colleagues[10] have correlated this regional variation in signal intensity with obliquity of the collagen matrix cleavage planes on freeze fracture specimens. Xia and colleagues[11] have performed high-resolution correlations of cartilage T2 and fibril anisotropy measured with polarized light microscopy in canine humeral head samples. These studies confirmed the high degree of structural variation of the cartilage tissue with respect to location of the joint, and the sensitivity of cartilage T2 relaxation to the tissue architecture.

While routine clinical MR imaging provides a relative subjective assessment of cartilage T2 changes, quantitative cartilage T2 mapping techniques provide objective data that can be useful in research studies and longitudinal trials where small differences must be compared between populations or over time. In vivo human cartilage T2 maps have been obtained from the adult[12] and pediatric femorotibial joint,[13] patellofemoral joint,[14] ankle,[15] hip,[16] and the proximal interphalangeal joint of the hand.[17]

T1rho

T1rho (T1ρ) is spin-lattice relaxation in the rotating frame and is similar to T2 relaxation except that there is an additional radio frequency (RF) pulse applied after the magnetization is tipped into transverse plane. The magnetization becomes aligned or "spin-locked" with the applied RF field. The signal decay is exponential with a time constant, T1ρ, and is typically calculated from multiple images by changing the duration of the spin-locking pulse. In liquids, T1, T2, and T1ρ relaxation times may be similar, but in tissue these values are typically different (T2 < T1ρ < T1). The measurements of T1ρ probe molecular fluctuations in the kHz range because of the dependence on the RF-generated magnetic field (B1), whereas T2 probes fluctuations in the MHz range because of the dependence on the static magnetic field (B0).

Duvvuri and colleagues[18] first described measurement of T1ρ relaxation in articular cartilage, demonstrating that T1ρ was greater in proteoglycan-depleted bovine cartilage than in normal cartilage samples. This finding was supported in a later study that also showed that the characteristic depth dependence in proteoglycan could be inferred from the depth dependence of T1ρ, seen to be higher in the superficial zone relative to the middle zone.[19] Also using a model of enzymatically degraded bovine cartilage, Regatte and colleagues[20] found that T1ρ-weighted MR imaging is more sensitive to proteoglycan depletion than T2-weighted MR imaging. These data suggested that T1ρ might be a useful metric in assessing OA, particularly for early degeneration, when significant changes in proteoglycan are thought to occur.

A few studies have explored T1ρ in human tissue. One of the first reports by Koskinen and colleagues,[21] involving spin-lock imaging of cadaveric patellae at 0.1 T, demonstrated increased T1ρ as a function of degeneration. Two years later, Mlynarik and colleagues[22] measured T2 and T1ρ, and T1 with Gd-DTPA^{2-} (a modified dGEMRIC method) in articular cartilage specimens following joint replacement to determine the effects of proteoglycan depletion on proton MR imaging relaxation times. T1ρ relaxation time was similar to T2 in both magnitude and spatial variation across the cartilage, with regions of fibrillation having higher times than nonfibrillated regions. T1ρ did not, however, correspond with either the T1 with Gd-DTPA^{2-} images, nor to the proteoglycan distbribution seen histologically. This observation was supported by a later study of human articular cartilage that revealed considerable contrast in T1ρ and T2 that could not be explained entirely by differences in proteoglycan concentration or collagen architecture.[23] Thus, it appears that there are several factors that contribute to variations in T1ρ, including collagen fiber orientation, and concentration of collagen,

proteoglycan, and possibly other macromolecules. Whereas it may never be possible to specifically identify the macromolecular difference (or change) that underlies a difference (or change) in T1ρ, it may well be that the general (nonspecific) sensitivity of T1ρ to differences in cartilage matrix will be shown empirically to provide valuable etiologic, diagnostic, and/or prognostic information relative to OA.

In vivo measurement of T1ρ at 1.5 T was first demonstrated in the femoropatellar joint of healthy adults,[24] and subsequently developed to assure that energy deposition falls within acceptable limits.[25] T1ρ has also been shown in the wrist[26] and meniscus.[27] These feasibility studies suggest that T1ρ is more sensitive than T2 at identifying chondral defects, has superior signal-to-noise ratio than T2-weighted images, and also has improved fluid and fat signal suppression (**Fig. 2**).

Sodium

Sodium MR imaging of cartilage was first demonstrated as a means of imaging the GAG content.[28] The use of sodium MR imaging to image GAG distribution is based on the fact that mobile ions in the interstitial fluid distribute such that their concentration is dependent on the concentration of macromolecular charge (ie, the charge "fixed" to macromolecules of the extracellular matrix). As noted above, the carboxyl and sulfate moieties of cartilage GAGs are ionized under physiologic conditions. Extensive physicochemical studies

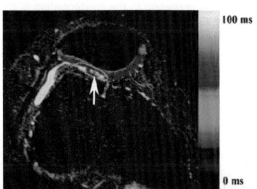

100 ms

0 ms

Fig. 2. T1ρ map obtained on axial fat-suppressed T2-weighted MR imaging. T1ρ image demonstrates similar variation across the cartilage depth similar to that seen by T2 map. The dynamic range for T1ρ is broader than for T2 and might be useful in clinical assessment of changes with osteoarthritis. A "lesion" possibly representing early degeneration is shown in the oval (*arrow*). (*Reproduced from* Borthakur A, Mellon E, Niyogi S, et al. Sodium and T1(rho) MRI for molecular and diagnostic imaging of articular cartilage. NMR Biomed 2006;19(7):781–821; with permission.)

have demonstrated that, in cartilage, the charge on the GAG macromolecules accounts for essentially all the charge in cartilage.[29] Because the GAG is negatively charged, the concentration of sodium in the interstitial fluid is greater than in surrounding synovial fluid or bone. With normal GAG concentrations of 5%–7% (and corresponding concentration of fixed charge of around –300 mmol), the interstitial sodium concentration is normally in excess of 300 mM, a very substantial difference from the 150 mM sodium concentration of synovial fluid. Therefore, the tissue with the highest signal intensity in a sodium image of the knee joint is the cartilage. Furthermore, within cartilage, sodium is higher in normal (GAG-rich) cartilage and lower in areas of cartilage depleted of the negatively charged GAG (**Fig. 3**).

The advantage of sodium MR imaging is that sodium is naturally occurring in cartilage, and the sodium signal in cartilage is high compared with background. The disadvantage is that sodium MR imaging requires specialized hardware, and the signal-to-noise (and hence resolution) of sodium imaging is significantly lower than that of proton MR imaging.

Delayed Gadolinium-Enhanced Magnetic Resonance Imaging of Cartilage

The delayed gadolinium-enhanced MR imaging of cartilage (dGEMRIC) method, developed as a measure of GAG, is also based on the general principle that ions in the interstitial fluid distribute in cartilage in relation to the concentration of the charged GAG molecules. Therefore, the anionic contrast agent Gd-DTPA^{2-} (Magnevist, Berlex, New Jersey), once penetrated into cartilage, distributes in inverse relation to the concentration of GAG. Because the concentration of Gd-DTPA^{2-} can be approximated from a T1 measurement, T1 distribution in a T1 map corresponds to the GAG distribution. This approach for imaging GAG distribution in cartilage is referred to as "dGEMRIC." The "delay" in dGEMRIC is needed to allow time for the Gd-DTPA^{2-} to penetrate the tissue. For in vitro studies, the cartilage is placed in a solution containing Gd-DTPA^{2-}, and sufficient time is left for the Gd-DTPA^{2-} to penetrate the full depth of cartilage, typically several hours to overnight, depending on cartilage thickness. Several studies of Gd-DTPA^{2-} transport into articular cartilages of the knee in vivo have indicated that the contrast agent penetrates cartilage from both the synovial–cartilage and bone–cartilage interfaces, and that 90 minutes is sufficient for penetration throughout the cartilage depth.[30] In practice, Gd-DTPA^{2-} is injected intravenously, the joint is moved for about 10 minutes, and then T1 imaging is performed about 90 minutes after injection,[31] although as few as 30 minutes has been used for hip studies.[32] T1 maps acquired in this way provide the "dGEMRIC index," and can then be used to approximate the Gd-DTPA^{2-} concentration distribution in cartilage. The Gd-DTPA^{2-} distribution presumably reflects the distribution of GAG; however, because an equilibrium state is never reached in vivo given the time-varying concentration of contrast agent in the blood, the T1 measurement after penetration of Gd-DTPA^{2-} is referred to as the "dGEMRIC index," allowing for the possibility that factors other than GAG concentration alone have an impact on the measurement. Variations in the dGEMRIC index have been noted in so-called "lesions" (**Fig. 4**), across populations, and with physiologic changes or interventions (see **Fig. 4** and discussion below), suggesting that it might be a sensitive index of physiologic state.

APPLICATIONS

Osteoarthritis is a multifactorial disease. In addition to systemic factors such as genetic

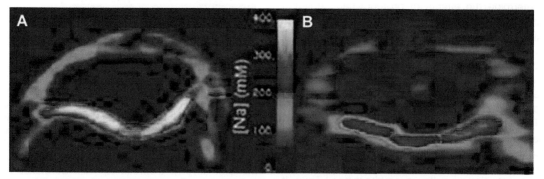

Fig. 3. (A) Axial sodium MR imaging shows high signal intensity in the cartilage. (B) Degenerated cartilage can have sodium concentration between 300 mM and 150 mM, making sodium very sensitive to cartilage disease. (*Reproduced from* Borthakur A, Mellon E, Niyogi S, et al. Sodium and T(1rho) MRI for molecular and diagnostic imaging of articular cartilage. NMR Biomed 2006;19(7):781–821; with permission.)

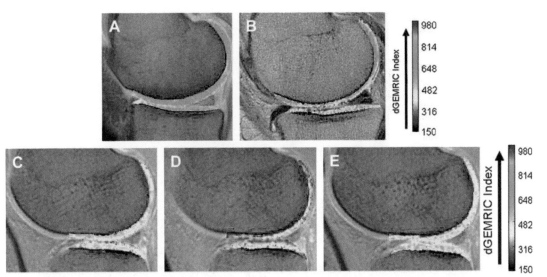

Fig. 4. Sagittal dGEMRIC MR imaging (T1Gd maps) show relatively homogeneous index (*A*), but show "lesions" even in grossly morphologically intact cartilage (*B*). Temporal changes in the dGEMRIC Index have been shown with physiologic events such as seen in the images of an individual (*C*) before running a marathon, (*D*) 1 day post-marathon, and (*E*) 1 week postmarathon.

predisposition, hormonal influences, inflammation, and nutritional factors, among others, early compositional and structural changes in cartilage are presumed to occur in response to local biomechanical factors. These local factors, in particular, are difficult to reproduce with animal or cell models of disease. Given the ability of MR imaging to noninvasively identify molecular compositional and structural changes in cartilage that precede loss of tissue in the human joint, MR imaging is likely to have a unique and important role in future research on cartilage physiology and the pathogenesis of OA, and eventually in clinical practice. However, without evidence that these early changes invariably progress to symptomatic OA and can be modified through treatment or lifestyle changes, one cannot yet articulate the areas where MR imaging diagnosis of early molecular changes may provide direct clinical benefit to the patient.

Identifying Early Changes in the Molecular Structure and Content of Cartilage

Biochemical and microstructural changes in the extracellular collagen matrix occur in response to cartilage maturation, aging, and in the early stages of OA. In a model of chondral injury originally described by Maroudas and colleagues,[3] fragmentation of the collagen network is one of the earliest irreversible changes that occur along the pathway leading to OA. Fractures in the collagen network reduce the normal constraint by the collagen matrix on the hydrated aggrecan, allowing the tissue to swell. As the tissue swells there is a small but measurable increase in water content and loss of the normally high interstitial swelling pressure that is essential for cartilage to withstand the high compressive load applied within the healthy joint. The working paradigm is that these forces influence cell behavior and degeneration, and, ultimately, loss of tissue when there is an imbalance whereby chondrocytes are no longer able to habituate to the forces applied to the cartilage.

Compared with T2 maps of normal cartilage (see **Fig. 1**), T2 maps of osteoathritic cartilage are more heterogeneous (**Fig. 5**). Although elevated T2 is most frequently associated with cartilage damage due to increased hydration, areas of low T2-weighted signal intensity are not infrequently observed in adjacent cartilage in the setting of subacute or chronic cartilage injury. The cause of this finding is unclear, but may be related to fragmentation of collagen fibrils exposing additional hydrophilic sites that could lead to more efficient T2 relaxation and greater magnetization transfer.

There does not appear to be a linear relationship between T2 and OA grade. Several studies have shown that T2 can be used to differentiate normal from mildly degenerated tissue, but cannot be used to differentiate between mild and more severe grades of OA. Integrating what we know about changes in disease, the current interpretation of the T2 changes is that a loss of collagen anisotropy with early damage produces an initial rise in cartilage T2; with further cartilage

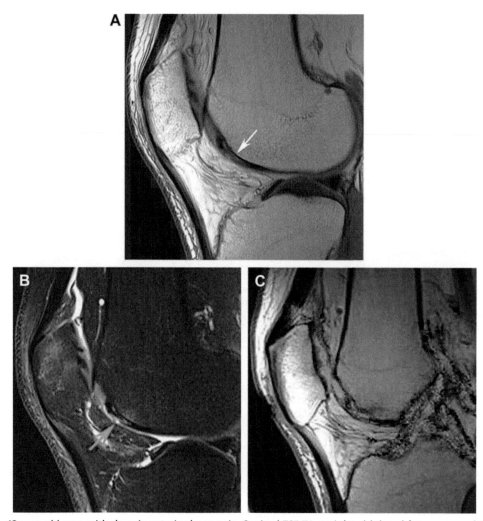

Fig. 5. 42-year-old-man with chronic anterior knee pain. Sagittal TSE T1- weighted (*A*) and fat-suppressed TSE T2-weighted (*B*) MR imaging demonstrates focal chondral delamination and heterogeneous signal in the femoral trochlea consistent with a chronic chondral injury (*arrow*). A small area of subchondral marrow edema is present in the adjacent femoral condyle. Quantitative cartilage T2 map (*C*) demonstrates loss of the normal spatial dependency in cartilage T2.

degradation there is an increase in T2 heterogeneity but no further elevation in T2. As such, it may ultimately be that cartilage T2 values will be useful to identify individuals with sites of early disruption of the collagen matrix, but may be inappropriate as a marker for radiologically observable disease progression.

Several studies have compared T1ρ changes with T2 to determine the relative sensitivity of these metrics. Li and colleagues[33] calculated T1ρ and T2 maps of articular cartilage in normal subjects and early OA subjects. T1ρ and T2 were increased in OA subjects and correlated to radiographic and MR imaging grading. The authors also suggest that T1ρ has a higher dynamic range than T2, as was demonstrated in OA cartilage

specimens,[34] and can be seen in **Fig. 6.** In subjects who had suffered an ACL injury, the lateral meniscus and the lateral femoral and tibial cartilage all showed enhanced T1ρ compared with uninjured controls.[35] Though the fate and clinical significance of these lesions remain unknown, studies such as these make it clear that,injury-associated changes in T1ρ can be observed even when standard MR imaging appears normal. Similarly, a case report following posttraumatic cartilage injury showed T1ρ "lesions" not seen with standard MR imaging confirmed by arthroscopy to be structural cartilage lesions.[36]

Evidence of early disease changes can be seen in metrics designed to be sensitive to GAG loss. Work by Maroudas,[3] among many others, through

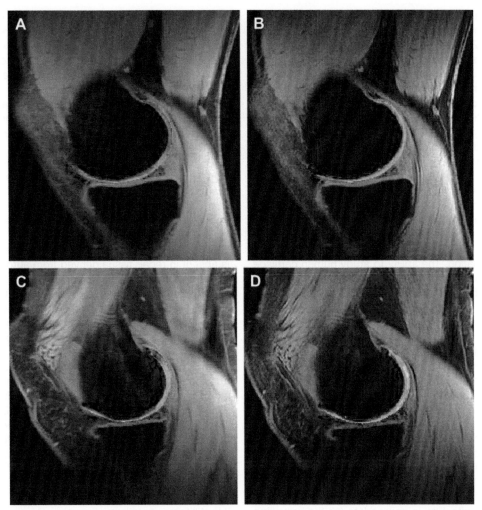

Fig. 6. Both T2 and T1rho are decreased in healthy subject (KL0) [(*A*) mean T2=27 ms; (*B*) mean T1rho=32 ms] when compared with OA subject (KL2) [(*C*) mean T2=34 ms; (*D*) mean T1rho=46 ms]; however, T1rho may have a larger dynamic range. (*Courtesy of* G. Blumenkrantz, San Francisco, CA.)

histologic and biochemical analysis of animal models, and through inferences derived from tissue excised during joint replacement, amputations, and autopsy, has suggested that one of the earliest, and potentially reversible, changes in the degenerative process is a reduction in tissue GAG. Consequently, the relative specificity and sensitivity of sodium MR imaging and dGEMRIC for the GAG component make it well suited to explore early changes in tissue GAG. Notably, in a group of subjects who had little or no radiographic evidence of OA in the knee or hip, there was a broad range of dGEMRIC index suggesting a commensurately broad range of functional capacity. The intriguing question is whether individuals progress from the higher dGEMRIC index group to the lower one before there are radiographically observable changes.

Relation to Biomechanical Function

The function of articulating joints is to absorb loads and enable low friction movement. The functional integrity of tissue is provided by the (fluid-filled) extracellular matrix. One can therefore imagine a stress test whereby the effect of increased load is detected by its impact on the matrix itself. This impact could be short-term, in which the effect is reflected in deformational changes in the tissue, or long-term, whereby the effect could include cell-mediated changes in the composition and architecture of the matrix.

Several studies have explored the possibility of using MR imaging techniques to study the mechanically-induced deformational changes in vivo. In initial feasibility studies, a decrease in cartilage T2 within the femorotibial joint was measured when static compression was applied to the leg within the magnet,[37] and in patellar cartilage following deep knee bends.[8] In an initial study using quantitative T2 mapping in humans, localized decreases in cartilage T2 were observed in the superficial 30% of femoral cartilage immediately after 30 minutes of running exercise.[38] These in vivo results in humans are consistent with prior studies in excised samples indicating greater compressibility of superficial cartilage[39] and changes in superficial collagen orientation with cyclical loading.[40] These observations indicate changes in cartilage T2 may be a potential method for obtaining regional information on cartilage deformation. The ability to study human cartilage response to physiologic loads provides an opportunity for new research toward understanding the role of cartilage biomechanics in cartilage physiology and pathogenesis of OA.

Sustained compression of excised cartilage plugs has been shown to lead to the expected increase in GAG concentration measured with sodium MR imaging.[28] We are not aware of any studies exploring the short-term changes in sodium imaging or dGEMRIC in response to loading in vivo. Indeed, conducting such studies is complicated by the need to allow sufficient time for the mobile ions (Na^+ or $Gd-DTPA^{2-}$) to redistribute in response to deformational changes.

Mechanical loading itself is presumed to modulate cell behavior such that the matrix composition and architecture is appropriate for the prevailing mechanical loading environment. A cross-sectional study of subjects with different exercise habits revealed that elite runners had a significantly higher dGEMRIC index than sedentary subjects,[41] supporting the hypothesis that higher loading environments are associated with higher GAG concentration. In further support of this hypothesis, a study involving exercise intervention showed an increase (decrease) in dGEMRIC index for subjects who increased (decreased) their exercise levels.[42] The degree to which exercise can influence cartilage composition and clinical outcome are as yet unknown; however, studies such as this offer the unprecedented opportunity to explore exercise conditions that may present benefit or risk to joint health.

Repair Processes

Perhaps one of the most intriguing and exciting results that have emerged from these newer methods for monitoring longitudinal changes in cartilage is in the demonstration that both implanted repair tissue and, perhaps more important, native cartilage have the capacity to reverse apparent degenerative or traumatic changes in vivo. These observations call into question the oft-cited claim that cartilage has limited capacity for repair, and presage a paradigm shift in our perspective of OA as a progressive, irreversible, degenerative process to one that is responsive to interventions that can prevent long-term irreversible changes.

Several studies have applied quantitative cartilage T2 mapping in evaluation of cartilage repair tissue in animal models[43] and humans.[44] White and colleagues[43] have shown that repair tissue from osteochondral transplantation that has hyaline cartilage histology retains the normal spatial dependency of T2, although this variation is absent in repair tissue derived from autologous chondrocyte implantation or microfracture techniques. Preliminary studies using matrix-induced autologous chondrocyte implantation suggest the biopolymer scaffolds may allow zonal differentiation of cartilage that more closely resembles the native tissue.[44]

A number of clinical studies have demonstrated an apparent improvement in the biochemical status of native cartilage over time. These include demonstration of an increase in the dGEMRIC index with exercise intervention,[42] after decrease due to traumatic injury,[45] and after surgical intervention.[46]

Predictive Value

It is still too early to know the value of any of these MR imaging measures to clinical decision making, but two recent studies are beginning to provide data along these lines. The first is in relation to hip dysplasia, a developmental malformation of the hip associated with a shallow acetabulum and early OA, often requiring total joint arthroplasty (TJA). One therapeutic strategy to delay TJA is to surgically modify the loading environment through a pelvic osteotomy. The osteotomy serves to rotate the shallow acetabulum so that it covers the femoral head, with the objective of improving joint mechanics, relieving pain, and preserving the joint. Unfortunately, surgical results are variable and appear to depend upon the extent of preexisting arthritis.[47] Presently, the measure of preexisting arthritis is limited to radiographic evidence. A pilot study was conducted to explore whether dGEMRIC could provide a better measure to guide the decision and timing for osteotomy. In a prospective cohort study, subject age, radiographic severity of arthritis, severity of dysplasia, and dGEMRIC index were investigated as metrics to predict early failure after osteotomy. Nine of 52 osteotomies failed, with the dGEMRIC index being the best predictor of failure (P<.002).[46] Though further studies are required, these data are the first to support the notion that an MR imaging technique designed to measure macromolecular status of cartilage has the potential to be used in the context of clinical decision making.

One recent study provides evidence that a low dGEMRIC index in radiographically normal knees might be predictive of subsequent development of radiographic OA.[48] Specifically, dGEMRIC images were taken of subjects having knee pain but no radiographic evidence of OA. Radiographs taken 6 years later revealed that some had developed radiographically apparent OA; subjects having a lower baseline dGEMRIC index were more likely to do so. This was a small study (17 knees in 15 subjects), but nevertheless provides the first evidence that knee pain and low dGEMRIC index may predict increased risk of OA.

Practical Aspects of Clinical Implementation

Technical considerations for human cartilage T2 mapping have been reviewed.[49] Pulse sequences for obtaining quantitative T2 maps, and software for generating color T2 maps are newly available in commercial software packages. Quantitative T2 maps are derived from multi-echo spin-echo imaging sequences by fitting the signal intensity of each pixel to a single exponential decay, although there is evidence to suggest that a multi-exponential decay model is more appropriate, particularly with more advanced tissue damage.[50] The calculated cartilage T2 is dependent on acquisition parameters[51] and the algorithm used in curve-fitting routine.[52] Bias in calculation of T2 can occur through the development of stimulated echoes produced by B1 inhomogeneity as well as magnetization transfer when multislice T2 maps are obtained.[51] Error from stimulated echoes can be reduced by excluding the initial echo from the T2 calculation. With current multi-slice multi-echo techniques, image acquisition times range from 5 to 10 minutes depending on spatial resolution.

To effectively demonstrate the depth-dependent spatial variation in cartilage T2 it is necessary to obtain high resolution T2 maps. For practical purposes, the resolution should be high enough to provide a minimum of six pixels across the cartilage plate. With current technology, in vivo T2 maps with this level of resolution are not feasible. To decrease image acquisition time, parallel imaging, rapid T2 mapping sequences,[53] hybrid gradient-echo/spin-echo,[54] and gradient-echo T2

mapping techniques have been explored, but to date have not been validated for routine use.

In addition to providing efficient T2 relaxation, the high concentration of collagen in the radial zone also decreases signal intensity through magnetization transfer produced by off-resonance irradiation. For collagen-rich tissues such as cartilage, incidental magnetization transfer reduces signal intensity by 15% to 20% as the number of slices and thus the amount of off-resonance irradiation increases. Because gradient-echo techniques use significantly less radiofrequency energy, there is less incidental magnetization transfer with gradient-echo techniques compared with spin-echo and fast spin-echo techniques.

Measuring T1ρ requires special pulse sequences on clinical scanners and therefore is typically only available at research institutions. No specific hardware is needed, but because the measurement is made by applying RF pulses, specific absorption rate (SAR) limits can be reached, especially when transmitting with the body coil and when using multiple RF pulses for data acquisition. However, the use of transmit/receive extremity coils can reduce the SAR.

Computation of T1ρ parameter maps requires multiple datasets with either varied spin-lock time, or varied RF, rendering this a time-consuming technique. Methods to decrease the T1ρ image acquisition time by half include partial k-space (keyhole) techniques;[55] similar techniques are used to reduce SAR.[56] Pakin and colleagues[57] combined three-dimensional imaging with parallel imaging at 3.0 T, demonstrating the ability to decrease both total acquisition time and SAR. The effects of parallel imaging on morphologic (cartilage volume and thickness) and quantitative parameter maps (T1ρ and T2) were also evaluated at 3.0 T with parallel-imaging techniques,[58] demonstrating a high intraclass correlation coefficient as a function of acceleration factor. Three-dimensional T1ρ-weighted imaging was first described by Borthakur and colleagues[59] in 2003 and applied to T1ρ mapping of human articular cartilage.[25]

After creating quantitative parameter maps, methods need to be developed to analyze the cartilage in two or three dimensions and to be able to follow the same subject longitudinally. Taking the average of a whole region of interest will have a large standard deviation due to the inherent spatial variation of the relaxation time from the subchondral bone to the articular surface. Recently, Carballido-Gamio and colleagues[16] have implemented methods to allow for intra- and intersubject comparison and mean T1ρ parameter maps over several individuals. Further refinement of these techniques will allow for population comparison studies.

dGEMRIC can be implemented clinically using standard 1.5 T or 3.0 T imaging hardware. Because of tradeoffs with respect to Gd-DTPA^{2-} relaxivity, there appears to be no particular advantage of 3.0 T over 1.5 T.[60] T1 maps are derived from a sequence of T1-weighted images acquired with an inversion recovery two- or three-dimensional pulse sequence.[61] More recently, fast mapping techniques such as Look-Locker and DESPOT (driven-equilibrium single-pulse observation of T1) have been applied to imaging T1 in cartilage for dGEMRIC applications.[62–65]

As noted, the pulse sequences for these molecular metrics of cartilage are generally not available as standard software packages on standard clinical MR imaging units. However, this situation is beginning to change, as acquisition and analysis packages have recently been introduced on several MR imaging systems (Cartigram from GE, and MapIT from Siemens) that calculate T2 and T1, T2 and T2* maps respectively and allow for fusion or overlay of the molecular metric on an anatomic reference image. Investigators interested in implementing such methods are encouraged to contact groups actively using these new systems to ensure the most up-to-date protocol.

Reproducibility for the molecular indices are beginning to be addressed; however, it is important to note that the MR imaging protocols are still undergoing significant flux and refinement, which will require reevaluation of reproducibility. In addition, and perhaps more important, the effect size of a given lifestyle, pharmacologic, or surgical intervention is not yet known, and therefore it is not clear what level of reproducibility is needed for a given application. For example, although a metric of T2, T1ρ, or dGEMRIC might be stable but at a diseased level in a knee with early OA, the level of improvement during an intervention trial is currently not predictable.

SUMMARY

The ability of MR imaging to see OA as a regional and responsive (ie, reversible) disease leads to new paradigms for developing, circumstances for applying, and means of imaging the therapeutic response to lifestyle, surgical, and disease-modifying drug interventions by providing a metric of the status of the cartilage in an individual on entry to the trial, as well as monitoring biologic effects that might be missed with radiographic monitoring alone. In the long run, alterations in these molecular and physiologic metrics must be correlated with clinically meaningful endpoints, such as improvement in pain, function, or delay in the need for surgical intervention.[66,67] In addition, though this review focuses on articular cartilage, future research must recognize that OA affects all the tissues of the joint, not only articular cartilage. The methods developed for articular cartilage, and the strategy for their development should provide a strong foundation for future development of methods to investigate other tissues. In summary, while development is still in its infancy, MR imaging methods for probing the macromolecular status of cartilage (and other joint tissues) remain very promising in offering information that is not available with standard approaches. As such, MR imaging has great potential to have a positive impact on the future development of disease-modifying strategies for OA.

REFERENCES

1. Billinghurst RC, Dahlberg L, Ionescu M, et al. Enhanced cleavage of type II collagen by collagenases in osteoarthritic articular cartilage. J Clin Invest 1997;99(7):1534–45.
2. Buckwalter JA, Martin J. Degenerative joint disease. Clin Symp 1995;47(2):1–32.
3. Maroudas AI. Balance between swelling pressure and collagen tension in normal and degenerate cartilage. Nature 1976;260(5554):808–9.
4. Weiss C, Rosenberg L, Helfet AJ. An ultrastructural study of normal young adult human articular cartilage. J Bone Joint Surg Am 1968;50(4):663–74.
5. Eisenberg SR, Grodzinsky AJ. Swelling of articular cartilage and other connective tissues: electromechanochemical forces. J Orthop Res 1985;3(2):148–59.
6. Frank EH, Grodzinsky AJ. Cartilage electromechanics. 1. Electrokinetic transduction and the effects of electrolyte pH and ionic strength. J Biomech 1987;20(6):615–27.
7. Lehner KB, Rechl HP, Gmeinwieser JK, et al. Structure, function, and degeneration of bovine hyaline cartilage: assessment with MR imaging in vitro. Radiology 1989;170(2):495–9.
8. Liess C, Lusse S, Karger N, et al. Detection of changes in cartilage water content using MRI T2-mapping in vivo. Osteoarthr Cartil 2002;10(12):907–13.
9. Mosher TJ, Smith H, Dardzinski BJ, et al. MR imaging and T2 mapping of femoral cartilage: in vivo determination of the magic angle effect. AJR Am J Roentgenol 2001;177(3):665–9.
10. Goodwin DW, Wadghiri YZ, Zhu H, et al. Macroscopic structure of articular cartilage of the tibial plateau: influence of a characteristic matrix

architecture on MRI appearance. AJR Am J Roentgenol 2004;182(2):311–8.

11. Xia Y, Moody JB, Alhadlaq H, et al. Characteristics of topographical heterogeneity of articular cartilage over the joint surface of a humeral head. Osteoarthr Cartil 2002;10(5):370–80.

12. Dardzinski BJ, Mosher TJ, Li S, et al. Spatial variation of T2 in human articular cartilage. Radiology 1997;205(2):546–50.

13. Dardzinski BJ, Laor T, Schmithorst VJ, et al. Mapping T2 relaxation time in the pediatric knee: feasibility with a clinical 1.5-T MR imaging system. Radiology 2002;225(1):233–9.

14. Koff MF, Amrami KK, Kaufman KR. Clinical evaluation of T2 values of patellar cartilage in patients with osteoarthritis. Osteoarthr Cartil 2007;15(2): 198–204.

15. Welsch GH, Mamisch TC, Weber M, et al. High-resolution morphological and biochemical imaging of articular cartilage of the ankle joint at 3.0 T using a new dedicated phased array coil: in vivo reproducibility study. Skeletal Radiol 2008;37(6):519–26.

16. Carballido-Gamio J, Link TM, Li X, et al. Feasibility and reproducibility of relaxometry, morphometric, and geometrical measurements of the hip joint with magnetic resonance imaging at 3T. J Magn Reson Imaging 2008;28(1):227–35.

17. Lazovic-Stojkovic J, Mosher TJ, Smith HE, et al. Interphalangeal joint cartilage: high-spatial-resolution in vivo MR T2 mapping—a feasibility study. Radiology 2004;233(1):292–6.

18. Duvvuri U, Reddy R, Patel SD, et al. T1rho-relaxation in articular cartilage: effects of enzymatic degradation. Magn Reson Med 1997;38(6):863–7.

19. Akella SV, Regatte RR, Gougoutas AJ, et al. Proteoglycan-induced changes in T1rho-relaxation of articular cartilage at 4T. Magn Reson Med 2001;46(3): 419–23.

20. Regatte RR, Akella SV, Borthakur A, et al. Proteoglycan depletion-induced changes in transverse relaxation maps of cartilage: comparison of T2 and T1rho. Acad Radiol 2002;9(12):1388–94.

21. Koskinen SK, Yla-Outinen H, Aho HJ, et al. Magnetization transfer and spin lock MR imaging of patellar cartilage degeneration at 0.1 T. Acta Radiol 1997; 38(6):1071–5.

22. Mlynarik V, Trattnig S, Huber M, et al. The role of relaxation times in monitoring proteoglycan depletion in articular cartilage. J Magn Reson Imaging 1999;10(4):497–502.

23. Menezes NM, Gray ML, Hartke JR, et al. T2 and T1rho MRI in articular cartilage systems. Magn Reson Med 2004;51(3):503–9.

24. Duvvuri U, Charagundla SR, Kudchodkar SB, et al. Human knee: in vivo T1(rho)-weighted MR imaging at 1.5 T–preliminary experience. Radiology 2001; 220(3):822–6.

25. Regatte RR, Akella SV, Wheaton AJ, et al. T1 rho-relaxation mapping of human femoral-tibial cartilage in vivo. J Magn Reson Imaging 2003;18(3):336–41.

26. Akella SV, Regatte RR, Borthakur A, et al. T1rho MR imaging of the human wrist in vivo. Acad Radiol 2003;10(6):614–9.

27. Rauscher I, Stahl R, Cheng J, et al. Meniscal measurements of T1rho and T2 at MR imaging in healthy subjects and patients with osteoarthritis. Radiology 2008;249(2):591–600.

28. Lesperance LM, Gray ML, Burstein D. Determination of fixed charge density in cartilage using nuclear magnetic resonance. J Orthop Res 1992;10(1):1–13.

29. Maroudas A. Physicochemical properties of cartilage in the light of ion exchange theory. Biophys J 1968;8(5):575–95.

30. Bashir A, Gray ML, Burstein D. Gd-DTPA2- as a measure of cartilage degradation. Magn Reson Med 1996;36(5):665–73.

31. Burstein D, Velyvis J, Scott KT, et al. Protocol issues for delayed Gd(DTPA)(2⁻)-enhanced MRI (dGEMRIC) for clinical evaluation of articular cartilage. Magn Reson Med 2001;45(1):36–41.

32. Kim YJ, Jaramillo D, Millis MB, et al. Assessment of early osteoarthritis in hip dysplasia with delayed gadolinium-enhanced magnetic resonance imaging of cartilage. J Bone Joint Surg Am 2003;85-A(10): 1987–92.

33. Li X, Benjamin Ma C, Link TM, et al. In vivo T(1rho) and T(2) mapping of articular cartilage in osteoarthritis of the knee using 3T MRI. Osteoarthr Cartil 2007;15(7):789–97.

34. Regatte RR, Akella SV, Lonner JH, et al. T1rho relaxation mapping in human osteoarthritis (OA) cartilage: comparison of T1rho with T2. J Magn Reson Imaging 2006;23(4):547–53.

35. Bolbos RI, Link TM, Ma CB, et al. T1rho relaxation time of the meniscus and its relationship with T1rho of adjacent cartilage in knees with acute ACL injuries at 3 T. Osteoarthr Cartil 2009;17(1): 12–8.

36. Lozano J, Li X, Link TM, et al. Detection of posttraumatic cartilage injury using quantitative T1rho magnetic resonance imaging. A report of two cases with arthroscopic findings. J Bone Joint Surg Am 2006;88(6):1349–52.

37. Nag D, Liney GP, Gillespie P, et al. Quantification of T(2) relaxation changes in articular cartilage with in situ mechanical loading of the knee. J Magn Reson Imaging 2004;19(3):317–22.

38. Mosher TJ, Smith HE, Collins C, et al. Change in knee cartilage T2 at MR imaging after running: a feasibility study. Radiology 2005;234(1):245–9.

39. Guilak F, Ratcliffe A, Mow VC. Chondrocyte deformation and local tissue strain in articular cartilage: a confocal microscopy study. J Orthop Res 1995; 13(3):410–21.

40. Kaab MJ, Ito K, Clark JM, et al. Deformation of artic-ular cartilage collagen structure under static and cyclic loading. J Orthop Res 1998;16(6):743–51.

41. Tiderius CJ, Svensson J, Leander P, et al. dGEMRIC (delayed gadolinium-enhanced MRI of cartilage) indicates adaptive capacity of human knee carti-lage. Magn Reson Med 2004;51(2):286–90.

42. Roos EM, Dahlberg L. Positive effects of moderate exercise on glycosaminoglycan content in knee cartilage: a four-month, randomized, controlled trial in patients at risk of osteoarthritis. Arthritis Rheum 2005;52(11):3507–14.

43. White LM, Sussman MS, Hurtig M, et al. Cartilage T2 assessment: differentiation of normal hyaline carti-lage and reparative tissue after arthroscopic carti-lage repair in equine subjects. Radiology 2006; 241(2):407–14.

44. Welsch GH, Mamisch TC, Domayer SE, et al. Cartilage T2 assessment at 3-T MR imaging: in vivo differentiation of normal hyaline cartilage from reparative tissue after two cartilage repair procedures–initial experience. Radiology 2008; 247(1):154–61.

45. Young AA, Stanwell P, Williams A, et al. Glycos-aminoglycan content of knee cartilage following posterior cruciate ligament rupture demonstrated by delayed gadolinium-enhanced magnetic reso-nance imaging of cartilage (dGEMRIC). A case report. J Bone Joint Surg Am 2005;87(12): 2763–7.

46. Cunningham T, Jessel R, Zurakowski D, et al. De-layed gadolinium-enhanced magnetic resonance imaging of cartilage to predict early failure of Bern-ese periacetabular osteotomy for hip dysplasia. J Bone Joint Surg Am 2006;88(7):1540–8.

47. Minoda Y, Kadowaki T, Kim M. Total hip arthroplasty of dysplastic hip after previous Chiari pelvic osteot-omy. Arch Orthop Trauma Surg 2006;126(6): 394–400.

48. Owman H, Tiderius CJ, Neuman P, et al. Association between findings on delayed gadolinium-enhanced magnetic resonance imaging of cartilage and future knee osteoarthritis. Arthritis Rheum 2008;58(6): 1727–30.

49. Mosher TJ, Dardzinski BJ. Cartilage MRI T2 relaxa-tion time mapping: overview and applications. Semin Musculoskelet Radiol 2004;8(4):355–68.

50. Mosher TJ, Chen Q, Smith MB. 1H magnetic reso-nance spectroscopy of nanomelic chicken cartilage: effect of aggrecan depletion on cartilage T2. Osteo-arthr Cartil 2003;11(10):709–15.

51. Maier CF, Tan SG, Hariharan H, et al. T2 quantitation of articular cartilage at 1.5 T. J Magn Reson Imaging 2003;17(3):358–64.

52. Koff MF, Amrami KK, Felmlee JP, et al. Bias of carti-lage T2 values related to method of calculation. Magn Reson Imaging 2008;26(9):1236–43.

53. Deoni SC, Rutt BK, Peters TM. Rapid combined T1 and T2 mapping using gradient recalled acquisition in the steady state. Magn Reson Med 2003;49(3): 515–26.

54. Van Breuseghem I, Bosmans HT, Elst LV, et al. T2 mapping of human femorotibial cartilage with turbo mixed MR imaging at 1.5 T: feasibility. Radiology 2004;233(2):609–14.

55. Wheaton AJ, Borthakur A, Reddy R. Application of the keyhole technique to T1rho relaxation mapping. J Magn Reson Imaging 2003;18(6):745–9.

56. Wheaton AJ, Borthakur A, Corbo M, et al. Method for reduced SAR T1rho-weighted MRI. Magn Reson Med 2004;51(6):1096–102.

57. Pakin SK, Xu J, Schweitzer ME, et al. Rapid 3D-T1rho mapping of the knee joint at 3.0T with parallel imaging. Magn Reson Med 2006;56(3):563–71.

58. Zuo J, Li X, Banerjee S, et al. Parallel imaging of knee cartilage at 3 Tesla. J Magn Reson Imaging 2007;26(4):1001–9.

59. Borthakur A, Wheaton A, Charagundla SR, et al. Three-dimensional T1rho-weighted MRI at 1.5 Tesla. J Magn Reson Imaging 2003;17(6):730–6.

60. Williams A, Mikulis B, Krishnan N, et al. Suitability of T(1Gd) as the dGEMRIC index at 1.5T and 3.0T. Magn Reson Med 2007;58(4):830–4.

61. McKenzie CA, Williams A, Prasad PV, et al. Three-dimensional delayed gadolinium-enhanced MRI of cartilage (dGEMRIC) at 1.5T and 3.0T. J Magn Reson Imaging 2006;24(4):928–33.

62. Kimelman T, Vu A, Storey P, et al. Three-dimensional T1 mapping for dGEMRIC at 3.0 T using the Look-Locker method. Invest Radiol 2006;41(2):198–203.

63. Li W, Scheidegger R, Wu Y, et al. Accuracy of T1 measurement with 3-D Look-Locker technique for dGEMRIC. J Magn Reson Imaging 2008;27(3): 678–82.

64. Mamisch TC, Dudda M, Hughes T, et al. Comparison of delayed gadolinium enhanced MRI of cartilage (dGEMRIC) using inversion recovery and fast T1 mapping sequences. Magn Reson Med 2008; 60(4):768–73.

65. Wang L, Schweitzer ME, Padua A, et al. Rapid 3D-T(1) mapping of cartilage with variable flip angle and parallel imaging at 3.0T. J Magn Reson Imaging 2008;27(1):154–61.

66. Simon LS. Osteoarthritis, imaging and guidance for approval of a structural "indication". Osteoarthr Car-til 2006;14(Suppl A):A2–3.

67. Burstein D, Gray ML. Potential of molecular imaging of cartilage. Sports Med Arthrosc 2003;11:182–91.

MR Imaging of Intra- and Periarticular Soft Tissues and Subchondral Bone in Knee Osteoarthritis

Michel D. Crema, MD[a],*, Frank W. Roemer, MD[a,b],
Monica D. Marra, MD[a], Ali Guermazi, MD[a]

KEYWORDS
- Knee • Osteoarthritis • MR imaging
- Bone marrow lesions • Synovitis

Although deterioration of the hyaline articular cartilage and osteophyte formation are considered the hallmark features of knee osteoarthritis (OA), it is now widely accepted that OA is a disease of the whole joint including the subchondral bone, synovium, menisci, and ligaments.[1] For decades, radiography has been the main imaging tool to assess osteoarthritic knees.[2,3] However, conventional radiography is only able to depict the osseous joint structures. With magnetic resonance (MR) imaging now widely available, a major paradigm shift has occurred in highlighting the importance of tissues other than bone. Furthermore, hyaline cartilage has no innervation,[4] and sources of pain in patients who have knee OA may include the intrinsic joint structures mentioned above, as well as periarticular structures such as bursae.[5] This article discusses the role of MR imaging assessment of the subchondral bone, synovium, ligaments, and intra- and periarticular soft tissues in patients who have knee OA, focusing on available information on semiquantitative assessment of pathology of these tissues using MR imaging. The role of these alterations in predicting pain and structural progression is also discussed.

SUBCHONDRAL BONE ALTERATIONS

Subchondral bone alterations, including bone marrow edema-like lesions (BMLs), subchondral cyst-like lesions, and attrition, are frequently observed on MR imaging in OA patients. Alterations of the subchondral bone microstructure associated with the different stages of OA are discussed in this article on semiquantitative imaging in OA.

Bone Marrow Edema-Like Lesions

Bone marrow edema-like lesions (BMLs) are defined on MR imaging as noncystic subchondral areas of ill-defined hyperintensity on proton density–weighted, intermediate-weighted, T2-weighted or short tau inversion recovery (STIR) sequences and areas of hypointensity on T1-weighted spin-echo images[6–9] (Fig. 1). MR imaging assessment of BMLs should be performed only on such sequences, because gradient-recalled-echo (GRE)–type sequences such as spoiled gradient-echo at a steady state (SPGR), fast low angle shot (FLASH), three-point Dixon, double-echo steady state (DESS), and others are insensitive to marrow abnormality and may lead to underestimation of size of BMLs[9–11] (Fig. 2). BMLs may be accurately assessed and quantified using appropriate MR imaging sequences.[12,13] It is very important to distinguish degenerative BMLs from other marrow alterations of traumatic or nontraumatic origin,[14] as the differential diagnoses are very broad. These

[a] Quantitative Imaging Center, Department of Radiology, Boston University School of Medicine, 820 Harrison Avenue, FGH Building, 3rd Floor, Boston, MA 02118, USA
[b] Department of Radiology, Klinikum Augsburg, Stenglinstrasse 2, 86156 Augsburg, Germany
* Corresponding author.
E-mail address: michelcrema@gmail.com (M.D. Crema).

Radiol Clin N Am 47 (2009) 687–701
doi:10.1016/j.rcl.2009.04.001
0033-8389/09/$ – see front matter © 2009 Published by Elsevier Inc.

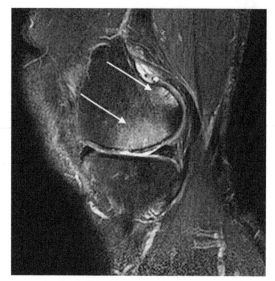

Fig. 1. Sagittal T2-weighted fat-suppressed (T2wFS) MR imaging shows a typical BML: subchondral ill-defined areas of high signal intensity located in the medial femoral condyle (*arrows*). Note adjacent irregular thinning of the articular cartilage in the weight-bearing region of the femur.

BMLs play an important role in predicting structural progression and pain incidence as well as fluctuation of symptoms.[17–22] The term "bone marrow edema-like lesion" or the synonymous "bone marrow lesion" (BML) is now widely accepted to describe these alterations, as edema appears to be only a minor constituent of these abnormalities.[6,23] In a study comparing the MR imaging features of the tibial plateau with histologic specimens in 16 subjects who had severe knee OA before joint replacement, Zanetti and colleagues[6] demonstrated that abnormal tissue appeared only in about half of the regions with MR imaging–detected BMLs. The most common abnormalities were bone marrow necrosis, fibrosis, and trabecular abnormalities. In a study comparing MR imaging features with histopathologic findings in 19 subjects after hip replacement, Taljanovic and colleagues[23] showed that microfractures in different stages of healing and bone marrow necrosis were found in 100% of subjects, and 85% had bone marrow fibrosis. These were the most common abnormalities found at histology, whereas only 40% of subjects had small amounts of edema.

Concerning the natural history of these lesions, BMLs represent a highly variable feature in patients who either have or are at risk for development of knee OA, as their size may increase or decrease over time.[18–20,24] Mechanical limb alignment is thought to directly affect location, prevalence, and change in BMLs, as medial knee BMLs occur mainly in individuals who have

degenerative lesions are frequently detected in conjunction with cartilage damage in the same region.[15,16] Knowing the specific MR imaging characteristics of such lesions is crucial for accurate detection and quantification of degenerative BMLs.

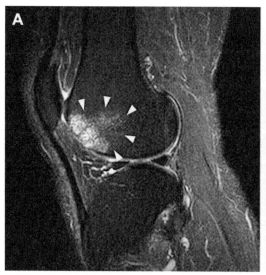
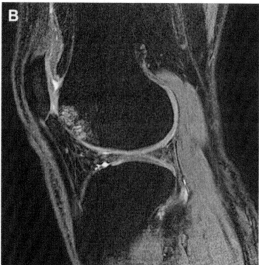

Fig. 2. Subchondral BML located in the lateral femoral trochlea. (*A*) T2wFS MR imaging demonstrates the full extension of the lesion (*arrowheads*). (*B*) 3D water-excitation DESS MR imaging at the same level clearly underestimates the size of this lesion, but distinctly shows the cystic parts of the lesion.

varus-aligned limbs, and lateral lesions occur mostly in those who have valgus-aligned limbs.[21] Furthermore, these lesions are associated with concomitant increased local bone density, suggesting that they may be secondary to long-term excess loading.[25]

Many studies have evaluated the role of BMLs in the progression of knee OA. In a longitudinal study evaluating the association between BMLs and radiographic progression, Felson and colleagues[21] demonstrated that BMLs were powerful predictors of risk of local structural deterioration. The fluctuation of BML size over time seems to have a direct effect on progression of disease assessed on a subregional basis. In a longitudinal MR imaging study, Roemer and colleagues[19] showed that subregions with incident and progressive BMLs demonstrated a higher risk of cartilage loss at follow-up and that absence of BMLs was associated with a lesser risk of cartilage loss in the same subregion. Hunter and colleagues[20] demonstrated that, compared with stable BMLs, enlarging lesions were strongly associated with cartilage loss at follow-up. Presence of BMLs was strongly associated with malalignment and the effect of these lesions on cartilage loss was diluted after adjustment for limb alignment. Another type of BML includes those localized in areas uncovered by articular cartilage, such as the interspinous region at the tibia and the femoral notch. These lesions, known as traction or insertional BMLs, are highly associated with anterior cruciate ligament tears, and may be a consequence of tensile stress on these ligaments[26] (Fig. 3). No relationship between lesions at the interspinous region and femoral notch and cartilage loss has been demonstrated so far.[26] However, lesions extending to the subchondral bone of the medial tibial plateau are associated with regional cartilage loss.

Data about the role of BMLs in predicting pain in patients who have knee OA is controversial. In a cross-sectional study, Felson and colleagues[17] demonstrated that subjects who had radiographic knee OA and pain were more likely to have BMLs than subjects who had no pain. Larger BMLs were found predominantly in the group experiencing pain. In a longitudinal study evaluating the relationship between fluctuation of BMLs and knee pain, Felson and colleagues[18] found that subjects who did not have frequent knee pain who then developed knee pain at follow-up were more likely to show an increase in BML size. In contrast, Kornaat and colleagues[24] found in a longitudinal study that changes in BMLs did not correlate with severity of pain as measured by WOMAC (Western Ontario and McMaster

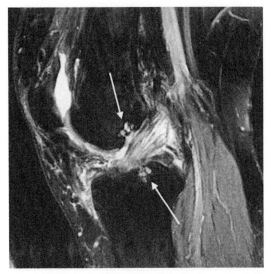

Fig. 3. Sagittal T2wFS MR imaging depicts a partially ruptured ACL. Note associated traction BMLs adjacent to the ligament's insertions at the femur and tibia (*arrows*).

Osteoarthritis) scores. Furthermore, subjects in whom BML size increased did not have a higher WOMAC score than subjects who had a decrease in BML size. Sowers and colleagues[27] found that frequency of BMLs was similar in both painful and painless knee OA, but larger BMLs were seen more frequently in subjects who had pain.

Subchondral Cyst-Like Lesions

Subchondral cyst-like lesions are a common finding in patients who have knee OA. These lesions have a characteristic appearance on MR imaging, demonstrating well-defined rounded areas of fluid-like signal intensity on nonenhanced imaging[6,28] (Fig. 4).

The term "subchondral cyst-like lesion" is probably more appropriate than "subchondral cyst," as no evidence of epithelial lining was detected in several histologic studies.[28–31] The etiology of subchondral cyst-like lesions is unknown. Two principal theories have been proposed: synovial fluid intrusion and bony contusion. The synovial fluid intrusion theory suggests that elevated intraarticular pressure may lead to the intrusion of joint fluid into the subchondral bone via fissured or ulcerated cartilage,[29,32] thus creating these lesions. The bony contusion theory suggests that subchondral cyst-like lesions are a consequence of traumatic bone necrosis following impact of two opposing articular surfaces.[30,33]

A recent cross-sectional study reported that subchondral cyst-like lesions were present in

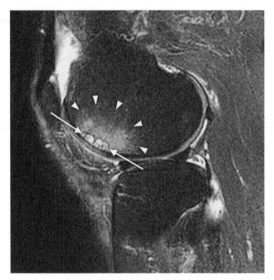

Fig. 4. Sagittal T2wFS MR imaging shows two areas of high signal intensity surrounded by a well-demarcated hypointense rim (*arrows*), representing subchondral cyst-like signal alterations. These are located directly subchondrally and are part of an ill-defined larger BML (*arrowheads*) in the lateral trochlea. Note intact adjacent cartilage.

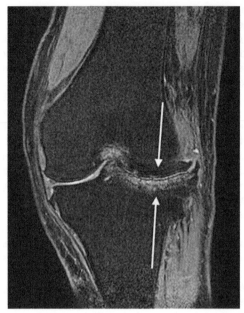

Fig. 5. Coronal GRE-type 3D water-excitation DESS MR imaging shows severe subchondral bone attrition in the lateral tibiofemoral compartment with flattening of the lateral femoral articular surface and depression of the lateral tibial plateau (*arrows*). Note also adjacent osteophytes.

subregions without full thickness cartilage defects in about half of the cases, a finding that does not support the synovial fluid intrusion theory.[34] Subchondral cysts are strongly associated with BMLs in the same subregion, and may develop within areas of noncystic BMLs,[34,35] which favors the bony contusion theory.

Two studies have found no association between the presence of subchondral cyst-like lesions and pain in subjects who have knee OA.[36,37]

Subchondral Bone Attrition

Subchondral bone attrition is defined as depression or flattening of the subchondral bony surface unrelated to gross fracture. It can be assessed on radiographs or semiquantitatively on MR imaging[12,38] (Fig. 5). Although attrition is usually observed in advanced knee OA, it may also appear in knees with mild OA that do not exhibit joint space narrowing on radiographs.[39]

The pathogenesis of subchondral bone attrition in knee OA is unknown. Subchondral microfracturing and remodeling due to alterations in mechanical loading, which are reflected as subchondral BMLs, may explain the presence and development of bone attrition in OA. A strong association between prevalent subchondral bone attrition and subchondral BMLs in the same subregion has been reported, and the association increased with BML size.[40] Furthermore, the risk of incident

subchondral bone attrition was elevated for subregions presenting baseline BMLs. Neogi and colleagues[41] showed that both prevalence and incidence of subchondral bone attrition are associated with knee malalignment, suggesting that attrition is a reflection of compartment-specific mechanical load. The same group[42] found that subchondral bone attrition is a good predictor of cartilage loss.

Attrition seems to play a role in predicting knee pain. In a recent cross-sectional study, Hernandez-Molina and colleagues[43] demonstrated that bone attrition was associated with knee pain, even after adjustment for other known factors linked to pain, suggesting an independent association of these features. Other studies have also suggested that subchondral bone attrition predicts knee pain.[37,38]

SYNOVITIS

Although synovitis in OA is thought to be a secondary phenomenon related to cartilage deterioration, its importance in the OA process is well recognized.[44–49] Degenerative joints usually demonstrate signs of synovitis, even in the early phase of disease.[50–52]

Several methods for detecting and quantifying synovitis with nonenhanced and contrast-enhanced

MR imaging are available. In a pathologic study conducted by Fernandez-Madrid and colleagues,[51] signal alterations in the Hoffa's fat pad correlated with mild chronic synovitis. This work led to the assumption that synovitis may be assessed on nonenhanced images, mainly proton density– or T2-weighted sequences, using signal alterations in the Hoffa's fat pad as a surrogate for whole-knee synovitis (Fig. 6).[45,46] Signal alterations in Hoffa's fat pad are a common finding on MR imaging of the knee and present a multitude of possible diagnoses (Fig. 7).[53] Roemer and colleagues[54] found that signal alterations in Hoffa's fat pad seen on noncontrast-enhanced sequences were a sensitive but not a specific sign of peripatellar synovitis, compared with contrast-enhanced sequences. Recently, another scoring system for the assessment of synovitis using nonenhanced scans has been introduced,[55] but it has not been tested against an established reference standard such as contrast-enhanced MR imaging or histology.[56] In a recent study comparing three scoring systems for evaluating synovitis and joint effusion on MR imaging, Loeuille and colleagues[57] found that only scoring of contrast-enhanced T1-weighted images correlated with microscopically proven synovitis. No correlation with microscopic synovitis was found when MR imaging was performed without contrast intravenous administration. Thus, ideally, synovitis should be assessed on contrast-enhanced T1-weighted MR imaging sequences, allowing evaluation of enhancement and thickening of the synovial membrane (Fig. 8).[58–60] Only contrast-enhanced images can differentiate between synovium and joint effusion. A new scoring system that uses contrast-enhanced T1-weighted sequences to assess synovitis at multiple sites in subjects who had knee OA was presented recently.[49] Synovial thickness was measured at the peripatellar region, around the cruciate ligaments and menisci, and around popliteal cysts and loose bodies if present, allowing assessment of synovitis at the whole knee joint. The reliability of the reading was good-to-excellent for the 11 different synovitis locations.

There is evidence that synovitis is not only a secondary phenomenon in subjects who have knee OA but also plays a role in progression of cartilage loss. In a longitudinal study with 422 subjects, Ayral and colleagues[47] assessed the medial perimeniscal synovium and the medial tibiofemoral cartilage using arthroscopy, and found that 123 subjects (29%) had a reactive aspect and 89 (21%) had an inflammatory aspect of the synovium. Interestingly, only the inflammatory synovitis group showed an association with cartilage loss at follow-up. Although histologic evaluation was not performed, previous studies have demonstrated a good correlation between arthroscopic and microscopic findings of synovitis.[61,62]

Synovial inflammation is believed to contribute to pain in patients who have knee OA, even though nociceptive fibers are inconsistently present within the synovial membrane.[4] Hill and colleagues[46]

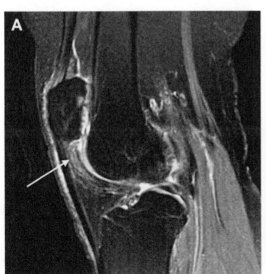
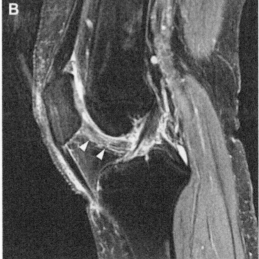

Fig. 6. Sagittal T2wFS MR imaging depicts signal alterations in the (A) infrapatellar (arrow) and (B) intercondylar (arrowheads) regions of Hoffa's fat pad. These are used as a surrogate for peripatellar synovitis in osteoarthritis trials.

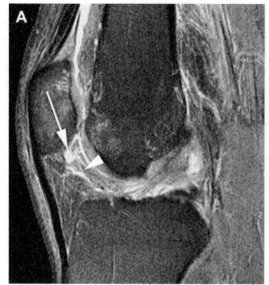
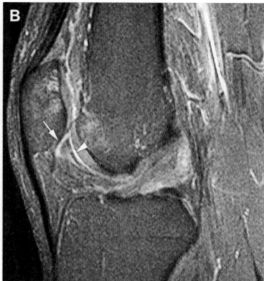

Fig. 7. Example of overestimation using signal changes in Hoffa's fat pad on nonenhanced images as a surrogate for synovitis. (*A*) Sagittal PDwFS image. Grade 2 infrapatellar signal change (*large arrow*) and grade 2 intercondylar signal change (*large arrowhead*). (*B*) Sagittal CE T1wFS image. Discrete grade 1 infrapatellar signal change (*enhancement–small arrow*) and discrete grade 1 intercondylar signal change (*enhancement–small arrowhead*).

showed that alterations in Hoffa's fat pad signal changes over time were modestly and directly correlated with changes in knee pain, but not with cartilage loss. Interestingly, the effect of these signal alterations on pain was independent of changes in joint effusion. In another cross-sectional study, the same group found that these alterations were far more common in subjects who had knee pain and radiographic OA than those who had radiographic OA and no pain.[45] However, both studies relied on noncontrast-enhanced MR imaging sequences. Recent studies assessing synovitis on contrast-enhanced MR imaging in subjects who either have or are at risk for knee OA demonstrated that high grade synovitis (graded from 0 to 2) was associated with knee pain compared with subjects who had no or low-grade synovitis.[48,49]

EFFUSION

Joint effusion is commonly detected in patients who have moderate-to-advanced knee OA,[45,63] and reflects synovial activation secondary to ligament injury, loose bodies, hyaline cartilage deterioration, and meniscal damage.[64] Joint effusion is ideally assessed and quantified on proton density–weighted, T2-weighted and STIR MR imaging sequences.[12,13] However, synovial thickening as seen in synovitis increases the total synovial volume in such sequences, and differentiating synovium and joint effusion on nonenhanced MR

imaging sequences is difficult (Fig. 9). The prevalence of joint effusion has a direct relationship with radiographic severity in the knee joint.[63] In a cohort of 1368 knees without radiographic knee OA, the prevalence of joint effusion was 33.7% and the large majority of effusions were

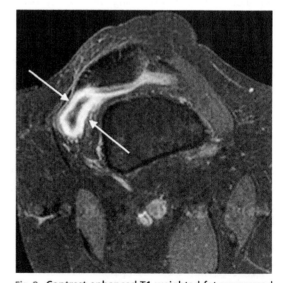

Fig. 8. Contrast-enhanced T1-weighted fat-suppressed (CE T1wFS) MR imaging demonstrates marked thickening and enhancement of the synovial membrane in the lateral parapatellar region. Note the adjacent low-signal intensity of the joint fluid well distinguished from the thickened synovium (*arrows*).

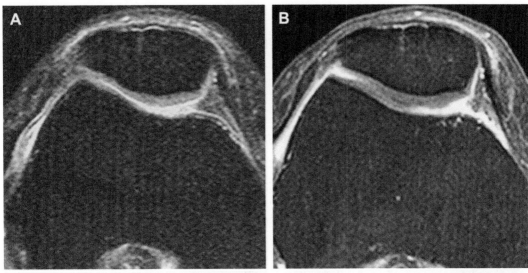

Fig. 9. Evaluation of synovial thickening and joint effusion on nonenhanced PDwFS and CE T1wFS MR imaging. (A) Axial PDwFS MR imaging shows high intensity fluid-equivalent signal in the patellofemoral joint space. (B) The axial CE T1wFS MR imaging demonstrates marked synovial thickening and enhancement in the same region. (Apparently the nonenhanced scan was not adequate for assessment.)

small.[64] Hill and colleagues[45] reported a high prevalence of joint effusion in individuals who had radiographic knee OA. Effusion was present in 91.7% of subjects who had radiographic OA and knee pain, and in 82.3% of those who had radiographic OA and no pain. In the same study, it was demonstrated that moderate and large effusions (graded from 0 to 3) were significantly more common among those who had knee pain. A significant association between grades of effusion (graded in conjunction with synovitis on nonenhanced MR imaging) with knee pain severity was found by Torres and colleagues[37] in a cohort of 143 subjects who had knee OA. The joint capsule contains pain fibers, and capsule distension associated with joint effusions may contribute to knee pain in OA.

CRUCIATE AND COLLATERAL LIGAMENTS

It is well recognized that traumatic complete *anterior cruciate ligament* (ACL) tears may lead to premature degeneration of the knee joint.[65–68] However, the role of traumatic incomplete ACL tears in predicting knee OA is unclear.[69] ACL disruption will inevitably cause alterations in knee kinematics, as the ACL is the primary restraint against tibial translation.[70] Furthermore, ACL failure increases the external adduction moment and consequently medial loading, increasing the risk of medial knee OA.[71] ACL tears are frequently associated with other relevant traumatic lesions in the knee such as meniscal tears and chondral/

osteochondral lesions, making the assessment of its role in knee degeneration more difficult.[72]

Incidental ACL tears are common among patients who have knee OA, with a reported prevalence ranging from 20 to 35%.[71,73,74] Patients who have knee OA and incidental ACL tears are often unable to recall significant knee injury. Degeneration within the ligament fibers, alterations in the notch width and depth, and the presence of notch osteophytes (Fig. 10) may predispose to ACL tears in patients who have knee OA.[75–78] Scoring methods to assess cruciate ligament tears in patients who have knee OA are available.[12,13] Usually, cruciate ligaments are scored as having a complete tear or not. In the BLOKS (Boston Leeds Osteoarthritis Knee Score) system[13] the presence of ligament repair is also noted. Evaluation of the cruciate ligaments in these scoring systems also includes assessment for tears and insertional or traction BMLs. Hernandez-Molina and colleagues[26] showed that traction BMLs, detected on MR imaging at the femoral and tibial insertions of the ACL, were strongly related to ACL pathology.

The role of ACL tears in predicting structural progression in patients who have knee OA remains unclear. In a recent longitudinal study, Amin and colleagues[79] found that the presence of an ACL tear at baseline increased the risk for cartilage loss in the medial compartment at 30-month follow-up. However, when adjustment for medial meniscal damage was performed, this effect was diluted. In a large cohort of 245 elderly subjects

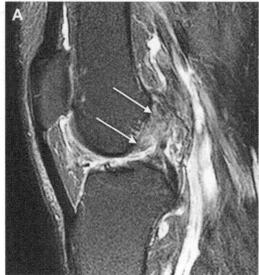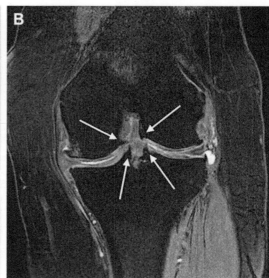

Fig. 10. (*A*) Sagittal T2wFS MR imaging shows a complete disruption of the ACL (*arrows*). (*B*) Coronal 3D water-excitation DESS MR imaging exhibits osteophytic formation around the femoral notch and the tibial spines (*arrows*), believed to be a risk factor for incidental nontraumatic ACL failure in patients who have knee OA.

(aged 70–79), the prevalence of any ligament tear in the knee was 27% in men and 30% in women, and a good correlation with cartilage loss was found.[80] However, no longitudinal assessment was performed.

The contribution of ACL tears to pain severity in patients who have knee OA is also unclear. Hill and colleagues[71] showed that complete ACL tears were common (22.8%) in a population with symptomatic knee OA and poor recall of knee trauma, and rare (2.7%) among those without knee symptoms. Another group reported that subjects who had a complete ACL tear tended to have greater knee pain at baseline, but no overall differences in pain severity were found after adjustment for potential confounders.[79] In both studies, the ACL was scored as pathologic when a complete tear was detected.

The **posterior cruciate ligament** (PCL) plays a role in the kinematics of the knee, mainly for the medial compartment, and a tear with a subsequent deficiency may increase the incidence of knee OA.[81,82] In a long follow-up study of 58 subjects who had isolated partial or complete PCL tears treated conservatively and evaluated after 2 to 19.3 years (mean 6.9 years), Patel and colleagues[83] found that 10 (17.2%) developed medial tibiofemoral radiographic OA. Incidental complete PCL tears are rare among patients who have knee OA.

Incidental **collateral ligaments** tears are infrequent among patients who have knee OA.[37] The WORMS (Whole-Organ Magnetic Resonance

Imaging Score) system allows assessment of collateral ligament tears in patients who have knee OA.[12] Collateral ligaments are scored as normal; thickened but continuous; or ruptured. In a small cohort of 30 subjects who had medial compartment knee OA without history of trauma and 30 age-matched subjects who had atraumatic knee pain but without OA, signal changes in or around the medial collateral ligament (MCL) (grade 1 and 2 lesions) were seen in 27 (90%) of the first group, but in only 2 (6.6%) from the control group,[84] suggesting that grade 1 and 2 MCL lesions may be related to medial knee OA in patients who have no history of trauma. The role of collateral ligament abnormalities in predicting structural progression and pain in patients who have OA is unknown.

PERIARTICULAR CYSTS AND BURSAE

A wide spectrum of periarticular cystic lesions may be encountered in knee OA.[85] Most cystic lesions around the knee are encapsulated fluid collections exhibiting low signal intensity on T1-weighted images and high signal intensity on T2-weighted images.[85,86]

Popliteal cysts ("Baker cysts") are not true cysts, but fluid in the semimembranosus–medial gastrocnemius bursa (**Fig. 11**). The extravasation of joint fluid through the posteromedial capsule between the medial head of the gastrocnemius and the semimembranosus tendon into the bursa located between these muscles seems to occur

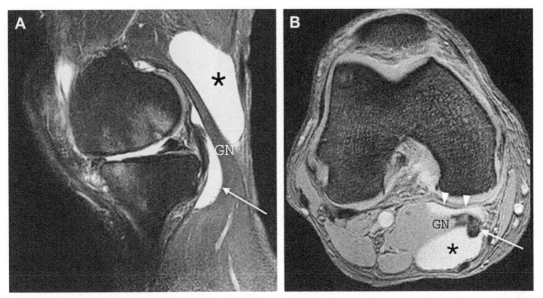

Fig. 11. Popliteal cyst ("Baker cyst") in a patient who has knee OA. Sagittal T2wFS spin-echo (A) and axial T2wFS gradient-echo (B) MR imaging shows fluid collection within the semimembranosus–gastrocnemius bursa ("Baker cyst", *asterisk*), extending posteriorly between the semimembranosus tendon (*arrow–B*) and the medial head of the gastrocnemius (GN). This bursa communicates with the knee joint via the subgastrocnemius bursa (*arrow–A*; *arrowheads–B*).

as a result of increased intraarticular pressure caused by joint effusions or altered biomechanics within the knee, as seen in meniscal tears or degenerative joint disease. Complications such as rupture of cysts and the presence of intracystic hemorrhage or loose bodies may also occur. Popliteal cysts are commonly detected in patients who have knee OA.[45,63,87] Hill and colleagues[45] found that the prevalence of these lesions was 43.2% in knees with moderate or larger effusions, compared with 22.7% in those with little or no effusion. In this study, presence of popliteal cysts was not associated with pain. However, different grades of synovitis may be present around

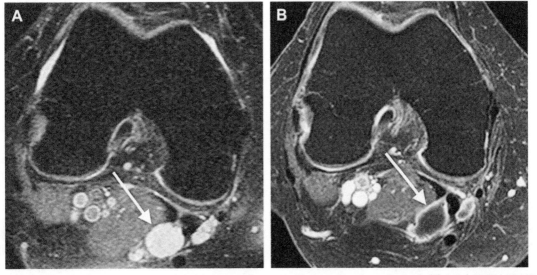

Fig. 12. Popliteal cyst. (A) Axial PDwFS MR imaging shows a typical popliteal cyst (*arrow*). (B) Axial CE T1wFS MR imaging demonstrates enhancement and thickening of the synovial membrane surrounding the popliteal cyst (*arrow*).

popliteal cysts[49] (**Fig. 12**). Moderate-to-large popliteal cysts are associated with incidental radiographic knee OA.[88]

A wide spectrum of bursitides may occur in patients who have knee OA.[85] ***Prepatellar bursitis*** (**Fig. 13**) may be seen in conjunction with knee OA, but its pathogenesis is thought not to be directly linked to degeneration. Overuse injury or chronic trauma of the subcutaneous tissues adjacent to the patella and to the proximal patellar tendon are the most common causes.[85] A less common site of bursitis is the **superficial infrapatellar bursa**, appearing on MR imaging as a fluid collection anterior to the tibial tubercle. A tiny amount of fluid within the **deep infrapatellar bursa** is frequently detected on MR imaging of the knee, including patients who have OA.[5] However, it may be considered a normal finding without clinical significance due to its high prevalence in asymptomatic subjects[5,89] (**Fig. 14**). ***Anserine bursitis*** (**Fig. 15**) may be detected in conjunction with knee OA, but its association with degeneration is controversial. Chronic anserine bursitis is thought to be most common in elderly patients who have degenerative disease or rheumatoid arthritis.[90] However, a recent case-control study found no association between prevalent anserine bursitis and radiographic knee OA.[91] Furthermore, anserine bursitis shows no significant association with incident knee pain or incident radiographic OA.[88]

Parameniscal cysts are though to be formed by fluid extravasation through a meniscal tear into the parameniscal soft tissue.[89] Most of these cysts result from horizontal tears, which are though to be of degenerative origin and are a common finding in knee OA[92–94] (**Fig. 16**). Lateral meniscal cysts (see **Fig. 16**) are associated with incident knee pain longitudinally.[88] ***Ganglion cysts***

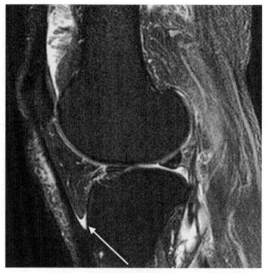

Fig. 14. Sagittal T2wFS MR imaging shows a tiny amount of fluid within the deep infrapatellar bursa (*arrow*), which is located between the distal patellar tendon and the anterior tibial surface. This finding is observed regularly in asymptomatic individuals, and should not be mistaken for bursitis.

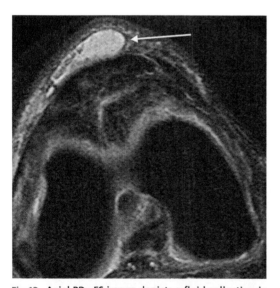

Fig. 13. Axial PDwFS image depicts a fluid collection in the subcutaneous fat anteriorly to the proximal patellar tendon, consistent with prepatellar bursitis (*arrows*).

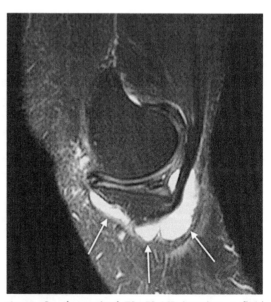

Fig. 15. On the sagittal T2wFS MR imaging, a fluid collection adjacent to the tibial insertion of the pes anserinus tendons is visualized, a finding consistent with anserine bursitis (*arrows*).

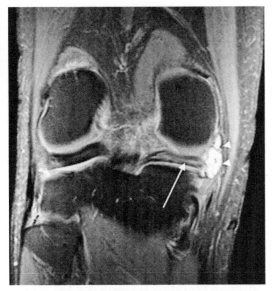

Fig. 16. Coronal T2wFS MR imaging shows a horizontal meniscal tear (*arrow*) and an adjacent parameniscal cyst originating from the posterior horn of the medial meniscus (*arrowheads*).

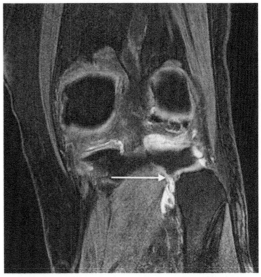

Fig. 18. Coronal 3D water-excitation DESS MR imaging shows a fusiform synovial cyst with its neck originating from the proximal tibiofibular joint (*arrow*).

(Fig. 17) around the knee are routinely detected on MR imaging examinations.[85] They may be seen in conjunction with OA, but accepted theories for ganglia formation are not directly related to OA.[95–97] *Tibiofibular synovial cysts* (Fig. 18) are more prevalent in patients who have knee effusion, because in 10% of adults the proximal tibiofibular joint communicates with the knee joint. The probable pathogenesis is increased pressure in the knee joint leading to dilatation of the tibiofibular joint capsule.[98] The reported prevalence in patients who have knee OA is low.[5] Other cystic lesions around the osteoarthritic knee are extremely rare.

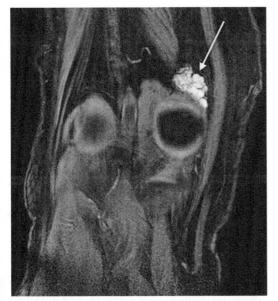

Fig. 17. Coronal 3D water-excitation DESS MR imaging sequence demonstrates an extraarticular multiloculated fluid collection adjacent to the posterior medial femoral condyle, consistent with an extraarticular ganglion cyst (*arrow*).

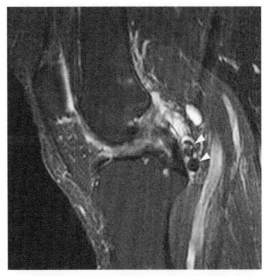

Fig. 19. Sagittal T2wFS MR imaging illustrates two intraarticular loose bodies (*arrowheads*) located between the posterior cruciate ligament and the posterior joint capsule.

LOOSE BODIES

Loose bodies are seen regularly in conjunction with knee OA, especially in severe cases. Chondral fragments, detached osteophytes, and meniscal fragments, for example, may originate loose bodies in knee OA. Synovial osteochondromatosis must also be considered.[99] The presence of loose bodies is related to internal knee derangement in patients who have OA.[100,101] They may trigger synovial inflammation as demonstrated by a recent study using contrast-enhanced MR imaging,[49] and are a common indication for arthroscopic treatment.[100,101] On MR imaging, loose bodies are best visualized in joints with prevalent effusion and may be delineated as solitary or multiple low signal intensity abnormalities within the joint (Fig. 19).

SUMMARY

Osteoarthritis of the knee is considered a disease of the whole joint. MR imaging has added much to our understanding of all the joint tissues involved in the disease process, such as the subchondral bone, synovium, ligaments, and periarticular soft tissues and their significance in explaining pain and structural progression. The use of appropriate MR imaging pulse sequences is crucial, allowing accurate assessment and quantification of these alterations. Reliable semi-quantitative scoring systems are available to assess and quantify subchondral bone, synovium, ligaments, and periarticular alterations. Contrast-enhanced MR imaging should be considered in the assessment of whole knee synovitis, as it enables accurate evaluation and quantification of synovial thickness.

REFERENCES

1. Felson DT. An update on the pathogenesis and epidemiology of osteoarthritis. Radiol Clin North Am 2004;42:1–9, v.
2. Kellgren JH, Lawrence JS. Radiological assessment of osteo-arthrosis. Ann Rheum Dis 1957;16: 494–502.
3. Emrani PS, Katz JN, Kessler CL, et al. Joint space narrowing and Kellgren-Lawrence progression in knee osteoarthritis: an analytic literature synthesis. Osteoarthritis Cartilage 2008;16: 873–82.
4. Dye SF, Vaupel GL, Dye CC. Conscious neurosensory mapping of the internal structures of the human knee without intraarticular anesthesia. Am J Sports Med 1998;26:773–7.
5. Hill CL, Gale DR, Chaisson CE, et al. Periarticular lesions detected on magnetic resonance imaging: prevalence in knees with and without symptoms. Arthritis Rheum 2003;48:2836–44.
6. Zanetti M, Bruder E, Romero J, et al. Bone marrow edema pattern in osteoarthritic knees: correlation between MR imaging and histologic findings. Radiology 2000;215:835–40.
7. Bergman AG, Willen HK, Lindstrand AL, et al. Osteoarthritis of the knee: correlation of subchondral MR signal abnormalities with histopathologic and radiographic features. Skeletal Radiol 1994;23: 445–8.
8. Yu JS, Cook PA. Magnetic resonance imaging (MRI) of the knee: a pattern approach for evaluating bone marrow edema. Crit Rev Diagn Imaging 1996;37:261–303.
9. Roemer FW, Hunter DJ, Guermazi A. MRI-based semiquantitative assessment of subchondral bone marrow lesions in osteoarthritis research. Osteoarthritis Cartilage 2008;17:414–5.
10. Peterfy CG, Gold G, Eckstein F, et al. MRI protocols for whole-organ assessment of the knee in osteoarthritis. Osteoarthritis Cartilage 2006;14(Suppl A): A95–111.
11. Yoshioka H, Stevens K, Hargreaves BA, et al. Magnetic resonance imaging of articular cartilage of the knee: comparison between fat-suppressed three-dimensional SPGR imaging, fat-suppressed FSE imaging, and fat-suppressed three-dimensional DEFT imaging, and correlation with arthroscopy. J Magn Reson Imaging 2004; 20:857–64.
12. Peterfy CG, Guermazi A, Zaim S, et al. Whole-Organ Magnetic Resonance Imaging Score (WORMS) of the knee in osteoarthritis. Osteoarthritis Cartilage 2004;12:177–90.
13. Hunter DJ, Lo GH, Gale D, et al. The reliability of a new scoring system for knee osteoarthritis MRI and the validity of bone marrow lesion assessment: BLOKS (Boston Leeds Osteoarthritis Knee Score). Ann Rheum Dis 2008;67:206–11.
14. Roemer FM, Frobell R, Hunter DJ, et al. MRI-detected subchondral bone marrow signal alterations of the knee joint: terminology, imaging appearance, relevance and radiological differential diagnosis. Osteoarthritis Cartilage 2009; [Epub ahead of print].
15. Baranyay FJ, Wang Y, Wluka AE, et al. Association of bone marrow lesions with knee structures and risk factors for bone marrow lesions in the knees of clinically healthy, community-based adults. Semin Arthritis Rheum 2007;37: 112–8.
16. Guymer E, Baranyay F, Wluka AE, et al. A study of the prevalence and associations of subchondral bone marrow lesions in the knees of healthy, middle-aged women. Osteoarthritis Cartilage 2007;15:1437–42.

17. Felson DT, Chaisson CE, Hill CL, et al. The association of bone marrow lesions with pain in knee osteoarthritis. Ann Intern Med 2001;134:541–9.

18. Felson DT, Niu J, Guermazi A, et al. Correlation of the development of knee pain with enlarging bone marrow lesions on magnetic resonance imaging. Arthritis Rheum 2007;56:2986–92.

19. Roemer FW, Guermazi A, Javaid MK, et al. Change in MRI-detected subchondral bone marrow lesions is associated with cartilage loss. The MOST study: a longitudinal multicenter study of knee osteoarthritis. Ann Rheum Dis 2008; [Epub ahead of print].

20. Hunter DJ, Zhang Y, Niu J, et al. Increase in bone marrow lesions associated with cartilage loss: a longitudinal magnetic resonance imaging study of knee osteoarthritis. Arthritis Rheum 2006;54: 1529–35.

21. Felson DT, McLaughlin S, Goggins J, et al. Bone marrow edema and its relation to progression of knee osteoarthritis. Ann Intern Med 2003;139: 330–6.

22. Zhang Y, Nevitt M, Niu J, et al. Reversible MRI features and knee pain fluctuation: the MOST study. Osteoarthritis Cartilage 2007;15(Suppl 3):C17.

23. Taljanovic MS, Graham AR, Benjamin JB, et al. Bone marrow edema pattern in advanced hip osteoarthritis: quantitative assessment with magnetic resonance imaging and correlation with clinical examination, radiographic findings, and histopathology. Skeletal Radiol 2008;37:423–31.

24. Kornaat PR, Kloppenburg M, Sharma R, et al. Bone marrow edema-like lesions change in volume in the majority of patients with osteoarthritis; associations with clinical features. Eur Radiol 2007;17:3073–8.

25. Lo GH, Hunter DJ, Zhang Y, et al. Bone marrow lesions in the knee are associated with increased local bone density. Arthritis Rheum 2005;52: 2814–21.

26. Hernandez-Molina G, Guermazi A, Niu J, et al. Central bone marrow lesions in symptomatic knee osteoarthritis and their relationship to anterior cruciate ligament tears and cartilage loss. Arthritis Rheum 2008;58:130–6.

27. Sowers MF, Hayes C, Jamadar D, et al. Magnetic resonance-detected subchondral bone marrow and cartilage defect characteristics associated with pain and X-ray-defined knee osteoarthritis. Osteoarthritis Cartilage 2003;11:387–93.

28. Pouders C, De Maeseneer M, Van Roy P, et al. Prevalence and MRI-anatomic correlation of bone cysts in osteoarthritic knees. AJR Am J Roentgenol 2008;190:17–21.

29. Landells JW. The bone cysts of osteoarthritis. J Bone Joint Surg Br 1953;35:643–9.

30. Rhaney K, Lamb DW. The cysts of osteoarthritis of the hip; a radiological and pathological study. J Bone Joint Surg Br 1955;37:663–75.

31. Resnick D, Niwayama G, Coutts RD. Subchondral cysts (geodes) in arthritic disorders: pathologic and radiographic appearance of the hip joint. AJR Am J Roentgenol 1977;128:799–806.

32. Freund E. The pathological significance of intra-articular pressure. Edinb Med J 1940;47: 192–203.

33. Ferguson AB Jr. The pathological changes in degenerative arthritis of the hip and treatment by rotational osteotomy. J Bone Joint Surg Am 1964; 46:1337–52.

34. Crema MD, Roemer FW, Marra MD, et al. MRI-detected bone marrow edema-like lesions are strongly associated with subchondral cysts in patients with or at risk for knee osteoarthritis: the MOST study. Osteoarthritis Cartilage 2008; 16(Suppl 4):160.

35. Carrino JA, Blum J, Parellada JA, et al. MRI of bone marrow edema-like signal in the pathogenesis of subchondral cysts. Osteoarthritis Cartilage 2006; 14:1081–5.

36. Kornaat PR, Bloem JL, Ceulemans RY, et al. Osteoarthritis of the knee: association between clinical features and MR imaging findings. Radiology 2006;239:811–7.

37. Torres L, Dunlop DD, Peterfy C, et al. The relationship between specific tissue lesions and pain severity in persons with knee osteoarthritis. Osteoarthritis Cartilage 2006;14:1033–40.

38. Dieppe PA, Reichenbach S, Williams S, et al. Assessing bone loss on radiographs of the knee in osteoarthritis: a cross-sectional study. Arthritis Rheum 2005;52:3536–41.

39. Reichenbach S, Guermazi A, Niu J, et al. Prevalence of bone attrition on knee radiographs and MRI in a community-based cohort. Osteoarthritis Cartilage 2008;16:1005–10.

40. Roemer FW. Tibiofemoral subchondral bone marrow lesions and the association with prevalent and incident subchondral bone attrition: the MOST study. Osteoarthr Cartil 2008;89:594–5.

41. Neogi T, Nevitt M, Niu J, et al. Subchondral bone attrition is a reflection of compartment-specific mechanical load: the MOST study. Osteoarthr Cartil 2008;16(Suppl 4):S140–1.

42. Neogi T, Zhang Y, Niu J, et al. Cartilage loss occurs in the same subregions as subchondral bone attrition: the MOST study. Osteoarthr Cartil 2008; 16(Suppl 4):S172–3.

43. Hernandez-Molina G, Neogi T, Hunter DJ, et al. The association of bone attrition with knee pain and other MRI features of osteoarthritis. Ann Rheum Dis 2007; [Epub ahead of print].

44. Pelletier JP, Martel-Pelletier J, Abramson SB. Osteoarthritis, an inflammatory disease: potential implication for the selection of new therapeutic targets. Arthritis Rheum 2001;44:1237–47.

45. Hill CL, Gale DG, Chaisson CE, et al. Knee effusions, popliteal cysts, and synovial thickening: association with knee pain in osteoarthritis. J Rheumatol 2001;28:1330–7.

46. Hill CL, Hunter DJ, Niu J, et al. Synovitis detected on magnetic resonance imaging and its relation to pain and cartilage loss in knee osteoarthritis. Ann Rheum Dis 2007;66:1599–603.

47. Ayral X, Pickering EH, Woodworth TG, et al. Synovitis: a potential predictive factor of structural progression of medial tibiofemoral knee osteoarthritis – results of a 1 year longitudinal arthroscopic study in 422 patients. Osteoarthritis Cartilage 2005;13:361–7.

48. Marra MD, Roemer FW, Crema MD, et al. Peripatellar synovitis in osteoarthritis: comparison of non-enhanced and enhanced magnetic resonance imaging (MRI) and its association with peripatellar knee pain: the MOST study. Osteoarthritis Cartilage 2008;16(Suppl 4):S167.

49. Guermazi A, Roemer FW, Crema MD, et al. Assessment of synovitis in knee osteoarthritis on contrast-enhanced MRI using a novel comprehensive semiquantitative scoring system. Arthritis Rheum 2008;58:S696–7.

50. Loeuille D, Chary-Valckenaere I, Champigneulle J, et al. Macroscopic and microscopic features of synovial membrane inflammation in the osteoarthritic knee: correlating magnetic resonance imaging findings with disease severity. Arthritis Rheum 2005;52:3492–501.

51. Fernandez-Madrid F, Karvonen RL, Teitge RA, et al. Synovial thickening detected by MR imaging in osteoarthritis of the knee confirmed by biopsy as synovitis. Magn Reson Imaging 1995;13:177–83.

52. Lindblad S, Hedfors E. Arthroscopic and immunohistologic characterization of knee joint synovitis in osteoarthritis. Arthritis Rheum 1987;30:1081–8.

53. Saddik D, McNally EG, Richardson M. MRI of Hoffa's fat pad. Skeletal Radiol 2004;33:433–44.

54. Roemer FW, Guermazi A, Zhang Y, et al. Evaluation of Hoffa's fat pad findings on non-contrast enhanced MR imaging as a measure of patellofemoral knee synovitis in osteoarthritis. AJR Am J Roentgenol, in print.

55. Pelletier JP, Raynauld JP, Abram F, et al. A new non-invasive method to assess synovitis severity in relation to symptoms and cartilage volume loss in knee osteoarthritis patients using MRI. Osteoarthritis Cartilage 2008;16(Suppl 3):S8–13.

56. Roemer FW, Hunter DJ, Guermazi A. Semiquantitative assessment of synovitis in osteoarthritis on non contrast-enhanced MR imaging. Osteoarthritis Cartilage 2008; [Epub ahead of print].

57. Loeuille D, Saulière N, Champigneulle J, et al. What is the most accurate MRI approach to assess synovitis and/or effusion in knee OA? Osteoarthritis Cartilage 2008;16(Suppl 4):176.

58. Ostergaard M, Hansen M, Stoltenberg M, et al. Magnetic resonance imaging-determined synovial membrane volume as a marker of disease activity and a predictor of progressive joint destruction in the wrists of patients with rheumatoid arthritis. Arthritis Rheum 1999;42:918–29.

59. Rhodes LA, Grainger AJ, Keenan AM, et al. The validation of simple scoring methods for evaluating compartment-specific synovitis detected by MRI in knee osteoarthritis. Rheumatology (Oxford) 2005; 44:1569–73.

60. Clunie G, Hall-Craggs MA, Paley MN, et al. Measurement of synovial lining volume by magnetic resonance imaging of the knee in chronic synovitis. Ann Rheum Dis 1997;56:526–34.

61. Lindblad S, Hedfors E. Intraarticular variation in synovitis. Local macroscopic and microscopic signs of inflammatory activity are significantly correlated. Arthritis Rheum 1985;28:977–86.

62. Kurosaka M, Ohno O, Hirohata K. Arthroscopic evaluation of synovitis in the knee joints. Arthroscopy 1991;7:162–70.

63. Fernandez-Madrid F, Karvonen RL, Teitge RA, et al. MR features of osteoarthritis of the knee. Magn Reson Imaging 1994;12:703–9.

64. Roemer FW, Guermazi A, Hunter DJ, et al. The association of meniscal damage with joint effusion in persons without radiographic osteoarthritis: the Framingham and MOST osteoarthritis studies. Osteoarthr Cartil 2008; [Epub ahead of print].

65. von Porat A, Roos EM, Roos H. High prevalence of osteoarthritis 14 years after an anterior cruciate ligament tear in male soccer players: a study of radiographic and patient relevant outcomes. Ann Rheum Dis 2004;63:269–73.

66. Maletius W, Messner K. Eighteen- to twenty-four-year follow-up after complete rupture of the anterior cruciate ligament. Am J Sports Med 1999;27:711–7.

67. Kannus P, Jarvinen M. Posttraumatic anterior cruciate ligament insufficiency as a cause of osteoarthritis in a knee joint. Clin Rheumatol 1989;8:251–60.

68. Nebelung W, Wuschech H. Thirty-five years of follow-up of anterior cruciate ligament-deficient knees in high-level athletes. Arthroscopy 2005;21:696–702.

69. Messner K, Maletius W. Eighteen- to twenty-five-year follow-up after acute partial anterior cruciate ligament rupture. Am J Sports Med 1999;27:455–9.

70. Dargel J, Gotter M, Mader K, et al. Biomechanics of the anterior cruciate ligament and implications for surgical reconstruction. Strategies Trauma Limb Reconstr 2007;2:1–12.

71. Hill CL, Seo GS, Gale D, et al. Cruciate ligament integrity in osteoarthritis of the knee. Arthritis Rheum 2005;52:794–9.

72. Crema MD, Marra MD, Guermazi A, et al. Relevant traumatic injury of the knee joint-MRI follow-up after 7-10 years. Eur J Radiol 2008; [Epub ahead of print].

73. Chan WP, Lang P, Stevens MP, et al. Osteoarthritis of the knee: comparison of radiography, CT, and MR imaging to assess extent and severity. AJR Am J Roentgenol 1991;157:799–806.

74. Link TM, Steinbach LS, Ghosh S, et al. Osteoarthritis: MR imaging findings in different stages of disease and correlation with clinical findings. Radiology 2003;226:373–81.

75. Cushner FD, La Rosa DF, Vigorita VJ, et al. A quantitative histologic comparison: ACL degeneration in the osteoarthritic knee. J Arthroplasty 2003;18:687–92.

76. Lee GC, Cushner FD, Vigoritta V, et al. Evaluation of the anterior cruciate ligament integrity and degenerative arthritic patterns in patients undergoing total knee arthroplasty. J Arthroplasty 2005;20: 59–65.

77. Wada M, Tatsuo H, Baba H, et al. Femoral intercondylar notch measurements in osteoarthritic knees. Rheumatology (Oxford) 1999;38:554–8.

78. Mullaji AB, Marawar SV, Simha M, et al. Cruciate ligaments in arthritic knees: a histologic study with radiologic correlation. J Arthroplasty 2008;23: 567–72.

79. Amin S, Guermazi A, Lavalley MP, et al. Complete anterior cruciate ligament tear and the risk for cartilage loss and progression of symptoms in men and women with knee osteoarthritis. Osteoarthritis Cartilage 2008;16:897–902.

80. Guermazi A, Taouli B, Lynch JA, et al. Prevalence of meniscus and ligament tears and their correlation with cartilage morphology and other MRI features in knee osteoarthritis (OA) in the elderly. The Health ABC Study. Arthritis Rheum 2002; 46(Suppl):S567.

81. Logan M, Williams A, Lavelle J, et al. The effect of posterior cruciate ligament deficiency on knee kinematics. Am J Sports Med 2004;32:1915–22.

82. Dejour H, Walch G, Peyrot J, et al. [The natural history of rupture of the posterior cruciate ligament]. Rev Chir Orthop Reparatrice Appar Mot 1988;74:35–43 [in French].

83. Patel DV, Allen AA, Warren RF, et al. The nonoperative treatment of acute, isolated (partial or complete) posterior cruciate ligament-deficient knees: an intermediate-term follow-up study. HSS J 2007;3: 137–46.

84. Bergin D, Keogh C, O'Connell M, et al. Atraumatic medial collateral ligament oedema in medial compartment knee osteoarthritis. Skeletal Radiol 2002;31:14–8.

85. Marra MD, Crema MD, Chung M, et al. MRI features of cystic lesions around the knee. Knee 2008;15:423–38.

86. Guermazi A, Zaim S, Taouli B, et al. MR findings in knee osteoarthritis. Eur Radiol 2003;13:1370–86.

87. Fam AG, Wilson SR, Holmberg S. Ultrasound evaluation of popliteal cysts on osteoarthritis of the knee. J Rheumatol 1982;9:428–34.

88. Guermazi A, Roemer FW, Niu J, et al. Periarticular cysts and their relation to symptoms in osteoarthritis: the MOST study. Osteoarthr Cartil 2007; 15(Suppl 3):C170–1.

89. Tschirch FT, Schmid MR, Pfirrmann CW, et al. Prevalence and size of meniscal cysts, ganglionic cysts, synovial cysts of the popliteal space, fluid-filled bursae, and other fluid collections in asymptomatic knees on MR imaging. AJR Am J Roentgenol 2003;180:1431–6.

90. McCarthy CL, McNally EG. The MRI appearance of cystic lesions around the knee. Skeletal Radiol 2004;33:187–209.

91. Alvarez-Nemegyei J. Risk factors for pes anserinus tendinitis/bursitis syndrome: a case control study. J Clin Rheumatol 2007;13:63–5.

92. Noble J, Hamblen DL. The pathology of the degenerate meniscus lesion. J Bone Joint Surg Br 1975; 57:180–6.

93. De Maeseneer M, Shahabpour M, Vanderdood K, et al. MR imaging of meniscal cysts: evaluation of location and extension using a three-layer approach. Eur J Radiol 2001;39:117–24.

94. Tyson LL, Daughters TC Jr, Ryu RK, et al. MRI appearance of meniscal cysts. Skeletal Radiol 1995;24:421–4.

95. Feldman F, Johnston A. Intraosseous ganglion. Am J Roentgenol Radium Ther Nucl Med 1973;118: 328–43.

96. Kim JY, Jung SA, Sung MS, et al. Extra-articular soft tissue ganglion cyst around the knee: focus on the associated findings. Eur Radiol 2004;14:106–11.

97. Bui-Mansfield LT, Youngberg RA. Intraarticular ganglia of the knee: prevalence, presentation, etiology, and management. AJR Am J Roentgenol 1997;168:123–7.

98. Jerome D, McKendry R. Synovial cyst of the proximal tibiofibular joint. J Rheumatol 2000;27: 1096–8.

99. El Andaloussi Y, Fnini S, Hachimi K, et al. Osteochondromatosis of the popliteal bursa. Joint Bone Spine 2006;73:219–20.

100. Steadman JR, Ramappa AJ, Maxwell RB, et al. An arthroscopic treatment regimen for osteoarthritis of the knee. Arthroscopy 2007;23:948–55.

101. Stuart MJ, Lubowitz JH. What, if any, are the indications for arthroscopic debridement of the osteoarthritic knee? Arthroscopy 2006;22:238–9.

The Role of the Meniscus in Knee Osteoarthritis: a Cause or Consequence?

Martin Englund, MD, PhD[a,b,*], Ali Guermazi, MD[c],
Stefan L. Lohmander, MD, PhD[a]

KEYWORDS

- Osteoarthritis • Knee • Meniscus-menisci • Pain
- Symptoms • MR imaging • Radiography

The loss of joint cartilage is considered to be the structural hallmark of osteoarthritis (OA). The last few decades of research focused on the knee, however, have proved OA to be a whole-joint disorder involving other tissues, such as subchondral bone, ligaments, synovial membrane, muscle, and the menisci. All of them can be evaluated by modern imaging techniques, such as MR imaging. This article reviews recent advances in the understanding of the role of the meniscus and meniscus pathology in OA. The meniscus plays a critical protective role in each tibiofemoral compartment through its shock-absorbing and load-distributing properties. Described are typical meniscal lesions found in the osteoarthritic knee and their etiology and significance, and briefly reviewed are past and current treatment concepts, all important knowledge to the practicing musculoskeletal radiologist.

ANATOMY, HISTOLOGY, AND FUNCTIONS OF THE NORMAL MENISCI IN BRIEF

The menisci are two semicircular fibrocartilage structures positioned between the joint surfaces of the femur and tibia in the medial and lateral knee joint compartments. Each meniscus covers approximately two thirds of the corresponding articular surface of the tibia. In cross-section, both menisci are wedge-shaped with a thick peripheral base infiltrated by capillaries and nerves that penetrate 10% to 30% of the meniscus width.[1,2] The medial meniscus is firmly attached to the joint capsule, whereas the lateral meniscus is more mobile. Both of the menisci are attached to the tibia through the anterior and posterior horns. Here, circumferential matrix fibers continue as ligaments attached to the intercondylar bone.

A sparse population of fibrochondrocytes produces and maintains the meniscal matrix. In contrast to articular cartilage, which contains principally type II collagen and an abundance of proteoglycan, meniscal matrix collagen is approximately 98% type I, and the meniscus contains much less proteoglycan (<1%).[3] The tightly woven collagen fibers are arranged predominantly in a circumferential pattern. This main fiber orientation is important in providing strength and to hold the meniscus in place when loaded.

The main functions of the menisci are shock absorption and load transmission during dynamic knee joint movement and static loading.[4–6] When the knee is loaded, the tensile strength of the

Parts of this of this article appeared in *Rheumatic Disease Clinics of North America* (2008 Vol. 34, 3) and Medical Clinics of North America (2009 Vol. 92, 1).

[a] Musculoskeletal Sciences, Department of Orthopedics, Clinical Sciences Lund, Lund University Hospital, Klinikgatan 22, SE-221 85 Lund, Sweden

[b] Clinical Epidemiology Research and Training Unit, Boston University School of Medicine, 650 Albany Street, Suite X200, Boston, MA 02118, USA

[c] Department of Radiology, Boston University School of Medicine, 820 Harrison Avenue, FGH Building, 3rd Floor, Boston, MA 02118, USA

* Corresponding author. Musculoskeletal Sciences, Department of Orthopedics, Lund University Hospital, Klinikgatan 22, SE-221 85 Lund, Sweden.

E-mail address: martin.englund@med.lu.se (M. Englund).

Radiol Clin N Am 47 (2009) 703–712
doi:10.1016/j.rcl.2009.03.003
0033-8389/09/$ – see front matter © 2009 Elsevier Inc. All rights reserved.

meniscal matrix (hoop tension) counteracts extrusion of the meniscus, and the meniscus distributes stress over a large area of the articular cartilage; the healthy meniscus mainly responds to load with compression. Removal of all or part of the meniscus leads to focally increased joint cartilage strain under static loading, and to increased dynamic deformation in knee joint areas known to develop OA.[7,8] The meniscus has also been reported to contribute to joint stability, proprioception, and joint lubrication.[9–11]

DIFFERENT TYPES OF MENISCAL LESIONS IN KNEE OSTEOARTHRITIS

MR imaging is the preferred imaging modality for evaluating the menisci, and the procedure is an increasingly popular diagnostic procedure of meniscal lesions (Fig. 1). A proton density weighted sequence using short TE and optimized signal-to-noise ratio and both coronal and sagittal images are preferred.[12] The sensitivity and specificity is in the range of 82% to 96% based on patients undergoing arthroscopy (using arthroscopy as the gold standard), but in subjects with prior meniscal repair the evaluation is more complex.[13–16]

A number of typical morphologic tear patterns of the meniscus can be distinguished not only at direct visual inspection and probing at arthroscopy but also on MR imaging, and it is important carefully to describe these.[17,18] The tear patterns can be classified into two main types of lesion: traumatic and degenerative.[19–22] Traumatic lesions usually occur in younger active individuals

because of a distinct knee trauma to a previously healthy joint when the meniscus is trapped between the femoral condyle and the tibial plateau under excessive forces. The meniscus often splits vertically and parallel to the circumferentially oriented collagen fibers (longitudinal tear) or occasionally perpendicular to the circumferential fibers (radial tear) (Fig. 2). Such tears, often leading to meniscal surgery, are associated with increased risk of knee OA.[23,24]

Degenerative lesions, described as horizontal cleavages (Fig. 3), flap (oblique), or complex (Fig. 4) tears or meniscal maceration (Fig. 5) or destruction (Fig. 6) are, in contrast, often associated with older age and pre-existing or incipient osteoarthritic disease.[19–22] In a report using a sample from the general population of middle-aged and elderly in Framingham, Massachusetts, unselected for knee joint symptoms, investigators found meniscal damage (tear, maceration, previous resection, or destruction) in 35% of knees (95% confidence interval, 32–38).[25] The prevalence of meniscal damage in the right knee, as detected on MR imaging, ranged from 19% among women 50 to 59 years of age to 56% among men 70 to 90 years of age (Fig. 7). Most of the tears were classified as degenerative. Interestingly, prevalences were not materially lower when subjects who had had previous knee surgery were excluded. Further, in the Framingham study sample 82% of knees with radiographic OA had meniscal damage. In another report including asymptomatic subjects with a mean age of 65 years, a tear was found in 67% using MR imaging, whereas in patients with symptomatic knee OA,

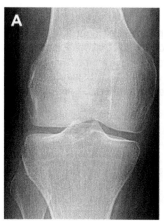
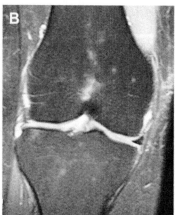
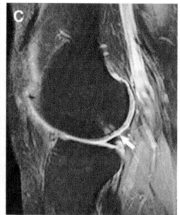

Fig. 1. This 38-year-old woman has undergone subtotal lateral meniscectomy in her right knee 16 years earlier. The last year she has experienced aching related to joint use, relieved by rest. The frontal knee radiograph (*A*) shows normal findings, whereas coronal T2-weighted MR imaging (*B*) reveals status after subtotal lateral meniscectomy, and sagittal image (*C*) shows reduced cartilage thickness and bone marrow edema (*arrow*). Findings are compatible with early stage knee OA. (*From* Englund et al. Meniscal tear: a feature of osteoarthritis. Acta Orthop Scand Suppl 2004;75:1–45; with permission.)

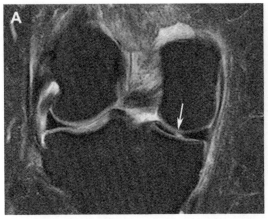
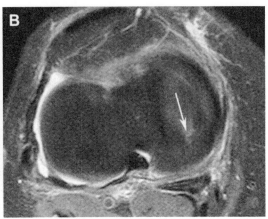

Fig. 2. Radial tear of the meniscus in a 52-year-old woman. (A) Coronal fat-suppressed proton density (PD) weighted MR imaging shows absence of the inner point of the medial meniscal triangle, typical for radial tear (*arrow*). There is a slight extrusion of the meniscus. (B) Axial fat-suppressed PD-weighted MR imaging shows the radial tear (*arrow*) starts at the free edge of the medial meniscus and extends peripherally.

a meniscal tear was found in 91%.[26] Other MR imaging studies support these findings of a high frequency of meniscal pathology in the middle-aged and elderly,[27] and similar findings have also been made in necropsy cases, where 60% of the subjects had a horizontal cleavage lesion.[20] The most frequent location is the posterior horn of the medial meniscus.[25] Also, even if a meniscal tear is not present on MR imaging, intrameniscal signal change (not classified as meniscal tear) is a frequent finding in the middle aged and elderly. Such linear or globular signal changes (**Fig. 8**) have been reported to represent mucoid degeneration and may represent a precursor to degenerative tears.[28,29]

Meniscal tears may be associated with knee joint symptoms, but actually not most lesions.[26] In the Framingham sample most subjects with a meniscal tear were without symptoms.[25] Still, in some patients a meniscal tear may cause severe discomfort or even locking of the knee because of a dislocated tear fragment, and surgical treatment becomes often necessary, particular in the young individual after knee trauma.

Although clinical radiologists normally describe meniscal pathology in detail in free text, sacrifices have to be made in clinical research with interest of practicality and feasibility. In research there are a number of semiquantitative meniscal classifications systems in use (eg, Whole-Organ MRI

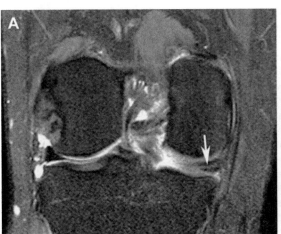
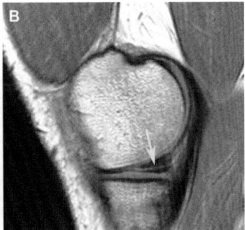

Fig. 3. Horizontal tear of the medial meniscus in a 47-year-old woman. Coronal fat-suppressed PD- weighted (A) and sagittal T1-weighted MR imaging (B) show almost horizontal tear (*arrow*) of the posterior horn of the medial meniscus with extension to meniscal undersurface.

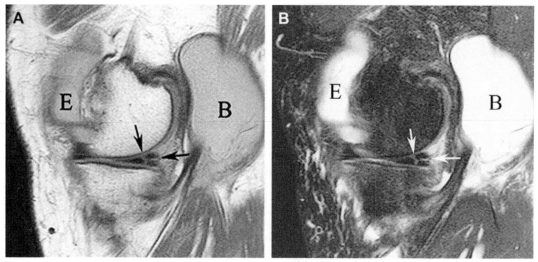

Fig. 4. Complex tear of the medial meniscus in a 53-year-old woman. Sagittal PD-weighted (*A*) and fat-suppressed T2-weighted (*B*) MR imaging show a complex tear (*arrows*) of the posterior horn of medial meniscus with longitudinal and horizontal cleavages. There are also a moderate joint effusion (E) and large partially ruptured Baker's cyst (B).

Score,[30] Knee OA Scoring System,[31] and the newly developed Boston-Leeds OA Knee Score).[32] These scoring systems have all been developed to quantify abnormalities of multiple knee joint structures involved in OA, but they also have limitations in meniscal scoring with respect to item content, separation of constructs, and sensitivity for change. For example, Whole-Organ MRI Score does not separate dislocated tears from partial resection (both scored as 3 on a 0–4 scale) and does not include meniscal positioning. Boston-Leeds OA Knee Score does not distinguish radial tears from longitudinal tears (both classified as vertical). Further, neither of the scoring methods takes account of the location of the tear with respect to capsular vicinity.

Measurements of meniscal height, articular cartilage covering or uncovering, and positioning based on coronal MR imaging have added new insights to meniscus pathology in OA.[33] Further, quantitative volume measurement of meniscal tissue (also based on MR imaging) is in development in line with the increasing research use of segmentation and volume determination of articular cartilage.[34–36] The main problem with these measurements is that they do not account for actual meniscal integrity. Hence, all three methods (semiquantitative scoring, morphologic measurements, and volume determination) are likely necessary tools for researchers to learn more about the role of the meniscus in knee OA.

MENISCAL DAMAGE: A CAUSE TO OR A CONSEQUENCE OF KNEE OSTEOARTHRITIS?

Normally configured menisci are rarely found in knees with OA; instead, they are often torn, macerated, or even totally destructed, which suggests a strong association between the disorder and the meniscus.[25,26,33] The relationship between

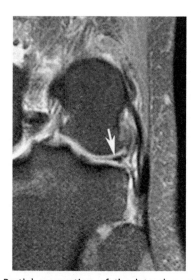

Fig. 5. Partial maceration of the lateral meniscus in a 61-year-old woman with no history of knee surgery. Coronal fat-suppressed PD-weighted MR imaging shows small body of the lateral meniscus (*arrow*) with loss of the normal triangular shape.

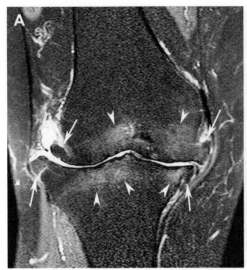
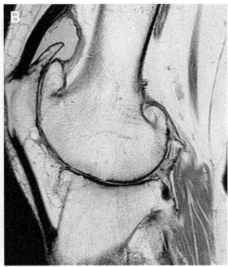

Fig. 6. Destruction of medial and lateral menisci in a 70-year-old woman with severe knee OA and no history of knee surgery. Coronal fat-suppressed (*A*) and sagittal PD-weighted (*B*) MR imaging show absence of both medial and lateral menisci. There is an extensive femoral and tibial osteophytosis (*arrows*), bone marrow lesions (*arrowheads*), cartilage loss, and bone attrition.

meniscal damage and knee OA, however, is complex. A meniscal lesion in a healthy knee may eventually lead to knee OA because of the loss of meniscal function, but knee OA may also lead to meniscal tears, which in turn may further accelerate the disease process.[37] The menisci and articular cartilage share many similar components and properties, and are exposed to similar stresses. The pathologic processes active in the early stage OA joint that eventually lead to the cartilage destruction characteristic of OA are not limited to the joint cartilage only, but are expected also to affect meniscus and ligament integrity. A

tear in a meniscus with degenerative changes is often associated with pre-existing structural changes in the articular cartilage that may represent early stage OA.[20] Patients with "meniscal" symptoms caused by a degenerative tear may constitute a subpopulation enriched in individuals with incipient OA.

In middle-aged or elderly persons, knees with meniscal lesions but without cartilage lesions are at much higher risk of radiographic knee OA than knees with intact menisci, suggesting that in many instances by MR imaging visible meniscal damage comes before visible cartilage changes.[38]

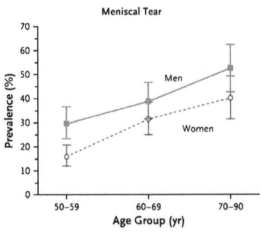
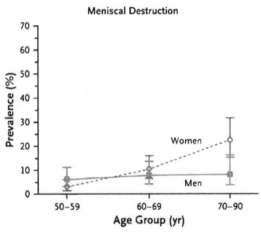

Fig. 7. Prevalence of meniscal damage in the right knee among the 426 men and 565 women from the general population of Framingham, Massachusetts. (*From* Englund M, Guermazi A, Gale D, et al. Incidental meniscal findings on knee MR imaging in middle-aged and elderly persons. N Engl J Med 2008;359:1108–15; with permission.)

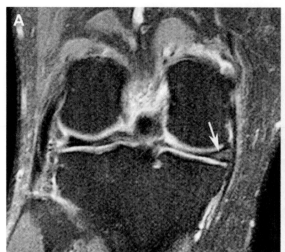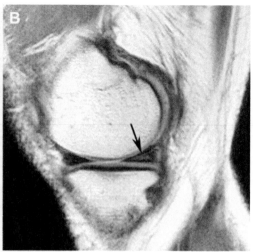

Fig. 8. Mucoid degeneration of meniscus. (*A*) Coronal fat-suppressed PD-weighted MR imaging shows an intrameniscal globular hypersignal (*arrow*) of the posterior horn of medial meniscus, which does not communicate with the articular surface. This corresponds to grade 1 mucoid meniscal degeneration. (*B*) Sagittal T1-weighted MR imaging shows primarily linear intrameniscal hypersignal (*arrow*) of the posterior horn of the medial meniscus, which does not communicate with the articular surface. This corresponds to grade 2 mucoid meniscal degeneration.

Shear stress and early proteolytic degradation of the meniscal matrix may result in decreased tensile strength. A meniscal tear could be the result of decreased ability of the compromised meniscus to withstand loads and force transmissions during normal knee joint loads. A lesion may develop spontaneously or in conjunction with minor knee trauma. Depending on how much functionality of the meniscus was lost because of the tear and any surgical resection, the OA development may then be further driven through increased biomechanical loading of the joint cartilage. Importantly, many patients may develop knee symptoms and be referred to an orthopedic surgeon, perhaps because a meniscal tear was found during a knee MR imaging examination. The meniscal tear itself in this age category is only weakly associated with knee symptoms, however, whereas other features of OA, visible or not, may be so associated.[25,39] The indication based on MR imaging findings, such as these for meniscus surgery, is questionable.[40–42]

Meniscal extrusion is also common among the middle aged and elderly, and is often another sign of a degraded or torn meniscus and existing OA (**Fig. 9**).[43,44] Meniscal tears predispose to meniscal extrusion, probably by interrupting the circumferential hoop collagen fiber orientation. Meniscal extrusion may also contribute to increased joint space narrowing seen on radiographs, and meniscal tear and displacement are strong determinants of the rate of cartilage loss in knee OA.[33,45,46]

GENES AND ENVIRONMENT INTERACT

A degenerative meniscal lesion was more frequently found in patients with radiographic hand OA, and subjects with bilateral knee OA had radiographic hand OA more frequently than did subjects with unilateral knee OA.[47] These findings provided additional support for an interaction between genetic and environmental risk factors in OA, although metabolic effects cannot be excluded. Worse outcome after lateral meniscectomy compared with medial has been shown in several studies. The lateral meniscus carries higher loads in the knee compared with the medial meniscus. Consequently, if removed, the slightly convex lateral tibial plateau is exposed to relatively more cartilage contact stress,[4,5] which may further facilitate the OA process, compared with the more concave medial tibial plateau after removal of the medial meniscus.[23,48–52] This may provide yet another example of the interaction of local environmental factors with the inherent risk of the individual.

PAST, PRESENT, AND FUTURE TREATMENT STRATEGIES OF A TORN MENISCUS

Interestingly, the first report known was of a meniscal repair. In 1883, a British surgeon successfully sutured a torn medial meniscus.[53] Four years later, however, he published yet another report, where he justified total removal of the meniscus rather than repair, and that view prevailed for over 80 years.[54] In the late 1940s, Fairbank[24]

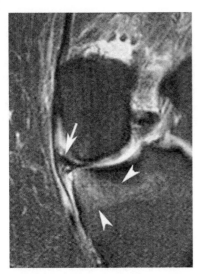

Fig. 9. Meniscal extrusion in a 57-year-old woman. Coronal fat-suppressed PD-weighted MR imaging shows subluxation of the body of the medial meniscus (*arrow*). There is also a grade 1 meniscal mucoid degeneration and important cartilage loss of the outer aspect of the medial tibiofemoral joint and bone marrow lesion of the medial tibial plateau (*arrowheads*).

speculated that frequent radiographic changes found after total meniscectomy were caused by the loss of the load-protective function of the menisci, resulting in remodeling of the joint. Total removal of the menisci was considered a mostly benign procedure, however, for at least another 20 years. From the late 1960s to the 1980s an increasing number of follow-up reports of meniscectomy were published, all indicating a high frequency of radiographic OA and reduced knee function.[48,51,52,55–60] Lack of standardized radiographic assessment and outcome measures, however, precluded consistent quantification of the OA risk.[61] In 1998, a study showed a sixfold increase in the risk of radiographic OA 21 years after total meniscectomy, compared with controls matched for age and gender.[62]

It was not until the 1970s, when arthroscopic technique was introduced, that interest increased in excising only the damaged portion of the meniscus. In the same period of time, several biomechanical studies reported on the load-bearing and shock-absorbing functions of the menisci.[4–6,63,64] There are several short-term benefits of the arthroscopic technique of surgery and partial meniscal resection in terms of length of hospital stay, rehabilitation, and so forth.[65–67] Further, with a substantial portion of the circumferentially oriented matrix fibers intact in the residual meniscus, hoop tension may still develop to counteract meniscal extrusion when the knee is loaded.

Substantial function may remain in the residual meniscus in shock absorption and load transmission yielding a lower risk of radiographic changes related to OA than total meniscectomy.[23] The frequency of symptomatic knee OA was not substantially lowered, however, which suggested that partial removal of the meniscus was not the final answer.[68]

In consequence, for younger individuals with traumatic injury to the meniscus, meniscal repair is presently advocated when the lesion is located in the vicinity of the vascularized zone (with the potential to heal). Interestingly, clinicians are back to where it all started in 1883. Rehabilitation after repair is much more demanding than after meniscal resection, however, and the long-term outcome of meniscal repair compared with partial meniscectomy with respect to OA is still unknown.[69,70] In practice meniscal resection is the most frequently performed procedure by orthopedic surgeons in the United States.[71]

Meniscal replacement using allogenic, xenogenic, or artificial materials has been tried in younger individuals who have undergone total meniscectomy. Transplant survival is variable, however, and long-term results using standardized outcomes are lacking.[68,72] Even so, because there is evidence that meniscal damage without surgery otherwise leads to radiographic OA, it is conceivable that treatments aimed at restoring meniscal function may lower this risk.[38] This remains to be shown, however, in randomized, appropriately controlled trials. Such treatments seem attractive in particular for younger individuals with a severely torn meniscus, but are hardly the answer to the one third of middle-aged older adult knees with meniscal damage in the general population.[25,26]

Today, middle-aged and older patients with knee pain and meniscal lesions represent a great challenge for the health professional. Incidental meniscal findings on MR imaging are frequent,[25] and it is difficult to discriminate between symptoms caused by a meniscal tear and symptoms of early stage knee OA.[73] The weak evidence base for many of the current treatments suggests that this therapeutic area is in great need of well-designed randomized controlled clinical trials to assess the true effects of arthroscopic meniscal resection, meniscal repair or transplant, or nonsurgical treatments compared with placebo or sham treatment.[40,41,42] For many patients in this category, based on the best evidence, medical treatment and structured exercise programs are as effective as arthroscopic surgery. Stratification with regard to lesion type, age, activity level, and other variables provides a challenge in trial design, but there is no shortage of patients. Blinding of patient and assessor, and ethical issues represent additional challenges.

SUMMARY

The menisci play a critical protective role for the knee joint through shock absorption and load distribution. Meniscal lesions are regular findings on MR imaging, especially in the osteoarthritic knee and in the form of horizontal, flap, and complex tears; maceration; or destruction. Asymptomatic lesions are common, however, and are frequent incidental findings on knee MR imaging of the middle-aged or older patient. This challenges the health professional in choosing the best treatment, both in the short- and long-term. A meniscal tear can lead to knee OA, but knee OA can also lead to a meniscal tear. A degenerative meniscal lesion, in the middle-aged or older patient, could suggest early stage knee OA and should be treated accordingly. Surgical resection of nonobstructive degenerate lesions may only remove evidence of the disorder while the OA and associated symptoms proceeds.

REFERENCES

1. Day B, Mackenzie WG, Shim SS, et al. The vascular and nerve supply of the human meniscus. Arthroscopy 1985;1(1):58–62.
2. Arnoczky SP, Warren RF. Microvasculature of the human meniscus. Am J Sports Med 1982;10(2):90–5.
3. Eyre DR, Wu JJ. Collagen of fibrocartilage: a distinctive molecular phenotype in bovine meniscus. FEBS Lett 1983;158(2):265–70.
4. Seedhom BB, Hargreaves DJ. Transmission of the load in the knee joint with special reference to the role of the meniscus. Part I + II. Eng Med 1979;4:207–28.
5. Walker PS, Erkman MJ. The role of the menisci in force transmission across the knee. Clin Orthop 1975;(109):184–92.
6. Kurosawa H, Fukubayashi T, Nakajima H. Load-bearing mode of the knee joint: physical behavior of the knee joint with or without menisci. Clin Orthop 1980;(149):283–90.
7. Song Y, Greve JM, Carter DR, et al. Meniscectomy alters the dynamic deformational behavior and cumulative strain of tibial articular cartilage in knee joints subjected to cyclic loads. Osteoarthritis Cartilage 2008;16(12):1545–54.
8. Song Y, Greve JM, Carter DR, et al. Articular cartilage MR imaging and thickness mapping of a loaded knee joint before and after meniscectomy. Osteoarthritis Cartilage 2006;14(8):728–37.
9. Levy IM, Torzilli PA, Warren RF. The effect of medial meniscectomy on anterior-posterior motion of the knee. J Bone Joint Surg Am 1982;64(6):883–8.
10. Levy IM, Torzilli PA, Gould JD, et al. The effect of lateral meniscectomy on motion of the knee. J Bone Joint Surg Am 1989;71(3):401–6.
11. Assimakopoulos AP, Katonis PG, Agapitos MV, et al. The innervation of the human meniscus. Clin Orthop 1992;(275):232–6.
12. Fox MG. MR imaging of the meniscus: review, current trends, and clinical implications. Radiol Clin North Am 2007;45(6):1033–53, vii.
13. Cheung LP, Li KC, Hollett MD, et al. Meniscal tears of the knee: accuracy of detection with fast spin-echo MR imaging and arthroscopic correlation in 293 patients. Radiology 1997;203(2):508–12.
14. De Smet AA, Tuite MJ. Use of the two-slice-touch rule for the MRI diagnosis of meniscal tears. AJR Am J Roentgenol 2006;187(4):911–4.
15. Escobedo EM, Hunter JC, Zink-Brody GC, et al. Usefulness of turbo spin-echo MR imaging in the evaluation of meniscal tears: comparison with a conventional spin-echo sequence. AJR Am J Roentgenol 1996;167(5):1223–7.
16. Vande Berg BC, Malghem J, Poilvache P, et al. Meniscal tears with fragments displaced in notch and recesses of knee: MR imaging with arthroscopic comparison. Radiology 2005;234(3):842–50.
17. Jee WH, McCauley TR, Kim JM, et al. Meniscal tear configurations: categorization with MR imaging. AJR Am J Roentgenol 2003;180(1):93–7.
18. Newman AP, Daniels AU, Burks RT. Principles and decision making in meniscal surgery. Arthroscopy 1993;9(1):33–51.
19. Poehling GG, Ruch DS, Chabon SJ. The landscape of meniscal injuries. Clin Sports Med 1990;9(3):539–49.
20. Noble J, Hamblen DL. The pathology of the degenerate meniscus lesion. J Bone Joint Surg Br 1975;57(2):180–6.
21. Noble J. Lesions of the menisci: autopsy incidence in adults less than fifty-five years old. J Bone Joint Surg Am 1977;59(4):480–3.
22. Smillie IS. Surgical pathology of the menisci: injuries of the knee joint. 3rd edition. Baltimore (MD): The Williams and Wilkins Co.; 1962. p. 51–90.
23. Englund M, Lohmander LS. Risk factors for symptomatic knee osteoarthritis fifteen to twenty-two years after meniscectomy. Arthritis Rheum 2004;50(9):2811–9.
24. Fairbank TJ. Knee joint changes after meniscectomy. J Bone Joint Surg Br 1948;30:164–70.
25. Englund M, Guermazi A, Gale D, et al. Incidental meniscal findings on knee MRI in middle-aged and elderly persons. N Engl J Med 2008;359(11):1108–15.

26. Bhattacharyya T, Gale D, Dewire P, et al. The clinical importance of meniscal tears demonstrated by magnetic resonance imaging in osteoarthritis of the knee. J Bone Joint Surg Am 2003;85(1):4–9.

27. Ding C, Martel-Pelletier J, Pelletier JP, et al. Meniscal tear as an osteoarthritis risk factor in a largely non-osteoarthritic cohort: a cross-sectional study. J Rheumatol 2007;34(4):776–84.

28. Stoller DW, Martin C, Crues III JV, et al. Meniscal tears: pathologic correlation with MR imaging. Radiology 1987;163(3):731–5.

29. Hodler J, Haghighi P, Pathria MN, et al. Meniscal changes in the elderly: correlation of MR imaging and histologic findings. Radiology 1992;184(1):221–5.

30. Peterfy CG, Guermazi A, Zaim S, et al. Whole-Organ Magnetic Resonance Imaging Score (WORMS) of the knee in osteoarthritis. Osteoarthritis Cartilage 2004;12(3):177–90.

31. Kornaat PR, Ceulemans RY, Kroon HM, et al. MRI assessment of knee osteoarthritis: Knee Osteoarthritis Scoring System (KOSS): inter-observer and intra-observer reproducibility of a compartment-based scoring system. Skeletal Radiol 2005;34(2):95–102.

32. Hunter DJ, Lo GH, Gale D, et al. The reliability of a new scoring system for knee osteoarthritis MRI and the validity of bone marrow lesion assessment: BLOKS (Boston Leeds Osteoarthritis Knee Score). Ann Rheum Dis 2008;67(2):206–11.

33. Hunter DJ, Zhang YQ, Niu JB, et al. The association of meniscal pathologic changes with cartilage loss in symptomatic knee osteoarthritis. Arthritis Rheum 2006;54(3):795–801.

34. Bowers ME, Tung GA, Fleming BC, et al. Quantification of meniscal volume by segmentation of 3T magnetic resonance images. J Biomech 2007; 40(12):2811–5.

35. Kessler MA, Glaser C, Tittel S, et al. Volume changes in the menisci and articular cartilage of runners: an in vivo investigation based on 3-D magnetic resonance imaging. Am J Sports Med 2006;34(5):832–6.

36. Kessler MA, Glaser C, Tittel S, et al. Recovery of the menisci and articular cartilage of runners after cessation of exercise: additional aspects of in vivo investigation based on 3-dimensional magnetic resonance imaging. Am J Sports Med 2008;36(5): 966–70.

37. Roos H, Adalberth T, Dahlberg L, et al. Osteoarthritis of the knee after injury to the anterior cruciate ligament or meniscus: the influence of time and age. Osteoarthritis Cartilage 1995;3(4):261–7.

38. Englund M, Guermazi A, Roemer FW, et al. Meniscal tear in knees without surgery and the development of radiographic osteoarthritis: a nested case-control study within the prospective Multicenter Osteoarthritis (MOST) Study. Arthritis Rheum 2009;60:831–9.

39. Englund M, Niu J, Guermazi A, et al. Effect of meniscal damage on the development of frequent knee pain, aching, or stiffness. Arthritis Rheum 2007; 56(12):4048–54.

40. Herrlin S, Hallander M, Wange P, et al. Arthroscopic or conservative treatment of degenerative medial meniscal tears: a prospective randomised trial. Knee Surg Sports Traumatol Arthrosc 2007;15(4): 393–401.

41. Kirkley A, Birmingham TB, Litchfield RB, et al. A randomized trial of arthroscopic surgery for osteoarthritis of the knee. N Engl J Med 2008;359(11): 1097–107.

42. Moseley JB, O'Malley K, Petersen NJ, et al. A controlled trial of arthroscopic surgery for osteoarthritis of the knee. N Engl J Med 2002;347(2):81–8.

43. Adams JG, McAlindon T, Dimasi M, et al. Contribution of meniscal extrusion and cartilage loss to joint space narrowing in osteoarthritis. Clin Radiol 1999; 54(8):502–6.

44. Gale DR, Chaisson CE, Totterman SM, et al. Meniscal subluxation: association with osteoarthritis and joint space narrowing. Osteoarthritis Cartilage 1999;7(6):526–32.

45. Berthiaume MJ, Raynauld JP, Martel-Pelletier J, et al. Meniscal tear and extrusion are strongly associated with progression of symptomatic knee osteoarthritis as assessed by quantitative magnetic resonance imaging. Ann Rheum Dis 2005;64(4):556–63.

46. Ding C, Martel-Pelletier J, Pelletier JP, et al. Knee meniscal extrusion in a largely non-osteoarthritic cohort: association with greater loss of cartilage volume. Arthritis Res Ther 2007;9(2):R21.

47. Englund M, Paradowski PT, Lohmander LS. Association of radiographic hand osteoarthritis with radiographic knee osteoarthritis after meniscectomy. Arthritis Rheum 2004;50(2):469–75.

48. Allen PR, Denham RA, Swan AV. Late degenerative changes after meniscectomy: factors affecting the knee after operation. J Bone Joint Surg Br 1984; 66(5):666–71.

49. Chatain F, Adeleine P, Chambat P, et al. A comparative study of medial versus lateral arthroscopic partial meniscectomy on stable knees: 10-year minimum follow-up. Arthroscopy 2003;19(8): 842–9.

50. Hede A, Larsen E, Sandberg H. The long term outcome of open total and partial meniscectomy related to the quantity and site of the meniscus removed. Int Orthop 1992;16(2):122–5.

51. Johnson RJ, Kettelkamp DB, Clark W, et al. Factors effecting late results after meniscectomy. J Bone Joint Surg Am 1974;56(4):719–29.

52. Jørgensen U, Sonne-Holm S, Lauridsen F, et al. Long-term follow-up of meniscectomy in athletes: a prospective longitudinal study. J Bone Joint Surg Br 1987;69(1):80–3.

53. Annandale T. An operation for displaced semilunar cartilage. Br Med J 1885;1:779.

54. Annandale T. Excision of the internal semilunar cartilage, resulting in perfect restoration of the joint-movements. Br Med J 1889;1:291–2.

55. Gear MW. The late results of meniscectomy. Br J Surg 1967;54(4):270–2.

56. Tapper EM, Hoover NW. Late results after meniscectomy. J Bone Joint Surg Am 1969;51(3):517–26.

57. Noble J. Clinical features of the degenerate meniscus with the results of meniscectomy. Br J Surg 1975;62(12):977–81.

58. Noble J, Erat K. In defense of the meniscus: a prospective study of 200 meniscectomy patients. J Bone Joint Surg Br 1980;62(1):7–11.

59. Sonne-Holm S, Fledelius I, Ahn NC. Results after meniscectomy in 147 athletes. Acta Orthop Scand 1980;51(2):303–9.

60. Doherty M, Watt I, Dieppe P. Influence of primary generalised osteoarthritis on development of secondary osteoarthritis. Lancet 1983;2(8340):8–11.

61. Lohmander LS, Roos H. Knee ligament injury, surgery and osteoarthrosis: truth or consequences? Acta Orthop Scand 1994;65(6):605–9.

62. Roos H, Lauren M, Adalberth T, et al. Knee osteoarthritis after meniscectomy: prevalence of radiographic changes after twenty-one years, compared with matched controls. Arthritis Rheum 1998;41(4):687–93.

63. Shrive NG, O'Connor JJ, Goodfellow JW. Load-bearing in the knee joint. Clin Orthop 1978;(131): 279–87.

64. Fukubayashi T, Kurosawa H. The contact area and pressure distribution pattern of the knee: a study of normal and osteoarthrotic knee joints. Acta Orthop Scand 1980;51(6):871–9.

65. Dandy DJ. Early results of closed partial meniscectomy. Br Med J 1978;1(6120):1099–100.

66. Oretorp N, Gillquist J. Transcutaneous meniscectomy under arthroscopic control. Int Orthop 1979; 3(1):19–25.

67. Northmore-Ball MD, Dandy DJ, Jackson RW. Arthroscopic, open partial, and total meniscectomy: a comparative study. J Bone Joint Surg Br 1983; 65(4):400–4.

68. Lohmander LS, Englund PM, Dahl LL, et al. The long-term consequence of anterior cruciate ligament and meniscus injuries: osteoarthritis. Am J Sports Med 2007;35(10):1756–69.

69. Steenbrugge F, Verdonk R, Verstraete K, et al. Long-term assessment of arthroscopic meniscus repair: a 13-year follow-up study. Knee 2002;9(3): 181–7.

70. Rockborn P, Messner K. Long-term results of meniscus repair and meniscectomy: a 13-year functional and radiographic follow-up study. Knee Surg Sports Traumatol Arthrosc 2000;8(1):2–10.

71. Hall MJ, Lawrence L. Ambulatory surgery in the United States, 1996. Adv Data 1998; 1-16. Available at: http://www.cdc.gov/nchs/data/ad/ad300.pdf.

72. Noyes FR, Barber-Westin SD, Rankin M. Meniscal transplantation in symptomatic patients less than fifty years old. J Bone Joint Surg Am 2005;87(Suppl 1 Pt 2):149–65.

73. Dervin GF, Stiell IG, Wells GA, et al. Physicians' accuracy and interrator reliability for the diagnosis of unstable meniscal tears in patients having osteoarthritis of the knee. Can J Surg 2001;44(4): 267–74.

MRI of Hip Osteoarthritis and Implications for Surgery

Tallal C. Mamisch, MD[a,b,*], Christoph Zilkens, MD[c,d],
Klaus A. Siebenrock, MD, PhD[a], Bernd Bittersohl, MD[a,c],
Young-Jo Kim, MD, PhD[d], Stefan Werlen, MD[b]

KEYWORDS

- Osteoarthritis • Hip • Femoroacetabular impingement
- MRI • dGEMRIC • Surgery

Osteoarthritis (OA) of the hip is caused by a combination of intrinsic factors, such as joint anatomy, and extrinsic factors, such as body weight, injuries, diseases, and load.[1] Possible risk factors for OA are especially instability and impingement. Different surgical tequniques such as osteotomies of the pelvis and the femur,[2] surgical dislocation,[3] and hip arthroscopy[4,5] are being performed to delay or halt OA. Success of salvage hip procedures depends on the existing cartilage and joint damage prior to surgery; the likelihood of therapy failure rises with cases of advanced OA.[6–8]

For imaging of intra-articular pathology, MR imaging represents the best technique because of its ability to directly visualize cartilage, superior soft tissue contrast, and the prospect of multi-dimensional imaging. Opinions differ on the diagnostic efficacy of MR imaging and the question of which MR imaging technique is most appropriate. Many techniques showing similar promising data have been introduced for the knee.[9–12] Conditions within the hip are different, and the relatively thin hip cartilage and the spherical-shaped joint pose difficulties in the diagnosis of cartilage and labral injury. High MR imaging resolution and contrast-to-noise ratio between bone, cartilage, synovium, and soft tissue such as labrum and capsule are required.

There is an ongoing investigation for the optimal MR imaging technique for imaging of the hip.[13–15]

Currently, MR arthrography using intra-articular contrast material has been established as the standard method for imaging of labral lesions;[13,16–18] however, the diagnostic reliability of cartilage lesion remains moderate.[19,20] The diagnostic reliability of acetabular cartilage delamination by MR imaging is still challenenging.[21] The aim of this article is to discuss the current use of MR imaging in hip OA and its implications for surgery. As femoroacetabular impingement (FAI) becomes an increasingly important clinical diagnosis of the hip joint and is recognized as a precursor to the onset of hip OA, we will focus on this entity. Current standards, difficulties, and possible solutions using high-field MR imaging and future approaches are covered.

FEMOROACETABULAR IMPINGEMENT

During the past decade, FAI has gained increasing attentiveness as a possible trigger of hip OA. The incongruency of the hip (eg, after Perthes disease) might be denominated as static form of impingement, whereas more subtle anatomic deformities, in which the incongruency of the hip joint exists only in certain positions during motion, are the dynamic form of impingement.[4,22,23] Depending on the anatomic abnormality, there are two types of FAI: cam and pincer. In cam FAI, the cause of

a Department of Orthopedic Surgery, University of Bern, Freiburgstrasse, 3010 Bern, Switzerland
b Department of Radiology, Sonnenhof Clinics, 3010 Bern, Switzerland
c Department of Orthopedic Surgery, University of Düsseldorf, 41313 Düsseldorf, Germany
d Department of Orthopedic Surgery, Children's Hospital, Harvard Medical School, Boston, MA 02215, USA
* Corresponding author. Department of Orthopedic Surgery, University of Bern, Freiburgstrasse, 3010 Bern, Switzerland.
E-mail address: mamisch@bwh.harvard.edu (T.C. Mamisch).

Radiol Clin N Am 47 (2009) 713–722
doi:10.1016/j.rcl.2009.04.008
0033-8389/09/$ – see front matter © 2009 Elsevier Inc. All rights reserved.

impact is a nonspherical shape of the femoral head coming along with insufficient femoral head-neck offset. In cam FAI, shear forces lead to acetabular cartilage damage (Fig. 1), especially through forced flexion and internal rotation of the hip. In pincer FAI, the impact arises from acetabular over-coverage or other false configuration or shape of the acetabulum. The shape of the femoral head is spherical; however, the proximal femoral neck abuts frontally against the labrum and the acetabular rim. That way, the labrum is damaged primarily through recurrent trauma (Fig. 2) before a cartilage damage occurs.[24] Further causes for FAI are rotational anomalies with reduced femoral neck antetorsion and reduced acetabular version[25,26] or an overcorrection after periacetabular osteotomy (PAO), also called "Bernese disease."[27]

Untreated FAI can lead to premature OA of the hip.[28] To relieve symptoms such as limited range of motion and pain and further delay or halt the progression of OA, surgical treatment is necessary. Surgery includes reshaping of nonspherical femoral head in terms of cam, trimming the acetabular rim, or use of PAO in case of pincer FAI. The outcome of surgery depends on the quantity of pre-existing OA, with poor results occurring in patients with advanced degenerative changes. Follow-up examinations after open or arthroscopic FAI surgery showed favorable results, particularly in the subgroup of patients who did not have signs of advanced hip OA.[28] In patients who have FAI, it is important to identify early stages of cartilage degeneration to identify patients who could profit from osteo- or chondroplastic types of surgery.

Diagnosis of Femoroacetabular Impingement

Diagnosis of FAI is based on clinical findings and radiographic analysis, including MR arthrography.[29] Clinical symptoms of FAI include a slow onset of inguinal pain, which is usually pronounced with physical activities or prolonged sitting.[30] During physical examination this can be reproduced by the "impingement test," which examines hip pain produced by passive flexion, internal rotation, and adduction.[31] A positive impingement test result can be correlated to acetabular labrum lesions.[24] Radiographic assessment by means of standard anteroposterior and lateral views[32] is used to asses late stages of hip OA[33] and abnormal femoral head morphology,[34,35] specifically the pistol grip deformity.[36] Plain radiographic analysis is important in assessing acetabular version and coverage.

In cases of FAI, plain radiographs are often inadequate in terms of femoral head-neck junction morphology assessment and assessment of early-stage OA.[37] Because of the importance of detecting these early hip joint lesions in FAI, MR imaging assessment is quickly becoming the standard tool for diagnostic assessment.[16] It is becoming clear that standard coronal, axial, and sagittal MR imaging planes are less reliable than radially reconstructed planes perpendicular to the acetabular labrum in detecting early degenerative pathologies of the hip (Fig. 3).[16,38] For the assessment of the femoral head-neck morphology, radial reconstructions along the femoral neck axis[35,39,40] improve the understanding of the FAI pathomechanism and correlate well with the prediction of FAI and intraoperative findings.[41] This imaging technique

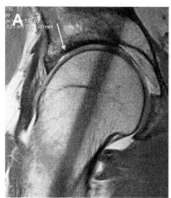
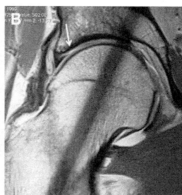
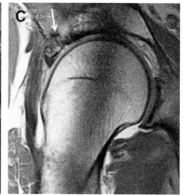

Fig. 1. (*A, B*) Radial turbo spin-echo proton density-weighted MR arthrography images at 3.0 T show cartilage damage (*arrow*) at the anterosuperior to superior portion of the acetabular rim caused by cam-type impingement. (*C*) Severe cartilage degeneration is associated with intact labrum and cystic deformation (*arrow*) of the acetabular rim.

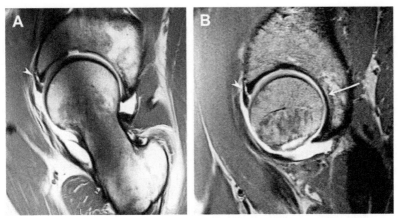

Fig. 2. (*A*) Radial and (*B*) sagittal turbo spin-echo proton density-weighted MR arthrography images at 3.0 T demonstrate labral tear in pincer-type impingement at the anterior position (*arrowhead*) and posterior femoroacetabular cartilage degeneration (*arrow*).

is increasingly recognized as an important tool for morphologic assessment of FAI and an improved technique to detect early labral and chondral damage in the hip.[29]

Measurements in Femoroacetabular Impingement

Different MR imaging parameters are defined for assessment of FAI, such as alpha angle,

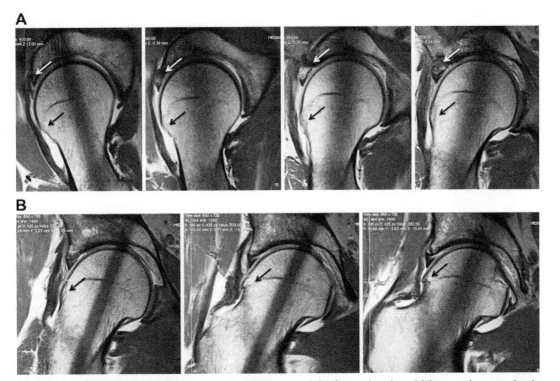

Fig. 3. Multiple (*A*) radial perpendicular reconstructions around the femoral neck and (*B*) coronal proton density-weighted MR imaging show loss of femoral head-neck offset from anterior to superior (*white arrows*). The radial reconstructions (*A*) also show a labral tear with exact anatomic localization at the anterosuperior position (*black arrows*).

head-neck-offset, acetabular depth, and acetabular version. According to Pfirrmann and colleagues,[21] the alpha angle can be measured between an axis parallel to the femoral neck passing through the narrowest portion of the femoral neck and an axis passing through the point at which the head contour passes into the metaphysis (Fig. 4). An angle of 55° or more is considered increased and pathologic. An interval of 30° among the radial reformats should be used to assess alpha angle. The offset can be determined based on the method described by Ito and colleagues.[39] It is the quotient of two lines defining the radius of the femoral head and the extension of the head-neck junction, which is defined by point at which the head contour passes into the metaphysis.

Offset is considered as reduced when it has a ratio of 1.2 or less. The acetabular coverage can be measured by assessing the acetabular depth within the axial reformat. The depth is expressed as distance between a line drawn among anterior and posterior acetabular horn and the center of the femoral head (Fig. 5). The acetabular version can be measured using two- or three-dimensional axial T1-weighted MR imaging through the acetabular roof as the anterior and posterior rims become apparent. The acetabular version is measured between the distance of the acetabular and posterior rim to the anterior and posterior axis of the pelvis, as shown in Fig. 6. Fig. 7 shows examples of different acetabular versions in patients with cam-type impingement (anteversion), mixed-type impingement (no version), and pincer-type impingement (retroversion).

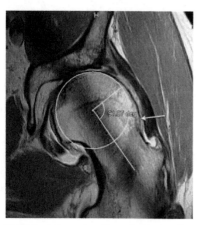

Fig. 4. Radial proton density-weighted reformatted MR imaging shows the assessment of increased alpha-angle (91°) at the anterosuperior position in a cam-type patient (*arrow*).

ASSESSMENT OF THE ACETABULAR LABRUM

For MR imaging assessment of the acetabular labrum, noncontrast techniques and arthrographic techniques are used. Based on comparison studies of different techniques in correlation to intraoperative findings, MR arthrography is more reliable in the diagnosis of acetabular labrum lesions. The contrast material, which is administered into the joint under fluoroscopic control, distends the capsule and allows better separation of the labrum and joint capsule. Labral tears may be better revealed through contrast filling into the clefts of the labrum. The diagnostic sensitivity of MR arthrography ranges from 90%[13] to 71%;[42] however, the interobserver reliability is only moderate.[20,42]

It is not possible to assess the thickness and orientation of the acetabular lesion when a two-dimensional MR imaging technique is used.[13,42] It is an invasive procedure that bears the risk of iatrogenic injury to adjacent neurovascular structures. Regarding staging and grading, most evaluation studies that have been described only determine location (anterosuperior, superolateral, and posterior) and whether a lesion is present.[42] The added grading classification of grades 1 to 3 used by Czerny and colleagues[43] depends on the degree of infiltration of the contrast agent into the acetabular labrum, a description of the tear, and changes of signal intensity, not yet correlated with structural changes of the acetabular labrum. In addition to staging there is still a lack of diagnosis for changes of the surface morphology, such as fibrillation, and changes on the junction between the acetabular cartilage and the acetabular labrum at 1.5 T.

ASSESSMENT OF ACETABULAR CARTILAGE

Compared to the well-established detection of osteonecrosis[44] and evaluation of the acetabular labrum, the role of cartilage lesion assessment is not well defined in the hip.[45] As in acetabular labrum diagnosis, noncontrast techniques and MR arthrography are used. Noncontrast techniques using two- and three-dimensional sequences analyze thickness measurement patterns for detection of the osteoarthritic changes.[46] Reported sensitivity for these measurements is 47% for grade 1 lesions and 49% for grade 2, which reveals low diagnostic efficiency and indicates that these measurements are more useful in follow-up studies.[46] Mintz and colleagues[47] tried to classify cartilage based on cartilage thickness and signal intensity changes according to the Outerbridge Score,[48] but the

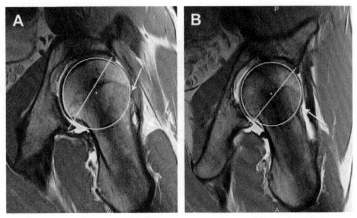

Fig. 5. Assessment of the acetabular depth according to Pfirrmann et al[21] in a radial position. Depth of the acetabulum was defined by the distance between the center of the femoral neck and the line that connects the anterior and posterior acetabular rim. Radial proton density-weighted reformatted MR imaging (A) shows the acetabulum is deeper the patient with pincer FAI and concave head-neck offset (arrow) (center of femoral head inside the acetabular fossa; acetabular depth negative) than in (B) the patient with cam FAI and loss of head-neck offset (arrow) (center of femoral head outside the acetabular fossa; acetabular depth positive).

results were unreliable. They compared only grades 1 to 3 lesions to no lesion (grade 0) for sensitivity and accuracy. The results are only comparable to thickness measurement studies with the same limitations. With the use of MR arthrography the detection of cartilage lesions could be improved,[20] but the classification within this study was done without staging or grading and the accuracy was only moderate (sensitivity of 47%). The analysis also was limited by low spatial resolution, particularly with regard to separated diagnosis of acetabular and femoral cartilage, restriction to two-dimensional imaging, and low signal-to-noise ratio caused by field strength of only 1.0 T or 1.5 T. High interobserver variability was reported.

Beaulé and colleagues[45] described cartilage delamination using MR arthrography and its correlation with intraoperative findings in four patients. Based on the subdivision of cartilage delamination by Beck and colleagues,[41] it was only possible to detect a cleavage (with a frayed edge). On the other hand, detection of debonding, in which the cartilage appears macroscopically sound but is mobile and simulates a carpet phenomenon that is observed intraoperatively anterosuperiorly in patients with FAI, was not possible. Overall, the cartilage diagnosis in the hip is limited so far, and no reliable staging and grading system has been established. The use of 3.0-T imaging in combination with MR arthrography in the future can overcome these limitations and improve cartilage diagnosis significantly (Fig. 8). Distinction of femoral and acetabular cartilage layer remains challenging because the cartilage of the femoroacetabular joint is thin and the

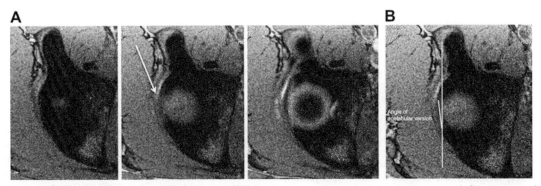

Fig. 6. Assessment of the acetabular version at the acetabular roof on axial three-dimensional, fat-suppressed, 2-mm slice thickness T1-weighted MR imaging shows (A, left to right) opening of the acetabulum (arrow) and (B) measurement of the acetabular version.

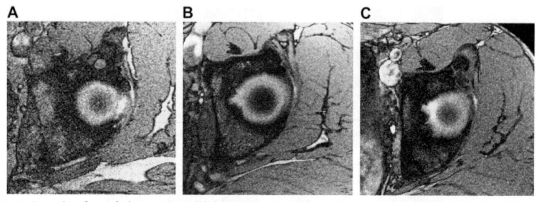

Fig. 7. Examples of acetabular version. Axial three-dimensional, fat-suppressed, 2-mm slice thickness T1-weighted MR imaging shows (*A*) cam-type hip with anteversion (12°), (*B*) mixed-type hip with neutral version (0°), and (*C*) pincer-type hip with retroversion (-9°).

cavity is circumferential, which makes it difficult to differentiate both cartilages from each other.

BIOCHEMICAL IMAGING

Articular cartilage is a highly structured tissue made up of chondrocytes and extracellular matrix composed of water, collagen fibers, negatively charged proteoglycan molecules, and glycosaminoglycans (GAG).[49,50] The collagen fibers network shows a specific arrangement. Fibers are oriented perpendicularly to the bone-cartilage interface within the radial zone (deepest zone); the orientation is oblique within the intermediate zone, and a parallel orientation is seen within the superficial zone. Not only does the orientation of collagen fibers differ between layers of cartilage but so does the concentration of proteoglycans, which

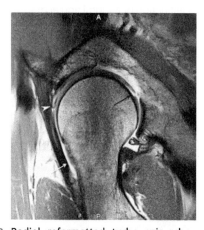

Fig. 8. Radial reformatted turbo spin-echo proton density-weighted MR imaging at 3.0 T in a patient with a cam-type impingement (*white arrow*) shows femoral cartilage lesion (*black arrow*) and intrasubstance lesion of the labrum (*white arrowhead*).

is superior within the intermediate zone, and the amount of water, which is greatest within the superficial zone.

During the progress of OA, cartilage constitution is altered (eg, in water content, collagen orientation, and proteoglycan/GAG content).[51] Biochemical MR imaging approaches, such as T1 mapping after gadolinium administration, T2 mapping, T2 magnetization transfer, and diffusion-weighted imaging sensitive for cartilage microstructure and biochemical content, may—in addition to morphologic evaluation—provide further insight into the progress of cartilage changing. One promising technique that was recently developed and applied to daily clinical routine is contrast-enhanced MR imaging, referred to as delayed gadolinium-enhanced MR imaging of cartilage (dGEMRIC). This technique is based on findings that GAG contributes a strong negative charge to the cartilage matrix. If a negatively charged contrast agent such as $Gd(DTPA)^{2-}$ is given time to distribute in the cartilage, it distributes in inverse proportion to the GAG content. By means of gadolinium-enhancement within cartilage and subsequent T1 quantification, T1 values can be used as an index for GAG concentration within cartilage. Because GAG seems to be lost early in cartilage degeneration, this technique may improve OA diagnosis at early stages.[12,52] dGEMRIC has been investigated in vitro,[53–55] in vivo,[56–60] and for follow-up of cartilage repair procedures.[61]

Kim and colleagues[52] investigated the applicability of dGEMRIC in hip dysplasia. In 68 hips (43 patients), the dGEMRIC index and joint space width were compared to radiographically and clinically relevant factors such as pain, severity of dysplasia, and age. The dGEMRIC index correlated significantly with pain ($r = -0.50$, $P < .0001$) and lateral center-edge angle as measure

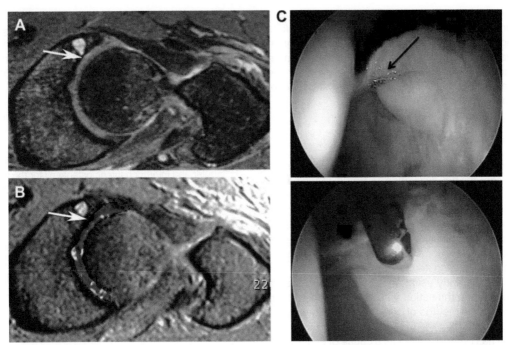

Fig. 9. A 36-year-old patient with cam-type impingement. (*A*) Axial T2-weighted MR imaging shows possible cartilage damage (*arrow*). (*B*) Axial dGEMRIC clearly shows an area of cartilage damage under the cyst (*arrow*). (*C*) Arthroscopic views demonstrate the cartilage lesion (*arrow*).

of severity of dysplasia (r = 0.52, P < .0001). In contrast, joint space width did not correlate with pain or severity of dysplasia. A statistically significant difference of the dGEMRIC index (P < .0001) among mild, moderate, and severe dysplasia could be observed. The average dGEMRIC index ranged from 570 ms (no dysplasia), to 550 ms (mild dysplasia), to 500 ms (moderate dysplasia), to 420 ms (severe dyplasia).

In another study, a cohort of 47 patients who underwent PAO for hip dysplasia was investigated prospectively.[62] In addition to patient age, radiographic severity of OA, and severity of dysplasia, the dGEMRIC index was evaluated. This study showed that PAO is an expedient tool to reduce pain and ameliorate joint function. Conversely, dGEMRIC was reported as the factor best applicable to identify possible failures of PAO preoperatively. The long-term follow-up of a cohort of patients after PAO with preoperatively low dGEMRIC index showed an increase of the dGEMRIC index postoperatively, which indicated that in defined and reversible stages of cartilage degeneration, OA might be reversible through disease-modifying procedures.[63]

Jessel and colleagues[64] used dGEMRIC to establish a prediction model in 96 hips (74 patients who had symptomatic dysplasia) and identified age, severity of dysplasia, and labral tear as

factors associated with significant hip OA. They showed that dGEMRIC might be able to identify patients who would develop significant hip OA and potentially would profit from a salvage procedure such as PAO. This finding was consistent with the other preliminary studies. Concerning the FAI group, Jessel and colleagues described 30 symptomatic patients (37 hips) who were treated with open surgery and were assessed by dGEMRIC preoperatively.[64] The dGEMRIC index (487 ± 70 ms) was significantly lower than in the control group (570 ± 90 ms). A statistically significant correlation could be established between dGEMRIC index and alpha angle (P < .05), although there was no correlation between age or gender of patients. They concluded that dGEMRIC index qualifies as a measure for the severity of cartilage damage in patients with FAI and reflects the severity of anatomic deformity. The results in the group of FAI patients are less consistent than in the group of dysplasia patients, which might be because of the complex nature of the deformity in FAI.

To reduce acquisition time, a gradient-echo approach for T1 mapping instead of multi-spin-echo using a dual flip angle technique to obtain T1 values has been developed. This technique has shown promising results in phantom experiments and in vivo for the evaluation of reparative cartilage within the knee after matrix-associated autologous chondrocyte transplantation at 3.0 T.[61] Besides a significant reduction of scanning time, the great advantage is the possibility to create three-dimensional maps of the hip cartilage that allow for the assessment of the complex special structure of damage pattern in FAI (Fig. 9).

SUMMARY

MR imaging represents the best available noninvasive tool for hip evaluation in terms of indication and planning for surgical treatment in OA. It still has limitations in diagnosing cartilage, especially in the early OA stage. The relatively thin cartilage, the spherical joint shape, and narrowness of tissue structures pose logistical difficulties and demand high MR imaging technology standards. So far, MR arthrography using an intra-articular contrast material in combination with radial reconstructed planes is the method of choice for hip assessment in early OA.

FAI has been identified as a cause of early-onset OA in the hip. Therapeutic strategies do exist but only achieve good results in hips without degenerative changes at the early stage. This finding emphasizes the need for diagnostic concepts that enable the detection of early cartilage and labral degeneration. Recent developments in high-resolution isotropic imaging, cartilage-specific MR imaging sequences, local gradient and radio frequency coils, and high field MR systems have improved diagnostic capabilities in terms of signal-to-noise ratio, contrast-to-noise ratio, and shorter acquisition times. In addition to morphologic MR imaging, biochemical MR imaging approaches that characterize cartilage microstructure and biochemical content will contribute to a better understanding of cartilage degeneration.

REFERENCES

1. Felson DT. An update on the pathogenesis and epidemiology of osteoarthritis. Radiol Clin North Am 2004;42(1):1–9, v.
2. Jäger M, Wild A, Westhoff B, et al. Femoroacetabular impingement caused by a femoral osseous head-neck bump deformity: clinical, radiological, and experimental results. J Orthop Sci 2004;9(3):256–63 [in German].
3. Ganz R, Gill TJ, Gautier E, et al. Surgical dislocation of the adult hip a technique with full access to the femoral head and acetabulum without the risk of avascular necrosis. J Bone Joint Surg Br 2001;83(8):1119–24.
4. Ganz R, Parvizi J, Beck M, et al. Femoroacetabular impingement: a cause for osteoarthritis of the hip. Clin Orthop Relat Res 2003;417:112–20.
5. Guanche CA, Bare AA. Arthroscopic treatment of femoroacetabular impingement. Arthroscopy 2006;22(1):95–106.
6. Murphy S, Tannast M, Kim YJ, et al. Debridement of the adult hip for femoroacetabular impingement: indications and preliminary clinical results. Clin Orthop Relat Res 2004;429:178–81.
7. Trousdale RT, Ekkernkamp A, Ganz R, et al. Periacetabular and intertrochanteric osteotomy for the treatment of osteoarthrosis in dysplastic hips. J Bone Joint Surg Am 1995;77(1):73–85.
8. Trumble SJ, Mayo KA, Mast JW. The periacetabular osteotomy: minimum 2 year followup in more than 100 hips. Clin Orthop Relat Res 1999;363:54–63.
9. Eckstein F. Noninvasive study of human cartilage structure by MRI. Methods Mol Med 2004;101:191–217.
10. Eckstein F, Glaser C. Measuring cartilage morphology with quantitative magnetic resonance imaging. Semin Musculoskelet Radiol 2004;8(4):329–53.
11. Koo S, Gold GE, Andriacchi TP. Considerations in measuring cartilage thickness using MRI: factors influencing reproducibility and accuracy. Osteoarthr Cartil 2005;13(9):782–9.
12. Recht MP, Goodwin DW, Winalski CS, et al. MRI of articular cartilage: revisiting current status and future directions. AJR Am J Roentgenol 2005;185(4):899–914.
13. Czerny C, Hofmann S, Neuhold A, et al. Lesions of the acetabular labrum: accuracy of MR imaging and MR arthrography in detection and staging. Radiology 1996;200(1):225–30.
14. Balkissoon A. MR imaging of cartilage: evaluation and comparison of MR imaging techniques. Top Magn Reson Imaging 1996;8(1):57–67.
15. Plotz GM, Brossmann J, Schunke M, et al. Magnetic resonance arthrography of the acetabular labrum: macroscopic and histological correlation in 20 cadavers. J Bone Joint Surg Br 2000;82(3):426–32.
16. Locher S, Werlen S, Leunig M, et al. [MR-Arthrography with radial sequences for visualization of early hip pathology not visible on plain radiographs]. Z Orthop Ihre Grenzgeb 2002;140(1):52–7 [in German].
17. Petersilge CA, Haque MA, Petersilge WJ, et al. Acetabular labral tears: evaluation with MR arthrography. Radiology 1996;200(1):231–5.
18. Petersilge CA. MR arthrography for evaluation of the acetabular labrum. Skeletal Radiol 2001;30(8):423–30.
19. Knuesel PR, Pfirrmann CW, Noetzli HP, et al. MR arthrography of the hip: diagnostic performance of a dedicated water-excitation 3D double-echo steady-state sequence to detect cartilage lesions. AJR Am J Roentgenol 2004;183(6):1729–35.

20. Schmid MR, Notzli HP, Zanetti M, et al. Cartilage lesions in the hip: diagnostic effectiveness of MR arthrography. Radiology 2003;226(2):382–6.

21. Pfirrmann CW, Mengiardi B, Dora C, et al. Cam and pincer femoroacetabular impingement: characteristic MR arthrographic findings in 50 patients. Radiology 2006;240(3):778–85.

22. Kim YJ, Bixby S, Mamisch TC, et al. Imaging structural abnormalities in the hip joint: instability and impingement as a cause of osteoarthritis. Semin Musculoskelet Radiol 2008;12(4):334–45.

23. Kim YJ. Nonarthroplasty hip surgery for early osteoarthritis. Rheum Dis Clin North Am 2008;34(3):803–14.

24. Leunig M, Beck M, Dora C, et al. [Femoroacetabular impingement: trigger for the development of osteoarthritis]. Orthopade 2005;35(1):77–84 [in German].

25. Reynolds D, Lucas J, Klaue K. Retroversion of the acetabulum: a cause of hip pain. J Bone Joint Surg Br 1999;81(2):281–8.

26. Dora C, Zurbach J, Hersche O, et al. Pathomorphologic characteristics of posttraumatic acetabular dysplasia. J Orthop Trauma 2000;14(7):483–9.

27. Dora C, Mascard E, Mladenov K, et al. Retroversion of the acetabular dome after Salter and triple pelvic osteotomy for congenital dislocation of the hip. J Pediatr Orthop B 2002;11(1):34–40.

28. Beck M, Kalhor M, Leunig M, et al. Hip morphology influences the pattern of damage to the acetabular cartilage: femoroacetabular impingement as a cause of early osteoarthritis of the hip. J Bone Joint Surg Br 2005;87(7):1012–8.

29. Kassarjian A, Yoon LS, Belzile E, et al. Triad of MR arthrographic findings in patients with cam-type femoroacetabular impingement. Radiology 2005;236(2):588–92.

30. Leunig M, Ganz R. [Femoroacetabular impingement: a common cause of hip complaints leading to arthrosis]. Unfallchirurg 2005;108(1):9–17 [in German].

31. MacDonald S, Garbuz D, Ganz R. Clinical evaluation of the symptomatic young adult hip. Semin Arthroplasty 1997;8:3–9.

32. Siebenrock KA, Schoeniger R, Ganz R. Anterior femoro-acetabular impingement due to acetabular retroversion: treatment with periacetabular osteotomy. J Bone Joint Surg Am 2003;85(2):278–86.

33. Kellgren JH, Lawrence JS. Radiological assessment of osteo-arthrosis. Ann Rheum Dis 1957;16:494–502.

34. Eijer H, Myers SR, Ganz R. Anterior femoroacetabular impingement after femoral neck fractures. J Orthop Trauma 2001;15(7):475–81.

35. Siebenrock KA, Wahab KH, Werlen S, et al. Abnormal extension of the femoral head epiphysis as a cause of cam impingement. Clin Orthop Relat Res 2004;418:54–60.

36. Stulberg SD, Cordell LD, Harris WH, et al. Unrecognized childhood hip disease: a major cause of idiopathic osteoarthritis of the hip. Proceedings of the Third Open Scientific Meeting of the Hip. St. Louis (MO); 1975; p. 212–28.

37. Locher S, Werlen S, Leunig M, et al. [Inadequate detectability of early stages of coxarthrosis with conventional roentgen images]. Z Orthop Ihre Grenzgeb 2001;139(1):70–4 [in German].

38. Kubo T, Horii M, Harada Y, et al. Radial-sequence magnetic resonance imaging in evaluation of acetabular labrum. J Orthop Sci 1999;4(5):328–32.

39. Ito K, Minka MA II, Leunig M, et al. Femoroacetabular impingement and the cam-effect: a MRI-based quantitative anatomical study of the femoral head-neck offset. J Bone Joint Surg Br 2001;83(2):171–6.

40. Leunig M, Werlen S, Ungersbock A, et al. Evaluation of the acetabular labrum by MR arthrography. J Bone Joint Surg Br 1997;79(2):230–4.

41. Beck M, Leunig M, Parvizi J, et al. Anterior femoroacetabular impingement: part II. Midterm results of surgical treatment. Clin Orthop Relat Res 2004;418:67–73.

42. Keeney JA, Peelle MW, Jackson J, et al. Magnetic resonance arthrography versus arthroscopy in the evaluation of articular hip pathology. Clin Orthop Relat Res 2004;429:163–9.

43. Czerny C, Kramer J, Neuhold A, et al. [Magnetic resonance imaging and magnetic resonance arthrography of the acetabular labrum: comparison with surgical findings]. Rofo 2001;173(8):702–7 [in German].

44. Mont MA, Hungerford DS. Non-traumatic avascular necrosis of the femoral head. J Bone Joint Surg Am 1995;77(3):459–74.

45. Beaulé PE, Zaragoza E, Copelan N. Magnetic resonance imaging with gadolinium arthrography to assess acetabular cartilage delamination: a report of four cases. J Bone Joint Surg Am 2004;86(10):2294–8.

46. Nishii T, Nakanishi K, Sugano N, et al. Articular cartilage evaluation in osteoarthritis of the hip with MR imaging under continuous leg traction. Magn Reson Imaging 1998;16(8):871–5.

47. Mintz DN, Hooper T, Connell D, et al. Magnetic resonance imaging of the hip: detection of labral and chondral abnormalities using noncontrast imaging. Arthroscopy 2005;21(4):385–93.

48. Outerbridge RE. The etiology of chondromalacia patellae. J Bone Joint Surg Br 1961;43:752–7.

49. Poole AR, Kojima T, Yasuda T, et al. Composition and structure of articular cartilage: a template for tissue repair. Clin Orthop Relat Res 2001;(Suppl 391):S26–33.

50. Cova M, Toffanin R. MR microscopy of hyaline cartilage: current status. Eur Radiol 2002;12(4):814–23.

51. Venn M, Maroudas A. Chemical composition and swelling of normal and osteoarthrotic femoral head cartilage. I. Chemical composition. Ann Rheum Dis 1977;36(2):121–9.

52. Kim YJ, Jaramillo D, Millis MB, et al. Assessment of early osteoarthritis in hip dysplasia with delayed gadolinium-enhanced magnetic resonance imaging of cartilage. J Bone Joint Surg Am 2003;85(10): 1987–92.

53. Woertler K, Buerger H, Moeller J, et al. Patellar articular cartilage lesions: in vitro MR imaging evaluation after placement in gadopentetate dimeglumine solution. Radiology 2004;230(3):768–73.

54. Mlynarik V, Trattnig S, Huber M, et al. The role of relaxation times in monitoring proteoglycan depletion in articular cartilage. J Magn Reson Imaging 1999;10(4):497–502.

55. Bashir A, Gray ML, Burstein D. Gd-DTPA2- as a measure of cartilage degradation. Magn Reson Med 1996;36(5):665–73.

56. Bashir A, Gray ML, Boutin RD, et al. Glycosaminoglycan in articular cartilage: in vivo assessment with delayed Gd(DTPA) (2-)-enhanced MR imaging. Radiology 1997;205(2):551–8.

57. Burstein D, Velyvis J, Scott KT, et al. Protocol issues for delayed Gd(DTPA) (2-)-enhanced MRI (dGEMRIC) for clinical evaluation of articular cartilage. Magn Reson Med 2001;45(1):36–41.

58. Tiderius C, Olsson L, de Verdier H, et al. Gd-DTPA2-enhanced MRI of femoral knee cartilage: a dose response study in healthy volunteers. Magn Reson Med 2001;46:1067–71.

59. Tiderius CJ, Olsson LE, Leander P, et al. Delayed gadolinium-enhanced MRI of cartilage (dGEMRIC) in early knee osteoarthritis. Magn Reson Med 2003;49(3):488–92.

60. Williams A, Gillis A, McKenzie C, et al. Glycosaminoglycan distribution in cartilage as determined by delayed gadolinium-enhanced MRI of cartilage (dGEMRIC): potential clinical applications. AJR Am J Roentgenol 2004;182(1):167–72.

61. Trattnig S, Marlovits S, Gebetsroither S, et al. Three-dimensional delayed gadolinium-enhanced MRI of cartilage (dGEMRIC) for in vivo evaluation of reparative cartilage after matrix-associated autologous chondrocyte transplantation at 3.0T: preliminary results. J Magn Reson Imaging 2007;26(4):974–82.

62. Cunningham T, Jessel R, Zurakowski D, et al. Delayed gadolinium-enhanced magnetic resonance imaging of cartilage to predict early failure of Bernese periacetabular osteotomy for hip dysplasia. J Bone Joint Surg Am 2006;88(7):1540–8.

63. Jessel R, Zurakowski D, Zilkens C, et al. Radiographic and patient factors associated with pre-radiographic osteoarthritis in hip dysplasia. J Bone Joint Surg Am 2009;91(5):1120–9.

64. Jessel R, Zilkens C, Tiderius C, et al. Assessment of osteoarthritis in hips with femoroacetabular impingement using delayed gadolinium enhanced MRI of cartilage. JMRM, accepted for publication.

Osteoarthritis of the Wrist and Hand, and Spine

Antoine Feydy, MD, PhD*, Etienne Pluot, MD, Henri Guerini, MD,
Jean-Luc Drapé, MD, PhD

KEYWORDS

- Osteoarthritis • Wrist • Hand • Finger
- Spine • Imaging • Grading

OSTEOARTHRITIS OF THE WRIST AND HAND

There is a striking difference between the rarity of osteoarthritis (OA) of the wrist and the rather high prevalence of OA of the fingers. OA in the fingers usually occurs following a trauma or as a result of ongoing metabolic joint diseases, especially calcium pyrophosphade dehydrate (CPPD) deposition disease, which is also called chondrocalcinosis. Finger OA is frequent in postmenopausal women and represents up to one third of the cases of peripheral OA, after OA of the knee and hip. Assessing the prevalence of hand OA (HOA) depends on the criteria supporting the diagnosis. The Framingham Study estimated the prevalence to be as high as 26% of women and 12% of men more than 70 years of age;[1] however, according to Kellgren and Lawrence,[2] radiographic definition HOA was identified in 67% of the women and 55% of the men in the Rotterdam Study, a population-based cohort study (age >55 years).[3] The prevalence of OA in distal interphalangeal and proximal interphalangeal joints in people older than 55 years of age reaches 20% and 5%, respectively. Trapezio-metacarpal (TMC) joint OA, which is also called rhizarthrosis, is present in 8% of the population more than 55 years of age. HOA remains a frequent complaint from patients, with the aesthetic harm resulting from deformity being a major concern in some patients. Pain is the main symptom of rhizarthrosis, ahead of deformity. Treatment of HOA should be individualized according to the localization of OA; risk factors (eg, age, sex, adverse mechanical factors); type of OA (eg, nodal, erosive, traumatic); presence of inflammation; severity of structural change; level of pain, disability, and restriction of quality of life; comorbidity and comedication (including OA at other sites); and the wishes and expectations of the patient.[4] Management of OA of the wrist and hand remains nonsurgical in most cases. Surgery should be discussed in case of failure of nonsurgical procedures in controlling the symptoms.

Demographics

Age is the main risk factor of developing HOA. The incidence of the condition increases after 45 years of age, ranging from 5% at 40 years to 65% after 80.[5] Mechanical overuse is classically the main predisposing factor to the development of HOA, but other factors such as gender, hormones, genetics, or obesity might be associated. Degenerative changes tend to be more severe in distal interphalangeal joints, especially of the index finger, than in proximal interphalangeal or carpometacarpal joints. HOA mostly occurs on the dominant hand.[6] Degenerative damages can be secondary to single or multiple preexisting traumatic injuries (eg, sprain, fracture), and men are most commonly affected.

The interphalangeal and TMC joints are the most common localization of HOA in women more than 55 years of age. Rhizarthrosis is rarely encountered in men younger than 50 years of age,

Department of Radiology B, Cochin Hospital, Paris Descartes University, 27 rue du Faubourg Saint Jacques, 75014 Paris, France
* Corresponding author.
E-mail address: antoine.feydy@cch.aphp.fr (A. Feydy).

Radiol Clin N Am 47 (2009) 723–759
doi:10.1016/j.rcl.2009.06.004
0033-8389/09/$ – see front matter © 2009 Published by Elsevier Inc.

whereas the condition is present in 8% of women of the same age group. Before 70 years of age, the prevalence of HOA in women exceeds that of men by 50%. The prevalence of finger OA is noticeably higher in women after early or induced menopause. The prevalence of TMC OA is dramatically increased in women after hysterectomy.[7] These differences of prevalence suggest a role of sexual hormones in the pathogenesis of HOA.[8] However, the exact role of estrogens remains unclear, even though their protective but rather deleterious actions have been described in the literature. Nevertheless, no correlation between HOA and administration of estrogens or a previous history of hysterectomy could be demonstrated in the Framingham Study.[9]

Genetic factors may also predispose a person to HOA, especially in women.[10] Mutations of genes that code for collagen II may increase the risk of developing early OA.[11] The role of human leukocyte antigen types in regard to the risk of OA remains much debated.[12,13]

Trapezio-metacarpal Joint Osteoarthritis (Rhizarthrosis)

Almost always bilateral, rhizarthrosis occurs in perimenopausal women and affects the dominant hand more severely. Rhizarthrosis should probably be called "peritrapezial OA" because the degenerative changes extend to the adjacent scapho-trapezial and trapezio-trapezoid joints.

Clinical presentation

Mechanical soreness of the base of the thumb and the thenar eminence is the main clinical sign of rhizarthrosis. The pattern of pain can also be inflammatory, and pain occurs when sleeping, although this pattern should raise the possibility of associated conditions, especially carpal tunnel syndrome, which is present in 40% of cases.[14] Clinical examination is reliable in distinguishing rhizarthrosis from the more proximal scapho-trapezial OA.

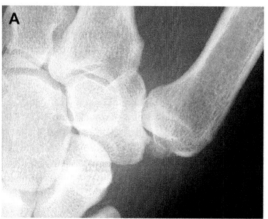
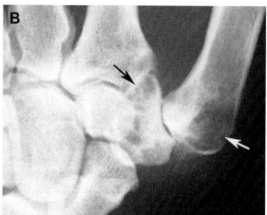
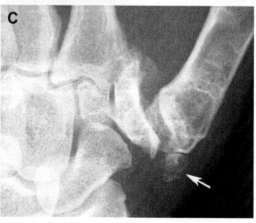

Fig. 1. Rhizarthrosis outcome. (A) PA radiograph of the wrist at baseline shows lateral TMC and slight trapezial osteophytosis with dysplasia. (B) Follow-up PA radiograph 3 years later demonstrates JSN and trapezial subchondral osteosclerosis with a large bone cyst of the trapezium and M1 (arrows). (C) PA radiograph at 12-year follow-up shows bone loss of the trapezium and loose bodies larger than 2 mm (arrow).

Radiographs

As in other localizations, there is no correlation between clinical presentation and radiographic findings. Specific posteroanterior (PA) and lateral views of the TMC joint must be obtained (using Kapandji's or Robert's views).[15] The radiographic features of rhizarthrosis are characterized by joint space narrowing (JSN) and deformity, the presence of osteophytes, and the development in the trapezium of subchondral sclerosis and geodes and subchondral cysts. Prominent destruction of the joint cartilage leads to subluxation of metacarpal (M1) laterally and enlargement of the first intermetacarpal space (**Fig. 1**). Secondary loose bodies may also occur. Dell's (**Box 1**) and Eaton's (**Box 2**) radiologic classifications are the most commonly used.[16] Dell's classification focuses only on the TMC joint, without the pre-OA stage. Eaton's classification includes a pre-OA stage and also the involvement of the scapho-trapezial, trapezio-trapezoid, and TMC joints.

The "trapezial tilt" can be assessed using PA Kapandji's or Robert's views (**Fig. 2**). The normal values are 125° and 42° ± 4°, respectively. Advanced TMC joint OA (Eaton III and IV) is associated with an increased trapezial tilt. Mild TMC joint arthritis with an increased trapezial tilt may be treated surgically. Dynamic PA views allow evaluation of the reversibility of the subluxation of M1 and assessment of the increased mobility of the trapezium bone in case of rhizarthrosis.

MR imaging

MR imaging may demonstrate extensive synovitis and bone marrow edema of the TMC joint (**Fig. 3**). Synovial expansions may develop toward the first intermetacarpal space. Bone cyst boundaries are more accurately defined using MR imaging than when using radiographs.

Scapho-trapezial Osteoarthritis

Scapho-trapezial OA is most commonly associated with rhizarthrosis. In cases of isolated OA of

> **Box 1**
> **Dell's classification of trapezio-metacarpal osteoarthritis**
>
> Stage I: Joint space narrowing without subluxation or osteophytes
>
> Stage II: Joint space narrowing, osteophytes, subtle subluxation
>
> Stage III: Joint space narrowing, osteophytes, subluxation or TMC dislocation
>
> Stage IV: As Stage III, plus geodes

> **Box 2**
> **Eaton's classification of trapezio-metacarpal osteoarthritis**
>
> Stage I: Normal or slightly widened TMC joint, normal articular contours, TMC subluxation (if present in up to one third of the articular surface)
>
> Stage II: Decreased TMC joint space, TMC subluxation (if present in up to one third of the articular surface), osteophytes or loose bodies less than 2 mm in diameter
>
> Stage III: Further decrease in TMC joint space, subchondral cysts or sclerosis, osteophytes or loose bodies 2 mm or more in diameter, TMC joint subluxation of one third or more of the articular surface
>
> Stage IV: Involvement of the scapho-trapezial joint or less commonly the trapezio-trapezoid or TMC joint to the index finger

the scapho-trapezial joint, this association would be highly suggestive of a crystal-related arthropathy, especially CPPD deposition disease. Scapho-trapezial OA is more frequent in women aged 50 or older. Asymptomatic forms are frequent. Radiographic features of the condition are seen in up to 7% of women and 2% of men.[17]

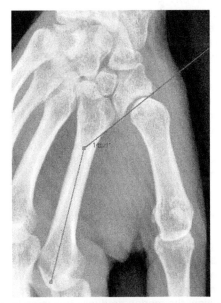

Fig. 2. Trapezial slope assessment. PA Kapandji's radiograph shows that the angle between the inferior joint surface of the trapezium and the long axis of M2 is significantly increased at greater than 140° and measures 142.7°.

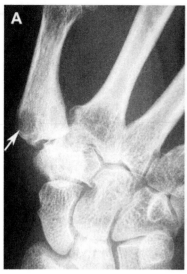
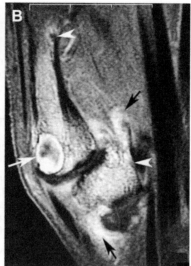

Fig. 3. Rhizarthrosis with extensive bone edema. (*A*) Radiograph shows a bone cyst of M1 (*arrow*) and trapezial osteosclerosis. (*B*) The coronal contrast-enhanced, fat-suppressed, T1-weighted MR image shows peripheral enhancement of the bone cyst (*white arrow*) and extensive bone edema (*arrowheads*) of the whole trapezium and most of the first metacarpal. There are synovial expansions (*black arrows*) superiorly and inferiorly toward the first intermetacarpal space.

Clinical presentation

In cases of CPPD deposition disease, OA of the scapho-trapezial joint is part of a multifocal form of OA. Initially, patients present with subtle tenderness exacerbated by thumb mobilization and a loss of strength of the pollici-digital pinch. A classic complication is represented by tenosynovitis of the flexor carpi radialis (FCR) tendon, which occurs because of the close relationship between the tendon and the scapho-trapezial joint.

Radiographs

A PA radiograph of the wrist and an oblique view of the semipronated wrist should be obtained to visualize the base of the thumb. Comparatives studies allow the detection of early joint space loss. Radiologic features are represented by JSN, subchondral sclerosis, subchondral geodes, osteophytes, and marked cortical irregularities at the distal aspect of the scaphoid, which can simulate erosions (Fig. 4). In later stages, the scaphoid bone tilts horizontally, which results in shortening of the carpus and secondary dorsal intercalated segmental instability.[18]

Ultrasound

The main ultrasonographic features of tendinopathy of the FCR tendon are characterized by enlargement of the tendon and hyporeflective areas replacing the normal fibrillar appearance of the tendon. Areas of tendon necrosis might appear as unreflective areas. In advanced stages of the condition, the tendon gradually becomes thinner, leading to partial or even full-thickness tears. Because of the oblique course of the tendon toward the deeper layers of the hand and its insertion on the base of M2, anisotropy provides

challenges to a thorough examination of the distal part of the tendon. Examinations may also be challenged by a probable hypertrophic tubercle of the scaphoid. A dynamic maneuver using palmar flexion of the wrist reduces the obliquity of the tendon and the associated anisotropy. Ultrasonic examination can also reveal cortical irregularities of the distal aspect of the scaphoid adjacent to the tendon sheath, joint effusion, and scapho-trapezial synovitis.

Arthrography and CT-arthrography

Arthrography obtained after midcarpal opacification may demonstrate an abnormal opacification of the FCR tendon sheath, indicating an abnormal

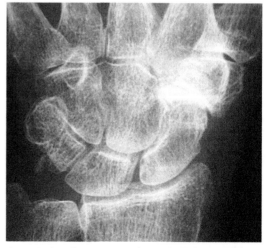

Fig. 4. Isolated, severe scapho-trapezial joint OA. PA radiograph shows complete JSN with subchondral bone sclerosis.

carpal capsular breach near the scapho-trapezial joint (Fig. 5). CT-arthrography best depicts the topography and severity of chondral lesions. Subchondral geodes are usually partially filled using intra-articular contrast.

MR imaging and MR-arthrography

MR imaging can be used to detect early scapho-trapezial OA before radiographic abnormalities are visible in demonstrating a subchondral bone edema (Fig. 6). The great advantage of MR imaging in comparison with ultrasound and CT-arthrography is the ability to show the scapho-trapezial joint and the adjacent soft tissues. In addition to demonstrating tenosynovitis of the FCR tendon and midsubstance tendinopathy, MR imaging is reliable in demonstrating joint effusion, synovitis, and extensive subchondral bone edema within the scapho-trapezial joint (Fig. 7). Intra-articular injection of gadolinium does not appear to improve the assessment of this joint and the surrounding soft tissues.

Radiocarpal Joint Osteoarthritis

Clinical presentation

Radiocarpal OA generally occurs secondary to wrist sprain (eg, scapho-lunate advanced collapse [SLAC] wrist), fracture, or necrosis involving a carpal bone (eg, scaphoid nonunion advanced

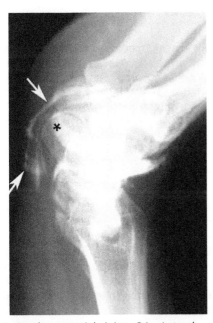

Fig. 5. Scapho-trapezial joint OA. Lateral arthrographic view with extension shows leakage of contrast medium toward the tendon sheath of the FCR tendon (*arrows*) in front of the distal tubercle of scaphoid (*).

collapse [SNAC] of the wrist), and it occurs much less frequently than OA in the fingers. The two most frequent types of OA in the wrist are SLAC (55%) and scaphotrapezio-trapezoid (STT) OA (20%). SLAC wrist involves the radio-scaphoid, luno-capitate, and scapho-capitate joints. STT OA involves the scapho-trapezial, scapho-trapezoid, and trapezio-trapezoid joints. SLAC wrist and STT OA can be associated with up to 10% of cases of OA of the wrist.

Radiographs

PA, lateral, and oblique views in neutral position should be obtained to best assess intra-carpal instabilities. Findings suggestive of OA are nonspecific, but the distribution of the lesions is stereotyped and classified as follows (Fig. 8):

> Grade 1: Limited radio-scaphoid OA to the lateral aspect of the joint
> Grade 2: Extensive OA of the radio-scaphoid joint
> Grade 3: Luno-capitate OA.

The scapho-capitate joint may also be severely damaged, leading to impaction of the capitate. The capitate then translates proximally toward the radius, which results in secondary narrowing of the hamato-lunate joint space (Fig. 9). This joint space loss is best diagnosed using PA views obtained with ulnar flexion of the wrist.

Radiographic evidence of CPPD deposition disease should not be overlooked because the triangular fibrocartilage complex, luno-triquetral ligament, and luno-triquetral cartilage are the most common sites of calcification around the wrist. Calcific deposits within hyaline cartilage appear to be thin, well-defined, and linear, following the contour of the subchondral plate.

CT-arthrography, MR imaging, and MR-arthrography

Radiographs are usually reliable to aid in the diagnosis of OA. Before any surgical treatment (eg, ligament repair, arthrodesis), a thorough assessment of the cartilage is often required. This is best demonstrated using CT-arthrography, MR imaging, or MR-arthrography, with the latter providing the highest degree of accuracy.

Classic features of chondropathy in the wrist are not specific, but the distribution of the chondral lesions is of utmost importance. More specific imaging findings of radiocarpal OA, such as the following, should be reported:

> Early subchondral edema of the distal tip of the radius, joint synovitis using MR imaging

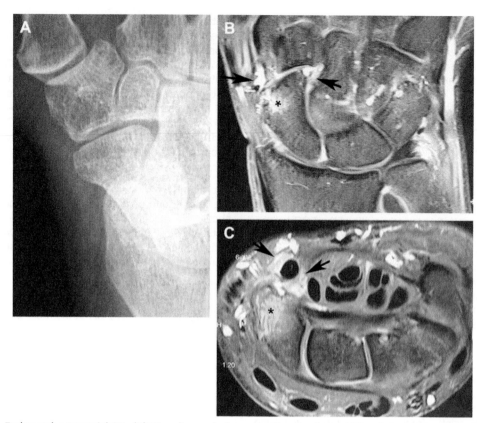

Fig. 6. Early scapho-trapezial OA. (*A*) PA radiograph shows no discrete abnormality of the scapho-trapezial joint. (*B*) Coronal and (*C*) axial contrast-enhanced, fat-suppressed, T1-weighted MR images show bone marrow edema of the distal scaphoid (*) with cortex irregularities and synovitis of the scapho-trapezio-trapezoid joint (*arrows*). Note on (*C*) the tenosynovitis of the FCR tendon (*arrows*).

and MR-arthrography that precedes the appearance of radiographic abnormalities.

- JSN, subchondral sclerosis and geodes, osteophytes using radiography and CT-arthrography. Osteophytes developed at the junction between the articular and nonarticular surfaces at the lateral edge of the scaphoid and the thinning of the radial styloid process are early signs of SLAC wrist.
- Chondral thinning, deepening of chondral fissures using CT-arthrography (Fig. 10), MR imaging, and MR-arthrography.
- In later stages, radio-carpal JSN and then luno-capitate JSN occur. When the cartilage surface between the capitate and hamate is worn out, impingement and secondary OA of the luno-hamate joint occurs.
- The radio-lunate joint is usually preserved until the late stages of the condition.

To date, there have been almost no studies in the literature comparing the accuracy of the different imaging modalities in detecting intracarpal chondral lesions. A recent study demonstrated a much better accuracy rate for CT-arthrography, supported by sensitivity and specificity of 100% compared with an average sensitivity of 10% to 30% and 30% to 40% using MR imaging and MR-arthrography, respectively.[19]

Distal Radio-ulnar Joint Osteoarthritis

Clinical presentation

Distal radio-ulnar joint OA usually occurs secondary to various types of trauma (ie, distal radio-ulnar joint dislocation, or fracture of both the distal radius and ulna). Pronation-supination is painful, markedly on the medial aspect of the wrist. The ulnar head is commonly subluxed dorsally. Any attempt to reduce this subluxation is painful and unstable.

Radiographs

Oblique views obtained in a neutral position show the dorsal displacement of the ulnar head. The pisiform bone should be centrally located between

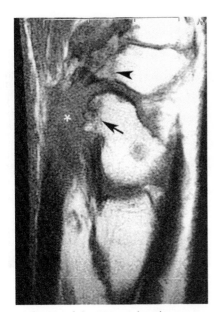

Fig. 7. Tendonitis of the FCR tendon due to severe sca-pho-trapezial OA. Sagittal T1-weighted MR image shows that the FCR tendon is enlarged with decreased signal (*) in front of bone spurs and bone marrow edema of the distal part of the scaphoid (*arrow*). Note also the degenerative lesions of the tubercle of the trapezium (*arrowhead*).

the palmar cortical lines of the scaphoid and capitate bones on oblique views. Other radiographic findings are bone sclerosis and geodes on the ulnar head and the sigmoid notch of the radius.

Ulno-carpal Joint Osteoarthritis

Ulnar impaction syndrome that is caused by a relatively long ulna leads to ulno-carpal OA. The presence of a relatively long ulna is either congenital or acquired following fractures complicated by vicious callus and shortening and angulation of the distal radius (Colles' fracture). Subsequent excessive load applied on the triangular ligament and the lunate and triquetrum bones induces mechanical pain located at the ulnar aspect of the wrist.

Radiographs
On PA views of a pronated wrist, the ulnar variance is positive, which indicates the presence of an excessively long ulna. The ulnar variance indicates the level of the distal ulna relative to the distal radius. Normal values range from −2 to 0 mm. Indirect signs of chondropathy (eg, sclerosis, geodes) are demonstrated on the medial part of the proximal aspect of the lunate and ulnar head (**Fig. 11**). Luno-triquetral joint diastasis and

disruption of Gilula's first arch related to a tear through the luno-triquetral ligament are also possible.

Arthrography, CT-arthrography, and MR imaging
The best imaging modality to reveal an ulnar impaction syndrome is MR imaging. It demonstrates a typical pattern of lesions, including medial and proximal chondral defect of the lunate, thinning and perforation of the triangular fibrocartilage complex associated with an excessively long ulna, and luno-triquetral ligament tears. The distribution of subchondral bone edema follows a typical pattern, and it is located at the medial and proximal part of the lunate, adjacent to chondral lesions. Subchondral edema in ulnar impaction syndrome tends to be less extensive than in Kienböck's disease, which is also more centrally located. Bone edema can also occur in the ulnar head and at the insertion of the luno-triquetral ligament. There seems to be a strong correlation between subchondral bone edema and the intensity of pain related to ulnar impaction syndrome. Noticeably, ulnar impaction syndrome can occur without abnormal ulnar variance and can be related to a sole dynamic impingement. In such cases, MR imaging is of great help to demonstrate associated signs (**Fig. 12**).

Piso-triquetral Joint Osteoarthritis

Clinical presentation
Diagnosing piso-triquetral joint OA is pretty straightforward and is mainly based on clinical examination. Patients present with typical ulnar-sided wrist pain, possibly associated with signs of ulnar nerve entrapment within Guyon's canal. Pain is exacerbated in ulnar or volar flexion.

Radiographs
In addition to PA and oblique views of the wrist, a carpal tunnel view and a 30° oblique view in supination must be obtained to correctly assess the joint space (**Fig. 13**).[20]

Ultrasound
Joint effusions, distension of the superior and inferior synovial recess, and a potential ganglion developing within Guyon's canal are well demonstrated using ultrasound (**Fig. 14**). Ulnar nerve displacement and any probable inflammatory appearance of the synovium are also detected. Steroids can be aspirated and injected into the joint using ultrasound guidance. The appearance of the flexor carpi ulnaris enthesis can also be depicted.

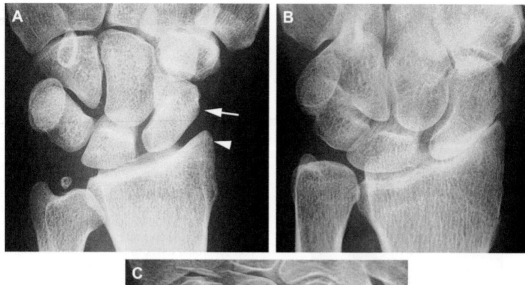

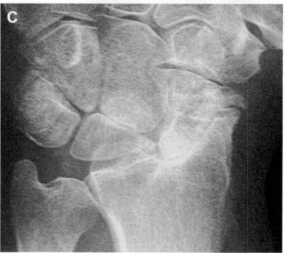

Fig. 8. SLAC wrist. PA radiographs show (*A*) Stage 1 with slight bone sclerosis of the radial styloid (*arrowhead*) and cortex irregularities of the scaphoid (*arrow*), (*B*) Stage 2, and (*C*) Stage 3. Note the scapho-lunate diastasis on each view.

MR imaging

MR imaging provides the same information as ultrasound but provides more accurate assessment of the joint line and any probable extensive subchondral bone edema (see Fig. 14).

Hamato-lunate Joint Osteoarthritis

Clinical presentation

Hamato-lunate impingement is a recently described, uncommon cause of ulnar-sided wrist pain.[21] A normal variant in a joint between the hamate and a medial facet of a Type II lunate may lead to a significantly high prevalence of chondromalacia (60%–82%).[22–24] In up to 50% of the population, the lunate has a medial facet that is separated from the distal facet that articulates with the hamate.[22] This

hamato-lunate facet measures 2 to 6 mm. Without such a medial facet (Type I lunate), the frequency of cartilage lesions in the proximal pole of the hamate is much lower (18%–27%). This type of chondral lesion may be responsible for ulnar-sided wrist pain and could be the result a chronic impingement caused by ulnar flexion of the wrist.[25]

Radiographs

Radiographs may show nothing but a Type II lunate at an early stage (Fig. 15). Focal areas of demineralization of the proximal hamate or subchondral geodes may also be seen.[26] The hamate facet is visible on plain films in only 64% to 72% of cases.[23]

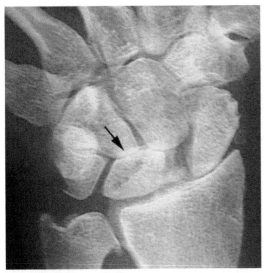

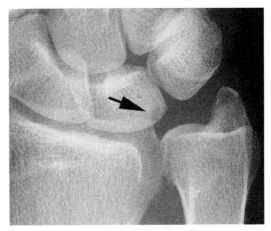

Fig. 11. Ulnocarpal impaction. PA radiograph shows positive ulnar index and subchondral bone cyst of the lunate (*arrow*).

Fig. 9. SLAC wrist. PA radiograph with ulnar tilt shows hamato-lunate JSN (*arrow*) and is more sensitive than the neutral view to depict this joint OA.

Infrequently, according to the intensity of symptoms, surgical resection of the proximal pole of the hamate may also be indicated.

CT-arthrography, MR imaging, and MR-arthrography

Both CT-arthrography and MR-arthrography clearly demonstrate chondral lesions (see **Fig. 15**).[27] MR imaging can depict bone marrow edema of the proximal part of the hamate (**Fig. 16**). The association between hamato-lunate OA and luno-triquetral ligament tears is debated. Most patients can be treated conservatively.

Finger Joint Osteoarthritis

Finger joints OA is a complex condition, as reflected by the wide and rather confusing terminology used in the literature to describe it. This terminology is summarized in **Table 1**.

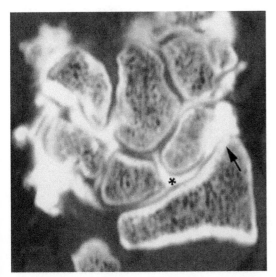

Fig. 10. SLAC wrist, Stage 1. Coronal CT-arthrography view shows cartilage thinning of the radial styloid (*arrow*) and tearing of the central part of the scapho-lunate ligament (*).

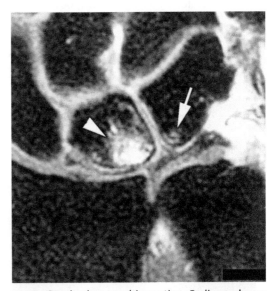

Fig. 12. Occult ulnocarpal impaction. Radiographs are negative, with a neutral ulnar index. Coronal STIR MR image shows degenerative thinning of the triangular ligament. There are also cartilage ulceration of the lunate with extensive bone edema (*arrowhead*) and bone edema of radial side of the triquetrum (*arrow*).

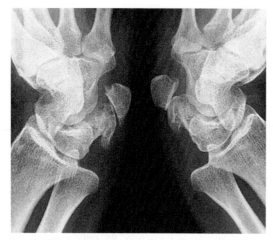

Fig. 13. Piso-triquetral joint OA. Comparative ulnar-side radiograph shows bilateral piso-triquetral joint OA.

Distal Interphalangeal Joint Osteoarthritis

Clinical presentation

The distal interphalangeal joints (DIPJs) are the sites most commonly affected by finger OA. The condition occurs predominantly in people 40 to 60 years of age, and it affects women four times more frequently than men. Osteophytes and thickening of the joint capsules and ligaments form two dorsolateral swellings, called Heberden's nodes, that are separated by a longitudinal groove. These nodes are hard swellings because of their bony structure and are usually painless. Secondary malalignment results from the involvement of the extensor tendon associated with ulnar inclination with or without torsion. Inflammatory changes around the nail are possible, sometimes associated with a mucoid cyst containing a translucent gelatinous fluid developed in the posterior nail fold. The cyst may also develop under the nail[28] and induce a compression of the nail root, leading to a longitudinal fissure of the nail plate.

The erosive form of finger OA was reported in 1961.[29] Initial clinical manifestations are usually striking, with pain and local inflammation of the DIPJ. Symptoms progressively involve the proximal interphalangeal joints (PIPJs). The metacarpophalangeal, TMC, and scapho-trapezial joints are less frequently affected in cases of erosive finger OA than in common OA (Fig. 17).

Joints are usually affected bilaterally and symmetrically, especially the index and ring fingers. Deformities are nonspecific but tend to evolve more frequently toward ankylosis. The relationship between conventional OA and erosive OA has been debated.[30] Erosive OA may represent a separate disease entity,[31] belong to one end of the spectrum of OA,[32] or represent a particularly aggressive subgroup of generalized OA.[30]

Radiographs

The diagnosis of DIPJ OA is usually confirmed on radiographs that exclude other conditions. Radiographic findings can be subtle initially, including indications of slight JSN or an asymmetrical

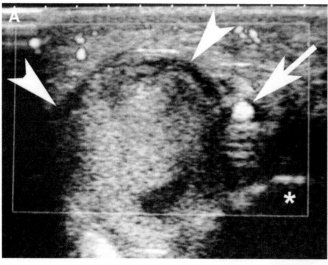
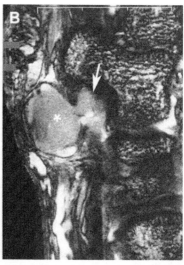

Fig. 14. Hemorrhagic ganglion of the Guyon's tunnel. (A) Axial ultrasound view shows echoic material within the ganglion cyst as the result of the hemorrhagic pattern (arrowheads), with a deep pedicle extending toward the pisiform bone (*). Ulnar artery (arrow). (B) Sagittal T2-weighted MR image shows that the ganglion has a relative central low signal as the result of hemorrhage (*). Note the deep pedicle (arrow) going to the piso-triquetral joint.

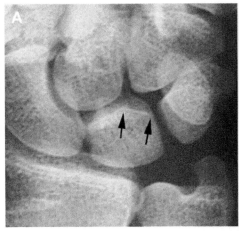
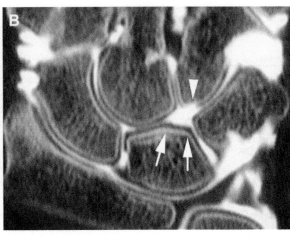

Fig. 15. Early hamato-lunate joint OA. (*A*) PA radiograph demonstrates a Type II lunate (*arrows*) without joint space or subchondral abnormality. (*B*) Coronal CT arthrography view shows cartilage ulceration of the proximal part of the hamate (*arrowhead*) and integrity of the lunate facet joint (*arrows*).

hypertrophic appearance of the middle phalanx head. More obvious signs, such as sclerosis, geodes, and osteophytes, appear later in the course of DIPJ OA. Lateral views are essential and may demonstrate a dorsal extension of the osteophytes developing from the base of the distal phalanx and bulging under the distal band of the extensor mechanism (Fig. 18). Thickening of the posterior nail fold suggests the probable presence of a mucoid cyst. Alternatively, a dorsal cortical bony erosion of the distal phalanx should raise the possibility of a subungueal mucoid cyst (Fig. 19). Osteophytes later develop laterally and therefore become more visible on anteroposterior views.

In erosive OA, the JSN is global, with an impacted appearance of the joint line due to central osteochondral erosions (Fig. 20). New bone formation (ie, subchondral bone sclerosis and osteophytes) does not differ from that in cases of common OA. The distal phalanx becomes cup shaped as the proximal phalanx becomes sharper (Fig. 21). The impaction of the joint is usually followed by malalignment. Thin, periarticular linear opacities are encountered.[33,34]

Ultrasound and MR imaging

On MR images, central erosions are seen at sites of cartilage loss and have more sharply angulated margins than marginal erosions, without evidence of associated synovitis.[35] Cross-sectional imaging can be informative in cases of nail plate fissure to confirm the presence of a compressive mass of the nail root. The space-occupying lesion can be an exuberant osteophytic growth or, more likely, a mucoid cyst. Both are related because a cyst

generally arises following an injury to the terminal band of the extensor mechanism caused by osteophytes. One should search for a pedicle tracking along the lateral border of the extensor tendon (Fig. 22). A cystic subungueal component is present in 20% of cases and may induce cortical scalloping. Extension of the cyst toward the finger pulp or infiltration of a proper digital nerve is rare. Ultrasound may be a suitable medium to investigate the relationship between erosive and non-erosive OA, although one study has found ultrasound to be less sensitive to erosions in cases of HOA than radiographs.[36] Symptomatic joints are more likely to demonstrate ultrasound-

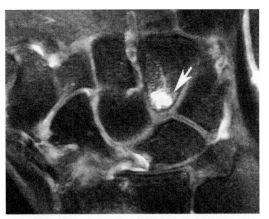

Fig. 16. Hamato-lunate joint OA. Coronal contrast-enhanced, fat-suppressed, T1-weighted MR image shows bone marrow edema of the proximal part of the hamate (*arrow*) with slight cortex irregularities. This is a Type II lunate.

Table 1
Terminology used in finger joints ostoeoarthritis

Terms	Definitions
Non-nodal OA	Clinical or radiographic IPJ OA without nodes
Heberden's and Bouchard's nodes	Posterolateral firm swellings at distal IPJ (Heberden's node) and proximal IPJ (Bouchard's node). Specific HOA clinical or radiologic abnormalities may not be present
Nodal OA	Heberden's or Bouchard's nodes with underlying clinical or radiologic IPJ OA
Generalized OA	HOA associated with other OA sites
Thumb-base OA	TMC joint with or without STT OA
Erosive OA	Subchondral bone erosion, cortical destruction, and subsequent reparative change, which may include bony ankylosis

Abbreviations: IPJ, interphalangeal joint; STT, scapho-trapezio-trapezoid joint.

detected changes of gray-scale synovitis, power Doppler signal, or osteophytes (Fig. 23).[37]

Proximal Interphalangeal Joint Osteoarthritis

Clinical presentation

PIPJ OA occurs less frequently than DIPJ OA, and both localizations are associated in 30% of cases. Nodes called Bouchard's nodes, which are similar to Heberden's nodes, appear around the PIPJs. Theses nodes are circumferential, fusiform, and without dorsal prominence. The lesions are often limited to a few joints, sometimes only one.

Compared with DIPJ OA, PIPJ OA is much less disabling and tends to respect the joints' range of motion.

Radiographs

Radiographic evidence of PIPJ is usually subtle and becomes visible late in the course of the disease (Fig. 24).

MR imaging

Marginal bone erosions are common in PIPJ OA and are often radiographically occult but well demonstrated using MR imaging. They are

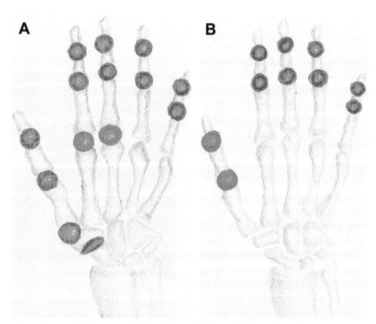

Fig. 17. Target sites of involvement (*blue spots*) for (*A*) hand OA and (*B*) erosive OA. Less commonly involved joints are indicated with *green spots*. (*Courtesy of* Rania Hito, MD, Boston, MA.)

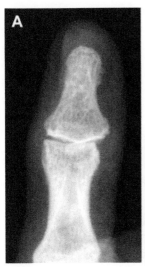
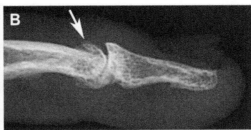

Fig. 18. Interphalangeal joint OA of the thumb. (*A*) PA radiograph shows focal JSN, subchondral bone sclerosis, and slight lateral subluxation. (*B*) Lateral radiograph demonstrates osteophytosis of the proximal phalanx with dorsal preponderance (*arrow*).

morphologically similar to the erosions of inflammatory arthritides such as rheumatoid and psoriatic arthritis. These erosions commonly occur close to the proximal enthesis site of the collateral ligaments in cases of OA. Synovitis and bone edema are usually present (Fig. 25).[35] A recent study compared OA with psoriatic arthritis using MR imaging and highlighted involvement of ligaments, tendons, and enthesis sites in both diseases.[38] Collateral ligament abnormalities influence the expression of the bony changes in the disease. These data are confirmed with histologic correlations in small joint OA and are in favor of a confirmation of whole-organ disease in OA.[39–41]

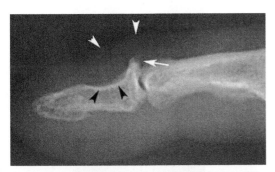

Fig. 19. Mucoid cyst of the interphalangeal joint of the thumb. Lateral radiograph shows OA with dorsal osteophytes (*white arrow*), thickening of the proximal nail fold (*white arrowheads*), and bone erosion of the dorsal cortex of the distal phalanx (*black arrowheads*) caused by the subungual component of the cyst.

The predictive value of bone edema for joint damage in OA is unknown.

Metacarpo-phalangeal Joint Osteoarthritis

Clinical presentation

OA of the metacarpo-phalangeal (MCP) joints is rare. MCP joint OA of the thumb is often secondary to traumatic injuries, especially sprains (eg, unhealed Stener's lesion). In cases of previously present MCP joint OA, ulnar drift is possible.[42] Symmetric OA involving the index and middle fingers should raise the possibility of crystal-related diseases, especially CPPD deposition disease.

Radiographs

AP and oblique radiographic views demonstrate classic findings of OA. Exuberant osteophytes leading to anchor-shaped metacarpal heads may be seen, affecting especially the index and middle fingers. Calcific deposits within hyaline cartilage and intrinsic wrist ligaments should suggest metabolic or crystal-related arthropathies (Fig. 26).

Diagnosis and Severity Assessment of Hand Osteoarthritis

The highly variable clinical and radiologic natural history of HOA and the large number of joints affected make it difficult to establish strict diagnostic criteria and reliable and reproducible tools to evaluate the severity of the disease. A number of criteria have been suggested.[43–45] There is no

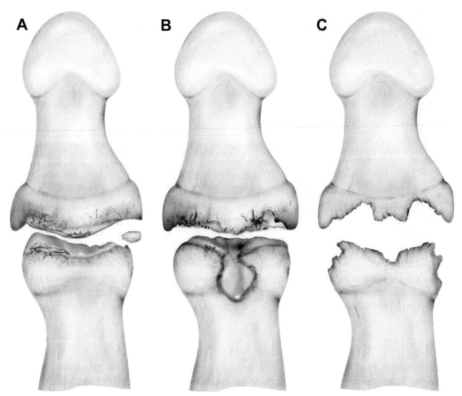

Fig. 20. Differential radiographic diagnosis of DIPJ OA. (*A*) OA: focal narrowing, marginal osteophyte, bone sclerosis, osteochondral bodies; (*B*) erosive OA: subchondral erosion; (*C*) psoriasis: proliferative marginal erosion, retained or increased bone density.

agreed upon gold standard for diagnosis of HAO. To date, the main reference cited for diagnosis of HOA is the list of the American College of Rheumatology criteria for classification of HOA (Box 3).[43] However, these criteria do not include radiologic data, so the inclusion of radiologic data in these criteria must be the ultimate objective of clinical and therapeutic studies. Most studies use the radiographic definition described by Kellgren and Lawrence.[3]

The European League Against Rheumatism (EULAR) OA Task Force developed recommendations for HOA diagnosis using an evidence-based format involving a systematic review of research evidence and expert consensus.[34] Ten propositions were agreed on after three anonymous Delphi rounds (Table 2).

Scoring

HOA represents a valuable model to evaluate structure-modifying treatments of OA. Analysis of clinical data and evaluation of the functional impact of HOA remain difficult. An algofunctional index can be established by adding a visual analog scale for pain and a method of indicating consumption of pain killers and nonsteroidal anti-

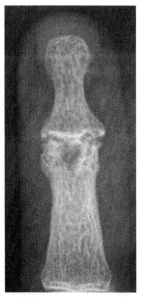

Fig. 21. Erosive OA of the DIPJ. PA radiograph shows subchondral erosion.

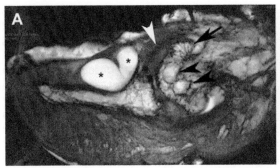
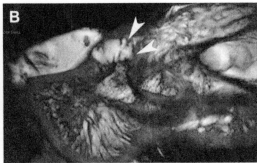

Fig. 22. Mucoid cyst of the DIPJ. (*A*) Midsagittal T2-weighted MR image shows the cyst, with a component in the proximal nail fold and a subungual component (*). Dorsal osteophyte (*black arrow*) lifting up the extensor tendon (*white arrowhead*). Subchondral bone cysts (*black arrowheads*). (*B*) Parasagittal T2-weighted MR image shows lateral pedicle beneath the extensor tendon (*white arrowheads*).

inflammatory drugs, or by using global evaluation conducted by the patient or the physician.[45]

Radiographs

The Osteoarthritis Research Society International recently published guidelines for the conduct of clinical trials of HOA, recommending conventional radiographs as the standard for assessing structural outcomes.[46] Various methods have been proposed to assess the radiologic severity of HOA and to score the progression of damage over time. These criteria are based on the use of radiography[7,43,47–52] or microfocal radiography.[53] An anteroposterior view of both hands on the same film is usually obtained, and the use of a 1:1 ratio of digitized radiographs is recommended. The quality of the radiographs does not seem to interfere greatly with the scoring. Only subchondral sclerosis assessment requires well-exposed radiographs. The use of either digitized or plain films for scoring does not seem to modify the quality of assessment.[54,55] The joint space width can be measured using automatic quantification and closely reflects semiquantitative scoring of JSN.[56] The grading system of Kellgren and Lawrence allows a wide range of interpretations for each grade, reducing interobserver reliability.[57,58] The intraobserver reliability is the determinant used to calculate the smallest detectable difference, and it accounts for the grading system's sensitivity to change.[59] Verbruggen and Veys[60] suggested an easy and reproducible scoring method that uses numeric scores for radiographs. The methods proposed differ by the number of hand joints and radiographic features scored (eg, osteophytes, JSN, subchondral bone sclerosis, bone cysts, erosion, and deformity); the respective importance attributed to each radiologic feature in the score; the method of scoring (eg, semiquantitative or global stage of

OA) and the summation. None of the proposed radiologic scales has proved to be better than others. Maheu and colleagues[61] compared, in the same sample of patients, the precision and sensitivity to change of four radiographic scoring methods proposed to assess the severity and progression of structural changes in HOA (Table 3). The Verbruggen and Kallman scales perform better with respect to reliability, and the Kallman method is slightly more sensitive to change.[61]

Ultrasound

Ultrasound is particularly useful to assess small superficial structures such as finger joints. The more complex anatomy and deeper structures of the wrist make ultrasound of the wrist less straightforward. The efficiency of ultrasound in the early diagnosis of synovitis and erosions in hands in cases of rheumatoid arthritis has been demonstrated.[62,63] A group of experts in OA, ultrasound, and outcome measures, working under the auspices of the Disease Characteristics in Hand

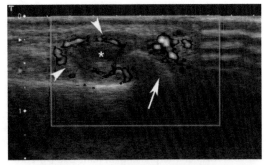

Fig. 23. DIPJ OA. Midsagittal ultrasound view shows dorsal osteophyte (*arrow*) with fluid effusion in the dorsal recess (*) and thickened synovium, using positive-power Doppler (*arrowheads*).

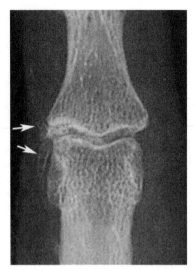

Fig. 24. Proximal interphalangeal joint OA. PA radiograph shows slight focal JSN with subchondral bone sclerosis, marginal osteophytes, and loose bodies (*arrows*).

OA Group, proposed a preliminary ultrasound hand scoring system.[64] Fifteen joints of the hand were examined: the first carpometacarpal joint, MCP joints 1 to 5, PIPJs 1 to 5, and DIPJs 2 to 5. Activity and damage criteria were scored: synovial hypertrophy and effusion, gray scale and power Doppler signal, and osteophytosis (Fig. 27).

Chondral defects or JSN cannot be reliably or meaningfully interpreted, despite these being

cardinal pathologic features of OA. Erosions are also excluded from the tool because of perceived problems with definition and reliability. Erosions can be difficult to detect because of overlying osteophytes. It may also be difficult to determine where focal erosions begin and where osteophytes end when the cortical surface is severely damaged. In a comparative study of patients who had symptomatic OA joints and a control group, neither the number of affected joints per individual nor the summative semiquantitative scores for synovitis per individual correlated with symptoms (eg, pain visual analog scale, global visual analog scale, or Australian/Canadian Osteoarthritis Hand Index).[37]

MR imaging

To date, no scoring method for HOA using MR imaging is available. The efficiency of MR imaging in rheumatoid arthritis has been extensively demonstrated (rheumatoid arthritis magnetic resonance imaging scoring). A similar approach could be adapted to HOA because it would be the best method to reveal subchondral bone edema among other abnormalities.

OSTEOARTHRITIS OF THE SPINE

Low back pain (LBP) is the second most common complaint encountered by primary care physicians. Chronic LBP is a major public health issue. Up to 80% of all individuals will experience LBP at some point in their lives. State-of-the-art

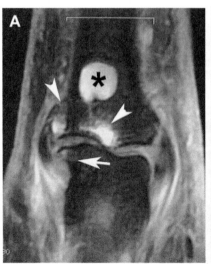
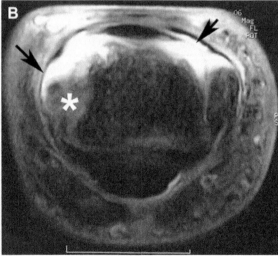

Fig. 25. Proximal interphalangeal joint OA. (*A*) Coronal T2-weighted MR image shows that both collateral ligaments are thickened, with bone erosion at the proximal attachment of the lateral collateral ligament (*arrow*). Bone marrow edema (*arrowheads*) and distant bone cyst (*) of the middle phalanx. (*B*) Axial contrast-enhanced, fat-suppressed, T1-weighted MR image shows thickened lateral collateral ligament (*) and synovitis of the dorsal recess (*arrows*).

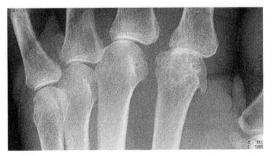

Fig. 26. Metacarpophangeal joint OA. Oblique radiograph shows exuberant osteophytes. The fact that the disease is limited to the second and third fingers should raise suspicion of a metabolic disease.

imaging provides excellent morphologic details on lumbar spine degenerative changes. With the wide use of MR imaging, it is now possible to examine the anatomy of the lumbar spine noninvasively, with excellent spatial and contrast resolution, in a short time. This has led to a better understanding of the frequency and spectrum of findings that can be present as part of the normal aging process without causing clinical symptoms. It is also now possible to distinguish accurately between mechanical causes of nerve-root compression that may result in radicular symptoms and normal imaging findings. The use of MR imaging allows for improved diagnostic imaging of lumbar ligaments, facet joints, and muscles. The main objective of imaging studies in the context of LBP or radicular

pain would be to support the clinical diagnosis by showing objective evidence of any kind of discopathy or facet joint arthropathy in a location consistent with the clinical findings. Abnormal findings have been reported by radiologists in asymptomatic subjects when using all imaging modalities, including radiography, myelography, discography, CT, and MR imaging. The terminology for disk abnormalities at imaging includes a variety of labels that can vary in meaning and importance from patient to patient and from location to location. The nomenclature to describe disk lesions has been greatly influenced by two factors: the concept of disk degeneration throughout life and the understanding of the physiopathology of clinically relevant disk disorders. Ideally, the nomenclature used for imaging should correspond to clinical entities and help orient the referring physician as to treatment.[65] The results of studies using MR imaging in asymptomatic volunteers support the notion that one must be careful before attributing causality to any abnormal finding in a symptomatic patient.[65–68] Finally, there is a trend to develop degenerative disk disease image-grading systems to further investigate the relationship between morphology, functional parameters, and clinical symptoms. This article focuses on the most recent and reliable MR imaging–based grading systems that are useful in cases of lumbar spine OA.[69]

Imaging Methods

Multiple imaging modalities are available, and include radiography, dynamic radiography, multidetector CT (MDCT), MR imaging, myelography with postmyelographic MDCT, and discography.[70–72]

Radiographs
Radiographs still play an important and preliminary role by providing an easy screening opportunity. They are cheap, universally available, and offer a good panoramic view of the lumbar spine, adding meaningful details on bone structures and the stability of the spine. Functional dynamic radiography remains the gold standard for the assessment of lumbar instability. Because of its simplicity, low cost, and availability, functional flexion-extension radiography is the most thoroughly studied and the most widely used method in the imaging diagnosis of lumbar intervertebral instability.[73]

MR imaging
MR imaging of the lumbar spine has become the initial imaging technique of choice in patients who have LBP or radicular pain. Usual clinical

---

Box 3
American College of Rheumatology classification criteria for osteoarthritis of the hand

Hand pain, aching, or stiffness

plus

Hard-tissue enlargement of two or more of 10 selected joints[a]

plus

Fewer than three swollen MCP joints

plus

Hard-tissue enlargement of two or more DIPJs

or

Deformity of two or more of 10 selected joints[a]The 10 selected joints are the second and third DIPJs, the second and third PIPJs, and the first carpometacarpal joints (of both hands).

Data from Altman R, Alarcon G, Appelrouth D, et al. The American College of Rheumatology criteria for the classification and reporting of osteoarthritis of the hand. Arthritis Rheum 1990;33:1601–10.

Table 2
Propositions and strength of recommendation for diagnosis of hand osteoarthritis European League Against Rheumatism (EULAR) Task Force

Proposition	LoE	SOR (95% CI)
1. Risk factors for HOA include female sex, more than 40 years of age, menopausal status, family history, obesity, higher bone density, greater forearm muscle strength, joint laxity, prior hand injury, and occupation- or recreation-related usage.	Ib–IIb	69 (54–84)
2. Typical symptoms of HOA are pain on usage and mild stiffness in the morning or when inactive affecting just one or a few joints at any one time; symptoms are often intermittent and target characteristic sites (eg, DIPJs, PIPJs, thumb base, index and middle MCP joints). With such typical features, a confident clinical diagnosis can be made in adults aged 40 or older.	IIb	85 (77–92)
3. Clinical hallmarks of HOA are Heberden's and Bouchard's nodes or bony enlargement with or without deformity (eg, lateral deviation of IPJs, subluxation and adduction of thumb base) affecting characteristic target joints (eg, DIPJs, PIPJs, thumb base, and index and middle MCP joints).	Ib–IV	80 (69–90)
4. Functional impairment in HOA may be as severe as in rheumatoid arthritis. Function should be carefully assessed and monitored using validated outcome measures.	IIb	57 (42–73)
5. Patients who have polyarticular HOA are at increased risk of knee OA, hip OA, and OA at other common target sites (generalized OA) and should be assessed and examined accordingly	IIa–IIb	77 (62–92)
6. Recognized subsets with different risk factors, associations, and outcomes (requiring different assessment and management) include IPJ OA (with or without nodes), thumb-base OA, and erosive OA. Each may be symptomatic or asymptomatic.	IIa–IIb	68 (56–79)
7. Erosive HOA targets IPJs and shows radiographic subchondral erosion, which may progress to marked bone and cartilage attrition, instability, and bony ankylosis. Typically, it has an abrupt onset, marked pain and functional impairment, inflammatory symptoms and signs (eg, stiffness, soft tissue swelling, erythema, paresthesia), mildly elevated CRP levels, and a worse outcome than nonerosive IPJ OA.	IIa–IIb	87 (81–93)

	LoE	SOR
8. The differential diagnosis for HOA is wide. The most common conditions to consider are psoriatic arthritis (which may target DIPJs or affect just one ray), rheumatoid arthritis (mainly targeting MCP joints, PIPJs, and wrists), gout (which may superimpose on preexisting HOA), and hemochromatosis (mainly targeting MCP joints and wrists).	Ib–IIb	81 (73–89)
9. Plain radiographs provide the gold standard for morphologic assessment of HOA. A PA radiograph of both hands on a single film or field of view is adequate for diagnosis. Classical features are JSN, osteophytes, subchondral bone sclerosis, and subchondral cysts, and subchondral erosion occurs in erosive HOA. The use of further imaging modalities is seldom indicated for diagnosis.	Ib–IIb	87 (81–93)
10. Blood tests are not required for diagnosis of HOA but may be required to exclude coexistent disease. In a patient who has HOA and has marked inflammatory symptoms or signs, especially involving atypical sites, blood tests should be undertaken to screen for additional inflammatory arthritides.	Ib–IIb	78 (63–92)

EULAR evidence hierarchy for diagnosis based on study design: Ia = meta-analysis of cohort studies; Ib = meta-analysis of case control studies; IIa = cohort studies; IIb = case control/cross-sectional comparative studies; III = noncomparative descriptive studies; IV = expert opinion.

Abbreviations: CRP, C-reactive protein; IPJ, interphalangeal joint; LoE, level of evidence (presented in a range on components assessed); SOR, strength of recommendation (on a visual analog scale; 0–100 mm, 0 = not recommended at all, 100 = fully recommended).

Data from Zhang W, Doherty M, Leeb BF, et al. EULAR evidence-based recommendations for the diagnosis of hand osteoarthritis: report of a task force of ESCISIT. Ann Rheum Dis 2009;68:8–17.

Table 3	
Four different hand osteoarthritis scoring systems assessed by Maheu and colleagues	
Scoring System	**Description**
Global scoring[49]	Reader decides whether the joint assessed is osteoarthritic (yes=1; no=0). A total of 32 joints are assessed (range 0–32)
Kellgren and Lawrence grading[3]	Each of the 30 joints examined are scored from 0 to 4, according to the presence and size of osteophytes and the presence of JSN. 0 = no OA; 1 = doubtful OA; 2 = definite minimal OA; 3 = moderate OA; and 4 = severe OA. The score ranges from 0 to 120.
Kallman radiographic scale[7]	Twenty-four joints (all but the MCP joints) are scored for six radiographic features, according to a seminumerical scale. Features: osteophytes (0–3), JSN (0–3), subchondral bone sclerosis (0–1), subchondral bone cysts (0–1), lateral bony deviation (>15°; 0–1), and bone erosion (0–1). The score ranges from 0 to 208.
Verbruggen numerical scoring system[50]	Semiquantitative grading scale of OA of the fingers. Of note, thumb-base joints (scapho-trapezial and TMC-I) are not considered in this score.

Abbreviation: JS, joint space.
Data from Maheu E, Altman RD, Bloch DA, et al. Design and conduct of clinical trials in patients with osteoarthritis of the hand: recommendations from a task force of the Osteoarthritis Research Society International. Osteoarthritis Cartilage 2006;14:303–22.

MR imaging has emphasized the use of orthogonal T1- and T2-weighted images for morphologic assessment of the discovertebral complex. The use of short TI inversion recovery (STIR) or fat-suppressed T2-weighted images has been added by many groups because these images are more sensitive to bone marrow and soft-tissue changes. Among the new MR imaging techniques currently available, only MR-neurography and dynamic MR imaging have expanded beyond the experimental phase and have demonstrated specific clinical utility in selected patients.[74] MR-neurography is based on three-dimensional, thin-section sequences. MR-neurography is capable of depicting a wide variety of pathologic conditions that involve the sciatic nerve, including compression related to degenerative disk disease or extraspinal lesions.[75] MR imaging is routinely performed with the patients supine and therefore with the spine unloaded. Recent technological advances have made possible the development of open MR imaging systems that allow an examination to be done with the patient in a seated or upright position. Dynamic MR imaging has been used to evaluate the occurrence of occult herniation, which may not be visible or be less visible when the patient is supine, to measure motion between spinal segments, and to measure the canal or foraminal diameter when the lumbar spine is subjected to axial loading.[76,77] In a study of 30 patients, Weishaupt and colleagues[78] showed

that positional (seated) MR imaging more frequently demonstrated minor neural compromise than did conventional MR imaging, but no convincing signs of canal or foraminal encroachments were found. The benefits from dynamic MR imaging seem small for the added machine time and patient discomfort. Further studies are required before the true management value of positional dynamic MR imaging can be determined, in part because of the various methods used.

CT

CT provides superior bone detail (Fig. 28) but is not quite as useful in depicting disk lesions when compared with multiplanar MR imaging. With the added value associated with high quality reformatted sagittal and coronal images, MDCT is useful for depiction of calcification and ossification of the spinal ligaments, spondylosis, facet joint changes with encroaching osteophytes, and scoliosis, and also for morphologic evaluation after myelography or discography. Exposure to radiation is an issue of MDCT, however.

Myelography

Myelography is rarely used, but is still useful in cases that are contraindicated for MR imaging. Myelography is usually combined with postmyelography MDCT. The combined study is complementary to MR imaging and may be useful in

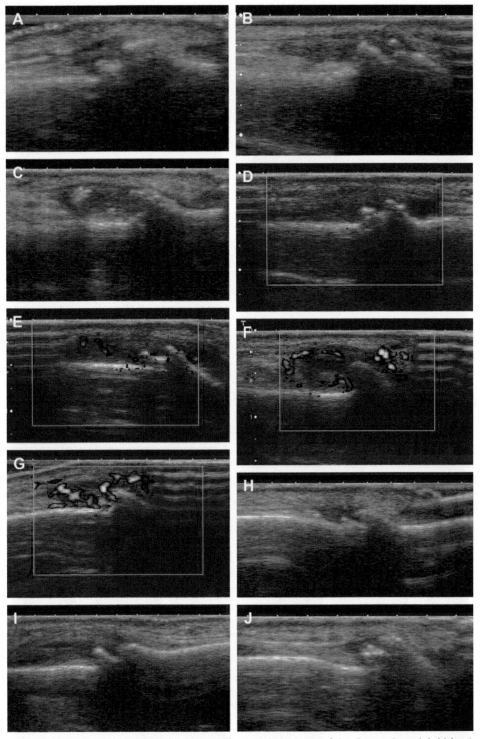

Fig. 27. Ultrasound scoring proposed by the Disease Characteristics in Hand OA Group. Synovial thickening with three grades: (*A*) mild, (*B*) moderate, and (*C*) severe. Power Doppler signal with four grades: (*D*) no signal, (*E*) mild, (*F*) moderate, and (*G*) severe. Osteophytes with three grades: (*H*) mild, (*I*) moderate, and (*J*) severe. (*Data from* Keen HI, Lavie F, Wakefield RJ, et al. The development of a preliminary ultrasonographic scoring system for features of hand osteoarthritis. Ann Rheum Dis 2008;67:651–5.)

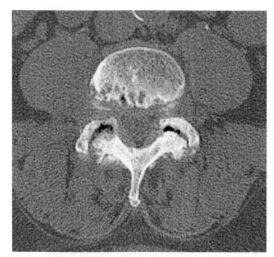

Fig. 28. Axial MDCT scan at the L4/5 level shows marked bilateral facet joint OA with erosive lesions and vacuum phenomenon. Note the erosive changes of the vertebral endplate.

surgical planning. Myelography offers a dynamic view of the lumbar spine that allows for comparison of supine and weight-bearing images (Fig. 29). However, myelography has the disadvantage of requiring lumbar puncture and intrathecal iodine contrast injection.

Discography

When other studies fail to localize the cause of pain, discography may occasionally be helpful if surgery is planned. Although the images often depict nonspecific age-related or degenerative changes, the injection itself may reproduce the patient's pain, which may have a diagnostic value.[79]

Degenerative Disk Disease

MR imaging is the most accurate anatomic method for assessing intervertebral disk disease. The signal intensity characteristics of the disk on T2-weighted images reflect changes caused by aging or degeneration.[74]

Annular tears, also properly called annular fissures, are probably a critical factor in the process of disk degenerative disease (Fig. 30). Annular tears are frequently found in an asymptomatic population.[68] The temporal evolution of annular fissures was studied in 56 patients, with an evaluation of the symptoms' evolution.[80] In this series, annular tears either did not change or improved spontaneously in a large proportion of cases over a period of time. Furthermore, there was no statistical correlation between annular tear changes and changes in patient's symptoms. Annular tears appear in the early stages of disk degeneration and are often seen in the absence of other identifiable morphologic changes of degeneration in the nucleus pulposus. Disks with annular tears are associated with a faster subsequent nuclear degeneration.[81]

Disk degeneration and disk herniation reporting and grading

A standardized nomenclature in the assessment of disk abnormalities is a prerequisite for comparison of data from different investigations. Disk degeneration is a continuum rather than a step-by-step process. As a result, any step-by-step grading

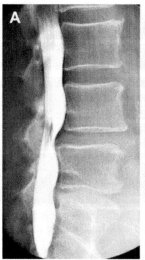
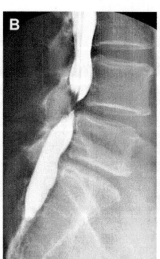
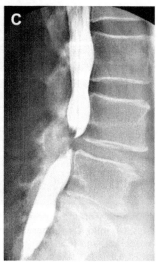

Fig. 29. Lumbar myelography in a 74-year-old man. Lateral radiographs in (A) flexion (B) neutral position, and (C) extension show degenerative spondylolisthesis at the L4/5 level, with a central stenosis. This dynamic stenosis is moderate in flexion and marked in neutral and extension positions.

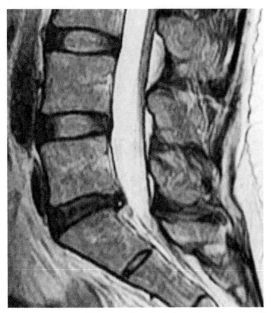

Fig. 30. 43-year-old man who had chronic LBP. Sagittal fast spin-echo, T2-weighted MR image shows a small annular tear of the L5/S1 disk space.

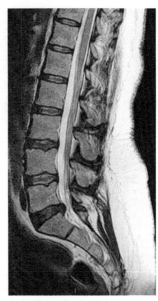

Fig. 31. 51-year-old woman who had chronic LBP. Sagittal fast spin-echo, T2-weighted MR image shows a degenerative L5/S1 disk with loss of signal intensity and convex posterior bulging.

system will by design contain ambiguity with respect to whether a disk should be graded as one particular level or another.

Millette[65] proposed a nomenclature and classification based on the expected anatomy and pathology of both the disk and adjacent vertebral bodies. Disks are classified as normal young disks, normal aging disks, scarred disks, annular tears, and herniated disks. This scheme can be applied to all imaging techniques, and the categories are not mutually exclusive. Mastering this classification requires some time and effort because assessment of multiple parameters is required to differentiate normal aging disks from truly degenerated or scarred disks. Finally, the reliability of this nomenclature has never been tested.

Herniation is defined as a localized displacement of disk material beyond the limits of the intervertebral disk space. The term "localized displacement" is in contrast to "generalized displacement," the latter being arbitrarily defined as encompassing more than 50% (180°) of the periphery of the disk.

Localized displacement in the axial (horizontal) plane can be focal, signifying that it encompassing less than 25% of the disk circumference, or broad based, meaning that it encompasses between 25 and 50% of the disk circumference. Presence of disk tissue circumferentially (50%–100%) beyond the edges of the ring apophyses may be called "bulging" (Fig. 31) and is not considered a form of herniation, nor are diffuse adaptive alterations of the disk contour secondary to adjacent deformity, such as may be present in severe scoliosis or spondylolisthesis.

The nomenclature recommendations of the combined task forces of the North American Spine Society, American Society of Spine Radiology, and American Society of Neuroradiology[82] (and those at http://www.asnr.org/spine_nomenclature) are as follows. Herniated disks may take the form of protrusions or extrusions, based on the shape of the displaced material. Protrusion is present if the greatest distance, in any plane, between the edges of the disk material beyond the disk space is less than the distance between the edges of the base in the same plane (Fig. 32). The base is defined as the cross-sectional area of disk material at the outer margin of the disk space of origin, in which disk material displaced beyond the disk space is continuous with disk material within the disk space. In the cranio-caudal direction, the length of the base cannot exceed, by definition, the height of the intervertebral space. Extrusion is present when, in at least one plane, any one distance between the edges of the disk material beyond the disk space is greater than the distance between the edges of the base in the same plane, or when no continuity exists between the disk material beyond the disk space and that within the disk space (Fig. 33). Extrusion may be further specified as being sequestration if the displaced disk material has lost completely any continuity with the parent disk. The term "migration" may be used to signify

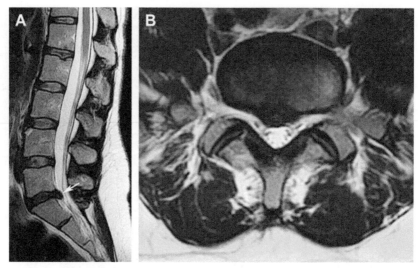

Fig. 32. 47-year-old man who had acute LBP. (*A*) Sagittal and (*B*) axial fast spin-echo, T2-weighted sagittal MR images show a protruded, herniated L5/S1 disk with a convex posterior margin (*arrow*). Protruded disk herniation is characterized by a broader base than the extension of disk material beyond the disk space.

displacement of disk material away from the site of extrusion, regardless of whether there is sequestration or not. In the axial plane, disk herniation is classified as being central, right-left central, right-left subarticular, right-left foraminal, or right-left extraforaminal.

These recommendations also apply to reporting. Reports should classify each disk that is examined into broad diagnostic categories. The statement of the degree of confidence is an important component of communication. The reader should characterize the impression as "definite"

if there is no doubt, "probable" if there is some doubt but the likelihood is greater than 50%, and "possible" if there is reason to consider the classification as accurate but the likelihood is less than 50%.

A specific classification system for lumbar disk degeneration based on routine MR imaging was developed by Pfirrmann and colleagues[83] That comprehensive five-level grading system was developed on the basis of the literature. Pfirrmann classification is based on the following MR imaging features: structure, distinction of

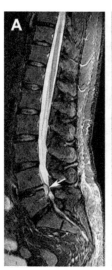
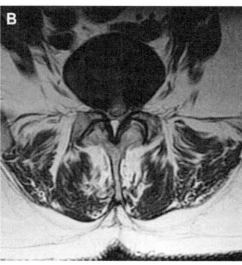

Fig. 33. 55-year-old woman who had acute radicular pain. (*A*) Sagittal and (*B*) axial STIR MR images show an extruded, herniated L4/5 disk with inferior migration (*arrow*). Extruded disk herniation is characterized by a base that is narrower than the distance of disk material extension beyond the disk space.

the nucleus and annulus, signal intensity, and height of intervertebral disk. Grading is performed using fast spin-echo T2-weighted sagittal images of the spine. The five grades are as follows:

- Grade I: The structure of the disk is homogeneous, with bright, hyperintense, white signal intensity and a normal disk height.
- Grade II: The structure of the disk is inhomogeneous, with hyperintense, white signal intensity. The distinction between the annulus and nucleus is clear, and the disk height is normal, with or without horizontal gray bands.
- Grade III: The structure of the disk is inhomogeneous, with intermediate, gray signal intensity. The distinction between the annulus and nucleus is unclear, and the disk height is normal or slightly decreased.
- Grade IV: The structure of the disk is inhomogeneous, with hypointense, dark gray signal intensity. The distinction between the annulus and nucleus is lost, and the disk height is normal or moderately decreased.
- Grade V: The structure of the disk is inhomogeneous, with hypointense, black signal intensity. The distinction between the annulus and nucleus is lost, and the disk space is collapsed.

This grading system focuses on the characteristics of disk structure. An algorithm to assess the grading was developed and optimized by reviewing lumbar MR images. The reliability of the algorithm in depicting intervertebral disk alterations was tested using MR images of 300 lumbar intervertebral disks in 60 patients. In that series, there were 14 images rated as Grade I, 82 as Grade II, 72 as Grade III, 68 as Grade IV, and 64 as Grade V disks. The κ coefficients for intra- and interobserver agreement were substantial to excellent. Complete agreement was obtained, on average, for 83.8% of all the disks. A difference of one grade occurred in 15.9% of all cases and a difference of two or more grades in 1.3% of all the cases. Pfirrmann and colleagues concluded that the grading system and algorithm allowed for reliable assessment of disk degeneration using routine sagittal T2-weighted MR images. They suggested combining the grading system with Modic classification for further specification of disk disease in cases with concomitant bone marrow changes. The useful, five-point, Pfirrmann grading system has been accepted and applied clinically. However, although it is discriminatory when applied to younger subjects,[84] it may not distinguish the severity of disk degeneration when applied to elderly subjects. A modified Pfirrmann grading system for lumbar intervertebral disk degeneration was therefore proposed recently.[84] That eight-level modified grading system for lumbar disk degeneration includes a description of the changes expected for each grade and a 24-image reference panel. The modified Pfirrmann grading system is useful at discriminating severity of disk degeneration in elderly subjects, and it can be applied with good intra- and interobserver agreement.

Herniation of the disk refers to localized displacement of the nucleus, cartilage, fragmented apophyseal bone, or fragmented annular tissue beyond the intervertebral disk space. Disk herniations of the same size may be asymptomatic in one patient and lead to severe nerve root compromise in another patient (Fig. 34). MR imaging reports usually focus on the morphology, location, and size of the herniated disk. The effects of disk herniation depend on the location and extent of the herniation relative to the diameter of the spinal canal. Therefore, a clinically relevant grading system for disk herniation must be based on the spatial relationship between herniated disk material and neural structures.

The system developed by Pfirrmann and colleagues[85] in grading compromise of the intraspinal, extradural lumbar nerve root consists of four grade categories, summarized as follows.

- Grade 0 (normal): No compromise of the nerve root is seen. There is no evident contact of disk material with the nerve root, and the epidural fat layer between the nerve root and the disk material is preserved.
- Grade 1 (contact): There is visible contact of disk material with the nerve root, and the normal epidural fat layer between the two is not evident. The nerve root has a normal position, and there is no dorsal deviation.
- Grade 2 (deviation): The nerve root is displaced dorsally by disk material.
- Grade 3 (compression): The nerve root is compressed between disk material and the wall of the spinal canal; it may appear flattened or be indistinguishable from disk material.

This grading system was tested in the interpretation of routine MR images of 500 lumbar nerve roots in 250 symptomatic patients. Intra- and interobserver reliability was assessed for three independent observers. In the 94 nerve roots that were

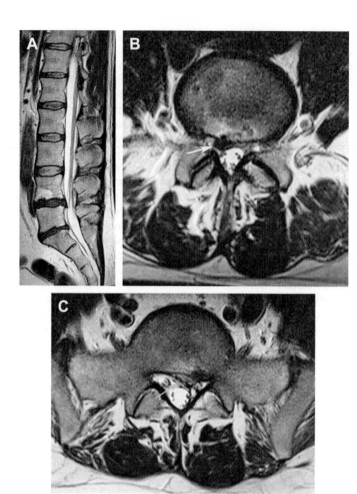

Fig. 34. 46-year-old man who had bilateral chronic radicular pain. Sagittal (*A*) and axial fast spin-echo, T2-weighted MR images show degenerative disk disease at the L4/5 (*B*) and L5/S1 (*C*) levels. (*B*) Right herniation at the L4/5 level (*white arrow*) with contact between disk material and the thecal sac. (*C*) Left herniation at the L5/S1 level (*red arrow*) with extruded disk material and deviation of the left S1 nerve root.

evaluated at surgery, surgical grading was correlated with image-based grading. Statistical results indicated substantial agreement between different readings by the same observer and between different observers. Correlation of image-based grading with surgical grading was high ($r = 0.86$).

Degenerative Bone Marrow Changes of Vertebral Endplates

Signal intensity changes in vertebral-body bone marrow adjacent to the endplates of degenerated disks are a common observation on MR images and appear to take three main forms according to Modic classification.[86]

- Type 1 changes demonstrate decreased signal intensity on T1-weighted images and increased signal intensity on T2-weighted images and have been identified in approximately 4% of patients scanned

for lumbar disease (**Fig. 35**). Histopathologic examination of sections of disks with Type I changes show disruption and fissuring of the endplate and vascularized fibrous tissues within the adjacent marrow. Rannou and colleagues[87] showed that low-grade inflammation indicated by high serum levels of high-sensitivity C-reactive protein in patients who have chronic LBP could point to Modic Type 1 signal changes. This supports the presence of a local inflammation phenomenon occurring at the vertebral endplate level.

- Type 2 changes are represented by increased signal intensity on T1-weighted images and isointense or slightly hyperintense signal intensity on T2-weighted images and have been identified in approximately 16% of patients using MR images (**Fig. 36**). Disks with Type II changes also

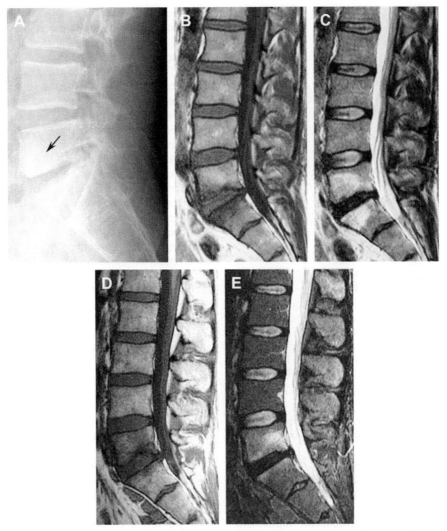

Fig. 35. 39-year-old man who had chronic back pain. (*A*) Lateral radiograph of the lumbar spine shows a moderate narrowing of the L5/S1 disk space, with an area of sclerosis of the anterior part of the L5 endplate (*arrow*). Initial (*B*) sagittal T1- and (*C*) T2-weighted MR images show extensive Type 1 Modic changes at the L5/S1 level, with erosive lesions of the L5 inferior endplate. At 6-month follow-up, (*D*) sagittal T1-weighted and (*E*) STIR MR images show that Modic Type 1 changes remained unchanged in the L5 inferior endplate, whereas they decreased in the S1 superior endplate. There was no significant change of the disk signal and morphology.

show evidence of endplate disruption, with yellow (lipid) bone marrow replacement in the adjacent vertebral body.

- Type 3 changes are represented by decreased signal intensity on both T1- and T2-weighted images and correlate with extensive bony sclerosis on plain radiographs (Fig. 37). The lack of signal in the Type 3 images reflects the relative absence of bone marrow in areas of advanced sclerosis.

The absence of Modic changes, which characterizes a normal anatomic appearance, has often been designated Modic Type 0. Longitudinal studies have shown that cases that show Modic Type 2 changes may be less stable than previously assumed.[88] Mixed Type 1-2 and 2-3 Modic changes have also been reported, suggesting that these changes can convert from one type to another and that they represent different stages of the same pathologic process.[89] Endplate Modic changes most often occur at the anterior aspect of the endplate, particularly at the L4/5 and L5/S1 levels. Fatty endplate changes are the most common. Modic changes occur more frequently with aging, which is evidence of their degenerative etiology.[90] Bony endplate sclerosis is often visible

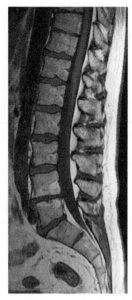

Fig. 36. 51-year-old woman who had moderate chronic LBP. Sagittal T1-weighted MR image shows reduced disk height at the L4/5 and L5/S1 levels associated with fatty Type 2 Modic changes of the vertebral endplates. At L4/5, the fatty changes involve the whole endplates; at L5/S1, the fatty changes involve only the anterior part of the endplates.

on MDCT images in cases of mixed Modic types, and not only in Type 3 changes, as previously assumed.[91]

A reliability study of the Modic classification system was performed by Jones and colleagues[92] using 50 spinal MR examination images. The individual intraobserver agreement was substantial or excellent. The overall interobserver agreement was excellent. There was complete agreement in 78% of the levels, a difference of one type in 14%, and a difference of two or more types in 8% of the levels. The study showed that Modic classification is both reliable and reproducible. It is simple and easy to apply for observers of varying clinical experience. This simplicity and reliability explains the diffusion and large use of the original Modic classification system in clinical research and practice.

Fayad and colleagues[93] determined the intra- and interobserver reliability of a modified Modic classification system, taking into consideration mixed signals. Pure edema endplate signal changes were classified as Modic Type 1, and pure fatty endplate changes as Modic Type 2. A mixture of types 1 and 2 but predominantly showing edema signal changes was classified as Modic 1-2 and a mixture of types 1 and 2 but predominantly showing fatty changes was classified as Modic 2-1. The intraobserver agreement

was excellent. The interobserver agreement was moderate to substantial. Interobserver reliability depended on the experience of the observer, thus highlighting the importance of a learning curve. The study showed that the modified Modic classification system is reliable and easy to apply for observers with different clinical experience.

The relationship of Modic Type 1 changes with disk degeneration was studied prospectively in 24 patients who had chronic LBP in a follow-up study lasting 18 to 74 months.[94] A relatively rapid progression of degenerative changes was found in association with the presence of and, in particular, the size and intensity of Modic Type 1 changes. Degenerative changes were already advanced at the baseline point in most disk that had an adjacent Modic Type 1, but were uncommon in those without. The progressive degenerative changes along with changes in an M1 were deforming to the discovertebral unit because irregularities and even defects developed in the subchondral bone at the endplate border, whereas central disk signal intensity changed and disk height strongly decreased as a result of a collapse of the disk. These results support the hypothesis that Modic Type 1 changes may be signs of a distinctive degenerative process in the discovertebral unit.

In summary, Modic changes are dynamic markers of the normal, age-related degenerative process that affects the lumbar spine (Fig. 38). Type 1 changes are likely to be inflammatory in origin and seem to be strongly associated with active low back symptoms and segmental instability of the lumbar spine.[95–97] In contrast, Type 2 changes are less clearly associated with low back symptoms and seem to indicate a more biomechanically stable state. Finally, the exact nature and pathogenic significance of Type 3 changes remains largely unknown.

Posterior Elements

With disk degeneration and loss of disk space height, there are increased stresses on the facet joints, with hypertrophy of the articular process (Fig. 39). Facet arthrosis can result in narrowing of the central canal, lateral recesses, and foramina, and it is an important component of lumbar stenosis (Fig. 40).[74] Degenerative spondylolisthesis is a spreading and displacement of a vertebral body anteriorly or posteriorly as the result of severe OA of the facet joints. It is frequent at the L4/5 level because of the more sagittal orientation of the joints there. Degenerative disk disease may predispose a person for or exacerbate this condition secondary to narrowing of the

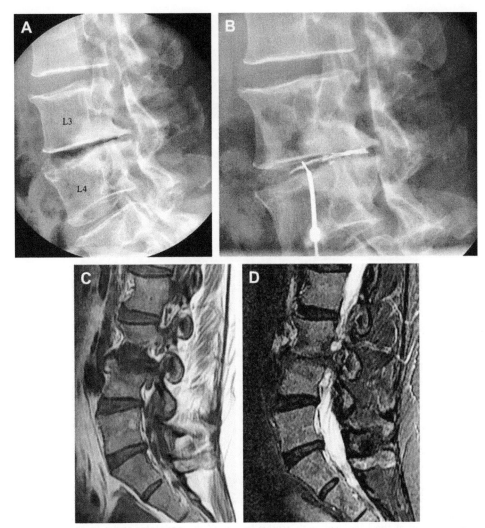

Fig. 37. 54-year-old woman who had chronic back pain. Radiographic images with oblique view (*A*) before and (*B*) after diskographic examination shows severe disk degeneration at L3/4 level with associated sclerosis of the posterior vertebral endplates. (*C*) Sagittal T1-weighted and (*D*) STIR MR images show Type 3 Modic changes at the L3/4 level.

disk space, which can produce subsequent malalignment of the articular processes and lead to rostrocaudal subluxation (Fig. 41). Radiographs are of limited value for the diagnosis of facet joint degenerative changes, and can be used only as a screening tool.[97] The abnormalities associated with OA can be best demonstrated and categorized using MDCT and MR imaging. There is moderate to good agreement between MR imaging and MDCT in this setting. If MR imaging examination is available, MDCT is not required for the assessment of facet joint OA in patients who have back pain and no previous surgery.[98]

Friedrich and colleagues[99] studied and described facet joint bone marrow changes associated with edema of the soft tissue surrounding the facet joints, which produce a condition that is referred to as facet joint edema. Lumbar spine MR imaging examinations with STIR, T1-, and T2-weighted images were performed in 145 consecutive patients who had back pain. Facet joint OA was graded using criteria adapted from Pathria and colleagues (Box 4).[100]

In 21 of the 145 patients (14%), bone marrow and surrounding soft tissue edema at the lumbar facet joints were reported: in 52.4% at L4/5, in 19% at L5/S1, in 14.3% at L4/5 and L5/S1, in 9.5% at L3/4 and L4/5, and in 4.8% at L3/4. OA of the facet joints was seen in all of the facet joints with edema. Disk degeneration was found at the level of the facet joint edema in 20 of the 21 patients. Twelve patients had anterolisthesis at

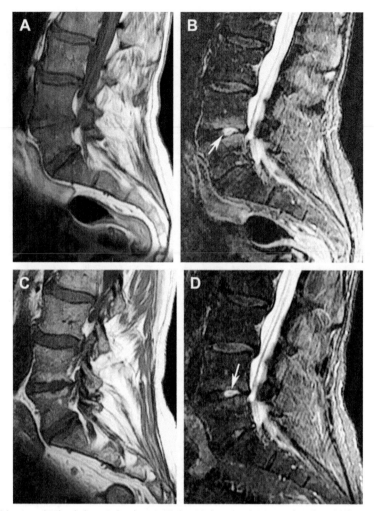

Fig. 38. 65-year-old man who had chronic back pain. (*A*) Initial sagittal T1-weighted and (*B*) STIR MR images show Type 1 Modic changes at the L4/5 level, with erosive lesions of the endplates and a bright central disk signal (*arrow*) on the STIR image. At 3-month follow-up, (*C*) sagittal T1-weighted and (*D*) STIR MR images show a change of signal of the endplates to Type 2 Modic classification, with a fatty signal of the endplates. There is no significant change of the disk signal (*arrow*) and morphology.

the segment that had facet joint edema. In summary, these findings support the fact that (a) degenerative changes of the facet joints occur mainly at the level of degenerative disk disease (functional unit), and (b) instability at a discovertebral level is associated with stress and overload for the facet joints. Lakadamyali and colleagues[101] studied sagittal STIR MR imaging findings in 372 patients who had nonradicular LBP and in 249 controls. All of the patients were diagnosed with pathologic changes in at least one of the posterior elements stabilizing the vertebral column. The incidences of facet joint effusion, interspinous ligament edema, neocyst formation, and paraspinal muscle edema were found to be statistically significantly higher in patients who had LBP than in controls. The most common

finding in these patients was facet joint effusion, which had a frequency of 85.5% compared with 45.8% in controls. Because of homogeneous fat-suppression and better depiction of soft-tissue edema, the use of STIR sequences is warranted for a good detection and visualization of these posterior changes.[101,102]

Reliability of MR Imaging Findings

Some prior work regarding observer performance in the interpretation of lumbosacral spine MR imaging data has been done in a variety of settings, including abnormalities of the intervertebral disk.[98,103] Recent imaging studies focused on disk contour and nondisk contour degenerative spine MR imaging findings. Van Rijn and

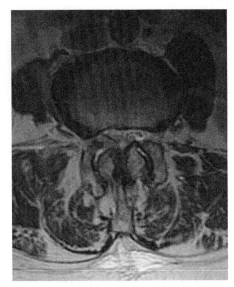

Fig. 39. 68-year-old man who had chronic back pain. Axial T2-weighted MR image at the L4/5 level shows marked, bilateral facet joint OA with hypertrophy, joint effusion, sagittalization, and stenosis of the spinal canal.

colleagues[104] assessed observer variation in MR image evaluation (disk contour findings) in patients suspected of having lumbar disk herniation. Two experienced neuroradiologists independently evaluated 59 consecutive patients who had lumbosacral radicular pain. Per patient, three levels (L3/4 through L5/S1) and the accompanying roots were evaluated on both sides. For each segment, the presence of a bulging disk or a herniation and compression of the root was reported.

Images were interpreted twice: once before and once after disclosure of clinical information. On average, more than 50% of interobserver variation in MR image evaluation of patients who had lumbosacral radicular pain was caused by disagreement on bulging disks. Knowledge of clinical information did not influence the detection of herniation, but it lowered the threshold for reporting bulging disks.[104] In addition to disk contour abnormalities, many spine degenerative findings depicted on MR images that involve the intervertebral disks, bone marrow, neuroforamina, spinal canal, and facet joints do exist and may be overlooked or poorly understood by those treating patients who have spine conditions. Results of prior investigations[98,103] suggest that the reliability of characterizing non–disk contour lumbar spine MR imaging findings is reasonable. Carrino and colleagues[105] were interested in the effectiveness of MR imaging findings as potential predictors of outcome. Thus, their work attempted to characterize inter- and intraobserver variability of qualitative, non–disk contour degenerative findings of the lumbar spine using MR imaging. The non–disk contour degenerative spine MR imaging findings assessed were spondylolisthesis, disk degeneration, marrow endplate abnormality (Modic changes), intervertebral disk posterior annular tears, and facet arthropathy. The 111 baseline MR imaging examinations were rated by four independent readers according to defined criteria for non–disk contour–related degenerative MR imaging findings, and a subgroup of 40 MR imaging examinations were rerated by the same readers. The interobserver agreement was good

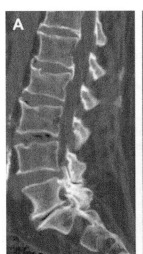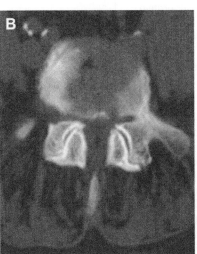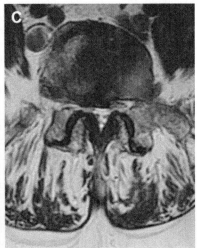

Fig. 40. Multilevel spinal OA in a 73-year-old man. (A) Sagittal and (B) axial MDCT scans show marked OA at the L5/S1 level with reduced disk height, disk vacuum phenomenon, and facet joint hypertrophy with bony spurs and foraminal stenosis. (C) Axial T2-weighted MR image at the L5/S1 level shows marked bilateral facet joint OA with hypertrophy and stenosis of the spinal canal. Note the bilateral fatty changes of the posterior spinal muscles.

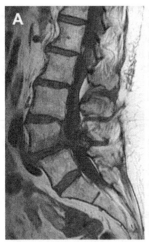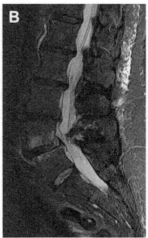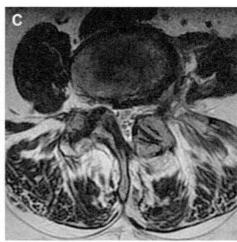

Fig. 41. Spinal OA in a 73-year-old woman. (*A*) Sagittal T1-weighted, (*B*) STIR, and (*C*) axial T2-weighted MR images at the L4/5 level show multilevel degenerative disk disease. There are also degenerative spondylolisthesis with vertebral endplates and Modic mixed 1-2 changes at the L4/5 level secondary to facet joint OA.

in rating disk degeneration and moderate in rating spondylolisthesis, Modic-type degenerative changes, facet arthropathy, and annular tears. The intraobserver agreement based on 40 MR imaging examination cases was good for rating spondylolisthesis, disk degeneration, Modic-type degenerative changes, facet arthropathy, and annular tears. Inter- and intraobserver agreement was moderate for rating the superior anteroposterior, inferior anteroposterior, superior craniocaudal, and inferior craniocaudal extents of Modic-type changes. Thus, some variability existed between readers despite standardized definitions and reader training. Carrino and colleagues concluded that non–disk contour degenerative lumbar spine MR imaging findings have sufficient reliability to potentially be used as predictors of clinical prognoses and outcomes if a rigorous MR imaging reader training paradigm is used.

Clinical Relevance of MR Imaging Findings on Spine Osteoarthritis

Any study looking at the natural history of degenerative disk disease, the prognostic value of imaging, or its effect on therapeutic decision making will be confounded by the high prevalence of morphologic changes in the asymptomatic population.[103,106] Jensen and colleagues[66] examined the prevalence of abnormal findings on MR images of the lumbar spine in 98 subjects without back pain. Thirty-six percent of the 98 asymptomatic subjects had normal disks at all levels. Fifty-two percent of the subjects had a bulge on at least one level, 27% had a protrusion, and 1% had an extrusion. Thirty-eight percent had an abnormality

of more than one intervertebral disk. The prevalence of bulges, but not of protrusions, increased with age. The most common nonintervertebral disk abnormalities were Schmorl's nodes, which were found in 19% of the subjects, annular defects in 14%, and facet arthropathy in 8%. The conclusions were that many people who did not have back pain did have disk bulges or protrusions but not extrusions. Given the high prevalence of these findings and of back pain, the discovery on MR images of bulges or protrusions in people who have LBP may frequently be coincidental. In

---

Box 4
Facet joint osteoarthritis grading system by Pathria and colleagues

Grade 0: Normal facet joint space (2–4 mm width)

Grade 1: Narrowing of the joint space (<2 mm) or small osteophytes or mild hypertrophy of the articular process

Grade 2: Narrowing of the joint space or small osteophytes or moderate hypertrophy of the articular process or mild subarticular bone erosions

Grade 3: Narrowing of the joint space or large osteophytes or severe hypertrophy of the articular process or severe subarticular bone erosions or subchondral cysts

Data from Luoma K, Vehmas T, Grönblad M, et al. Relationship of Modic type 1 change with disk degeneration: a prospective MRI study. Skeletal Radiol 2009;38:237–44.

an MR imaging study of 60 asymptomatic volunteers aged 20 to 50 years, Weishaupt and colleagues[67] concluded that disk bulging and protrusion and annular fissures are common findings in asymptomatic individuals younger than 50 years of age. However, disk extrusion and sequestration, nerve root compression, endplate abnormalities, and OA of the facet joints were rare and therefore may be predictive of LBP in symptomatic patients.[67] Recent studies show that Type 1 Modic endplate changes seem to be associated with a higher prevalence of active LBP symptoms.[11,24] Type 1 Modic endplate changes on MR images have positive predictive value in the presence of concordant pain provocation at provocative lumbar discography in a large sample population. However, no individual MR imaging finding is sufficient to predict pain provocation at discography.[79] The clinical importance of Type 2 Modic endplate changes remains unclear and limited.

SUMMARY

In summary, radiographs provide are a validated imaging technique to demonstrate morphologic changes of HOA. Diagnosis based on this single imaging modality (eg, for JSN or osteophytes) has limited value, whereas detection of associated clinical and radiographic changes dramatically improves diagnostic performance. Other imaging modalities (eg, ultrasound, MR imaging) are understudied, and their indications remain debated. Some imaging modalities are routinely indicated before wrist surgery (eg, CT-arthrography, MR imaging, MR-arthrography). Severity scores based on imaging findings mostly rely on plain films. In the future, one may assure that ultrasound and MR imaging will provide a better evaluation of established structural damages and the level of activity of the condition. All these imaging-based scoring methods should be cross-validated for cases of HAO with clinical status, including disease activity, function and performance, biomarkers, and long-term outcome. In the future, recently developed clinical and radiologic tools might help establish OA of the wrist and hand as a model of OA, along with OA of the hip or knee.

MR imaging is the best imaging technique to demonstrate the morphologic changes of lumbar spine OA, including disk and vertebral endplates changes, facet joint lesions, spinal canal narrowing, and nerve root compromise. Other imaging modalities such as MDCT may be useful in selected cases. The use of a standardized nomenclature and reader training are recommended to reduce the variability in MR image reporting and to improve intra- and interobserver agreement. All validated grading scores based on imaging findings now rely on MR imaging. In patients who have subacute or chronic back pain, the Modic classification is clinically useful, reliable, and relevant.

REFERENCES

1. Zhang Y, Niu J, Kelly-Hayes M, et al. Prevalence of symptomatic hand osteoarthritis and its impact on functional status among the elderly: the Framingham Study. Am J Epidemiol 2002;156:1021–7.
2. Dahaghin S, Bierma-Zeinstra SMA, Ginai AZ, et al. Prevalence and pattern of radiographic hand osteoarthritis and association with pain and disability (the Rotterdam Study). Ann Rheum Dis 2005;64:682–7.
3. Kellgren JH, Lawrence JS. Radiological assessment of osteoarthritis. Ann Rheum Dis 195;16: 494–502.
4. Zhang W, Doherty M, Leeb F, et al. EULAR evidence based recommendations for the management of hand osteoarthritis: report of a Task Force of the EULAR Standing Committee for International Clinical Studies Including Therapeutics (ESCISIT). Ann Rheum Dis 2007;66:377–88.
5. Hautefeuille P, Delcambre B, Duquesnoy B, et al. Etude clinique et épidémiologique des arthroses de la main. A partir de 500 observations sélectionnées dans un centre d'examen de santé. [Clinical and epidemiological study of osteoarthritis of the hand. Based on 500 cases selected from a Health Examination Center]. Rev Rhum Mal Osteoartic 1991;58:35–41 [in French].
6. Acheson RM, Chan YK, Clemet AR. New Haven Survey of Joint Diseases XII: distribution and symptoms of osteoarthritis in the hands with reference to handedness. Ann Rheum Dis 1970;29:275–86.
7. Kallman DA, Wigley FM, Scott WW, et al. New radiographic grading scales for osteoarthritis of the hand. Arthritis Rheum 1989;32:1584–91.
8. Spector TD, Brown GC, Silman AJ. Increased rates of prior hysterectomy and gynaecological operations in women with osteoarthritis. Br Med J 1988; 297:899–900.
9. Felson DT. The epidemiology of knee osteoarthritis: results from the Framingham Osteoarthritis Study. Semin Arthritis Rheum 1990;20:42–50.
10. Spector TD, Cicuttini F, Baker J, et al. Genetic influences on osteoarthritis in women: a twin study. Br Med J 1996;312:940–3.
11. Patotie A, Vaisanen P, Ott J, et al. Previous predisposition to familial osteoarthritis linked to type II collagen gene. Lancet 1989;1(8644):924–7.
12. Pattrick M, Manhire A, Ward AM, et al. B antigens and alpha 1-antitrypsin phenotypes in nodal and generalized osteoarthritis and erosive osteoarthritis. Ann Rheum Dis 1989;48:470–5.

13. Brodsky A, Appelboom A, Govaerts A, et al. HLA antigenes and Heberden nodes. Acta Rhumatol 1979;3:95–103.

14. Florak TM, Miller RJ, Pellegrini VT, et al. The prevalence of carpal tunnel syndrome in patients with basal joint arthritis of the thumb. J Hand Surg 1992;17:624–30.

15. Kapandji A, Moatti E, Raab C. La radiographie spécifique de l'articulation trapézométacarpienne. Sa technique, son intérêt [Specific radiography of the trapezo-metacarpal joint and its technique]. Ann Chir 1980;34:719–26 [in French].

16. Dell PC, Brushart TM, Smith RJ. Treatment of trapeziometacarpal arthritis: results of resection arthroplasty. J Hand Surg 1978;3:243–9.

17. Forestier J. L'ostéoarthrite sèche trapézométacarpienne (rhizarthrose du pouce). Presse Med 1937;45: 315–7 [in French].

18. Allieu Y, Chammas M, Cenac P. L'arthrose scapho-trapézo-trapézoïdienne isolée, une entité méconnue. Rhumatol Prat 1991;58:4–6 [in French].

19. Moser T, Dosch JC, Moussaoui A, et al. Wrist ligament tears: evaluation of MRI and combined MDCT and MR arthrography. AJR Am J Roentgenol 2007;188:1278–86.

20. Le Nen D. Arthrose pisotriquétrale. Maîtrise Orthop 1996;156:4–9 [in French].

21. Thurston AJ, Stanley JK. Hamato-lunate impingement: an uncommon cause of ulnar-sided wrist pain. Arthroscopy 2000;16:540–4.

22. Pfirmann CW, Theumann NH, Chung CB, et al. The hamatolunate facet: characterization and association with cartilage lesions—magnetic resonance arthrography and anatomic correlation in cadaveric wrists. Skeletal Radiol 2002;31:451–6.

23. Sagerman SD, Hauck RM, Palmer AK. Lunate morphology: can it be predicted with routine x-ray films? J Hand Surg [Am] 1995;20:38–41.

24. Viegas SF, Patterson RM, Eng M, et al. Wrist anatomy: incidence, distribution, and correlation of anatomic variations, tears and arthrosis. J Hand Surg [Am] 1993;18:463–75.

25. Nakamura K, Beppu M, Patterson RM, et al. Motion analysis in two dimensions of radial-ulnar deviation of type I versus type II lunates. J Hand Surg [Am] 2000;25:877–88.

26. Viegas SF, Wagner K, Patterson R, et al. Medial (hamate) facet of the lunate. J Hand Surg [Am] 1990;15:564–71.

27. Malik AM, Schweitzer ME, Culp RW, et al. MR imaging of the type II lunate bone: frequency, extent, and associated findings. AJR Am J Roentgenol 1999;173:335–8.

28. Delcambre B, Guyot-Drouot MH. Arthroses digitales et rhizarthrose [Joint osteoarthritis and rhizarthrosis]. Rev Prat 1996;46:2187–91 [in French].

29. Crain DC. Interphalangeal osteoarthritis characterized by painful inflammatory episodes resulting in deformity of the proximal and distal articulations. JAMA 1961;175:1044–53.

30. Punzi L, Ramonda R, Sfriso P. Erosive osteoarthritis. Best Pract Res Clin Rheumatol 2004;18:739–58.

31. Peter JB, Pearson CM, Marmor L. Erosive osteoarthritis of the hands. Arthritis Rheum 1966;9: 365–88.

32. Cobby M, Cushnaghan J, Creamer P, et al. Erosive osteoarthritis: is it a separate disease entity? Clin Radiol 1990;42:258–63.

33. Amadio PC, De Silva SP. Comparison of the results of trapeziometacarpal arthrodesis and arthroplasty in men with osteoarthritis of the trapeziometacarpal joint. Ann Chir Main 1990;9:358–63.

34. Zhang W, Doherty M, Leeb BF, et al. EULAR evidence-based recommendations for the diagnosis of hand osteoarthritis: report of a task force of ESCISIT. Ann Rheum Dis 2009;68:8–17.

35. Grainger AJ, Farrant JM, O'Connor PJ, et al. MR imaging of erosions in interphalangeal joint osteoarthritis: is all osteoarthritis erosive? Skeletal Radiol 2007;36:737–45.

36. Iagnocco A, Filippucci E, Ossandon A, et al. High resolution ultrasonography in detection of bone erosions in patients with hand osteoarthritis. J Rheumatol 2005;32:2381–3.

37. Keen HI, Wakefield RJ, Grainger AJ, et al. An ultrasonographic study of osteoarthritis of the hand: synovitis and its relationship to structural pathology and symptoms. Osteoarthritis Cartilage 2008;16:12–7.

38. Tan AL, Grainger AJ, Tanner SF, et al. A high-resolution magnetic resonance imaging study of distal interphalangeal joint arthropathy in psoriatic arthritis and osteoarthritis: are they the same? Arthritis Rheum 2006;54:1328–33.

39. Tan AL, Grainger AJ, Tanner SF, et al. High-resolution magnetic resonance imaging for the assessment of hand osteoarthritis. Arthritis Rheum 2005; 52:2355–65.

40. Tan AL, Toumi H, Benjamin M, et al. Combined high-resolution magnetic resonance imaging and histology to explore the role of ligaments and tendons in the phenotypic expression of early hand osteoarthritis. Ann Rheum Dis 2006;65: 1267–72.

41. Hunter DJ, Felson DT. Osteoarthritis. BMJ 2006; 332:639–42.

42. Williams WV, Cope R. Metacarpophalangeal arthropathy associated with manual labor. Arthritis Rheum 1987;30:1362–71.

43. Altman R, Alarcon G, Appelrouth D, et al. The American College of Rheumatology criteria for the classification and reporting of osteoarthritis of the hand. Arthritis Rheum 1990;33:1601–10.

44. Campion G, Dieppe P, Watt I. Heberden's nodes in osteoarthritis and rheumatoid arthritis. BMJ 1983; 287:1512.

45. Hart D, Spector T, Egger P, et al. Defining osteoarthritis of the hand for epidemiological studies: the Chingford Study. Ann Rheum Dis 1994;53:220–3.

46. Dreiser RL, Maheu E, Guillou GB, et al. Validation of an algofunctional index for osteoarthritis of the hand. Rev Rhum Engl Ed 1995;62(Suppl 1): 43S–53S.

47. Maheu E, Altman RD, Bloch DA, et al. Design and conduct of clinical trials in patients with osteoarthritis of the hand: recommendations from a task force of the Osteoarthritis Research Society International. Osteoarthritis Cartilage 2006;14:303–22.

48. Kallman DA, Wigley FM, Scott WW Jr, et al. The longitudinal course of hand osteoarthritis in a male population. Arthritis Rheum 1990;33: 1323–32.

49. Dougados M, Nguyen M, Mijiyawa M, et al. Reproducibility of X-ray analysis of hand osteoarthrosis. Rhumatologie 1990;42:287–91.

50. Verbruggen G, Veys EM. Erosive and non-erosive hand osteoarthritis. Use and limitations of two scoring systems. Osteoarthritis Cartilage 2000; 8(Suppl A):S45–54.

51. Lane NE, Kremer LB. Radiographic indices for osteoarthritis. Rheum Dis Clin North Am 1995;21: 379–94.

52. Kessler S, Dieppe P, Fuchs J, et al. Assessing the prevalence of hand osteoarthritis in epidemiological studies. The reliability of a radiological hand scale. Ann Rheum Dis 2000;59:289–92.

53. Buckland-Wright JC, Macfarlane DG, Lynch JA, et al. Quantitative microfocal radiographic assessment of progression in osteoarthritis of the hand. Arthritis Rheum 1990;33:57–65.

54. Richmond BJ, Powers C, Piraino DW, et al. Diagnostic efficacy of digitized images vs plain films: a study of the joints of the fingers. Am J Roentgenol 1992;158:437–41.

55. Swee RG, Gray JE, Beabout JW, et al. Screen film versus computed radiography imaging of the hand: a direct comparison. AJR Am J Roentgenol 1997;168:539–42.

56. Van 't Klooster R, Hendriks EA, Watt I, et al. Automatic quantification of osteoarthritis in hand radiographs: validation of a new method to measure joint space width. Osteoarthritis Cartilage 2008;16:18–25.

57. Spector TD, Cooper C. Radiographic assessment of osteoarthritis in population studies: whither Kellgren and Lawrence? Osteoarthritis Cartilage 1993;1:203–6.

58. Spector TD, Hochberg M. Methodological problems in the epidemiological study of osteoarthritis. Ann Rheum Dis 1994;53:143–6.

59. Ravaud P, Giraudeau B, Auleley GR, et al. Assessing smallest detectable change over time in continuous structural outcome measures: application to radiological change in knee osteoarthritis. J Clin Epidemiol 1999;52:1225–30.

60. Verbruggen G, Veys EM. Numerical scoring systems for the anatomic evolution of osteoarthritis of the finger joints. Arthritis Rheum 1996;39:308–20.

61. Maheu E, Cadet C, Gueneugues S, et al. Reproducibility and sensitivity to change of four scoring methods for the radiological assessment of osteoarthritis of the hand. Ann Rheum Dis 2007;66: 464–9.

62. Lopez-Ben R, Bernreuter WK, Moreland LW, et al. Ultrasound detection of bone erosions in rheumatoid arthritis: a comparison to routine radiographs of the hands and feet. Skeletal Radiol 2004;33: 80–4.

63. Szkudlarek M, Court-Payen M, Strandberg C, et al. Power Doppler ultrasonography for assessment of synovitis in the metacarpophalangeal joints of patients with rheumatoid arthritis: a comparison with dynamic magnetic resonance imaging. Arthritis Rheum 2001;44:2018–23.

64. Keen HI, Lavie F, Wakefield RJ, et al. The development of a preliminary ultrasonographic scoring system for features of hand osteoarthritis. Ann Rheum Dis 2008;67:651–5.

65. Millette PC. The proper terminology for reporting lumbar intervertebral disk disorders. AJNR Am J Neuroradiol 1997;18:1859–66.

66. Jensen MC, Brant-Zawadzki MN, Obuchowski N, et al. Magnetic resonance imaging of the lumbar spine in people without back pain. N Engl J Med. 1994;331:69–73.

67. Weishaupt D, Zanetti M, Hodler J, et al. MR imaging of the lumbar spine: prevalence of intervertebral disk extrusion and sequestration, nerve root compression, end plate abnormalities, and osteoarthritis of the facet joints in asymptomatic volunteers. Radiology 1998;209:661–6.

68. Stadnik TW, Lee RR, Coen HL, et al. Annular tears and disk herniation: prevalence and contrast enhancement on MR images in the absence of low back pain or sciatica. Radiology 1998;206: 49–55.

69. Kettler A, Wilke HJ. Review of existing grading systems for cervical or lumbar disk and facet joint degeneration. Eur Spine J 2006;15:705–18.

70. Brandt-Zawadzki M, Dennis SC, Gade GF, et al. Low back pain. Radiology 2000;217:321–30.

71. Gallucci M, Puglielli E, Splendiani A, et al. Degenerative disorders of the spine. Eur Radiol 2005;15: 591–8.

72. Bradley WG Jr. Low back pain. AJNR Am J Neuroradiol 2007;28:990–2.

73. Leone A, Guglielmi G, Cassar-Pullicino VN, et al. Lumbar intervertebral instability: a review. Radiology 2007;245:62–77.

74. Modic MT, Ross JS. Lumbar degenerative disk disease. Radiology 2007;245:43–61.

75. Moore KR, Tsuruda JS, Dailey AT. The value of MR neurography for evaluating extraspinal neuropathic leg pain: a pictorial essay. AJNR Am J Neuroradiol 2001;22:786–94.

76. Jinkins JR, Dworkin JS, Damadian RV. Upright, weight-bearing, dynamic-kinetic MRI of the spine: initial results. Eur Radiol 2005;15:1815–25.

77. Hiwatashi A, Danielson B, Moritani T, et al. Axial loading during MR imaging can influence treatment decision for symptomatic spinal stenosis. AJNR Am J Neuroradiol 2004;25:170–4.

78. Weishaupt D, Schmid MR, Zanetti M, et al. Positional MR imaging of the lumbar spine: does it demonstrate nerve root compromise not visible at conventional MR imaging? Radiology 2000;215:247–53.

79. Thompson KJ, Dagher AP, Eckel TS, et al. Modic changes on MR images as studied with provocative discography: clinical relevance—a retrospective study of 2457 disks. Radiology 2009;250: 849–55.

80. Mitra D, Cassar-Pullicino VN, McCall IW. Longitudinal study of high intensity zones on MR of lumbar intervertebral disks. Clin Radiol 2004;59: 1002–8.

81. Sharma A, Pilgram T, Wippold FJ. Association between annular tears and disk degeneration: a longitudinal study. AJNR Am J Neuroradiol 2009;30:500–6.

82. Fardon DF, Milette PC. Nomenclature and classification of lumbar disk pathology: recommendations of the combined task forces of the North American Spine Society, American Society of Spine Radiology, and American Society of Neuroradiology. Spine 2001;26:E93–113.

83. Pfirrmann CW, Metzdorf A, Zanetti M, et al. Magnetic resonance classification of lumbar intervertebral disk degeneration. Spine 2001;26:1873–8.

84. Griffith JF, Wang YX, Antonio GE, et al. Modified Pfirrmann grading system for lumbar intervertebral disk degeneration. Spine 2007;32:E708–12.

85. Pfirrmann CW, Dora C, Schmid MR, et al. MR image–based grading of lumbar nerve root compromise due to disk herniation: reliability study with surgical correlation. Radiology 2004;230:583–8.

86. Modic MT, Steinberg PM, Ross JS, et al. Degenerative disk disease: assessment of changes in vertebral body marrow with MR imaging. Radiology 1988;166:193–9.

87. Rannou F, Ouanes W, Boutron I, et al. High-sensitivity C-reactive protein in chronic low back pain with vertebral end-plate Modic signal changes. Arthritis Rheum 2007;57:1311–5.

88. Kuisma M, Karppinen J, Niinimäki J, et al. A three-year follow-up of lumbar spine endplate (Modic) changes. Spine 2006;31:1714–8.

89. Rahme R, Moussa R. The Modic vertebral endplate and marrow changes: pathologic significance and relation to low back pain and segmental instability of the lumbar spine. AJNR Am J Neuroradiol 2008;29:838–42.

90. Karchevsky M, Schweitzer ME, Carrino JA, et al. Reactive endplate marrow changes: a systematic morphologic and epidemiologic evaluation. Skeletal Radiol 2005;34:125–9.

91. Kuisma M, Karppinen J, Haapea M, et al. Modic changes in vertebral endplates: a comparison of MR imaging and multislice CT. Skeletal Radiol 2009;38:141–7.

92. Jones A, Clarke A, Freeman BJ, et al. The Modic classification: inter- and intraobserver error in clinical practice. Spine 2005;30:1867–9.

93. Fayad F, Lefevre-Colau MM, Drapé JL, et al. Reliability of a modified Modic classification of bone marrow changes in lumbar spine MRI. Joint Bone Spine 2009;76:286–9.

94. Luoma K, Vehmas T, Grönblad M, et al. Relationship of Modic type 1 change with disk degeneration: a prospective MRI study. Skeletal Radiol 2009;38:237–44.

95. Mitra D, Cassar-Pullicino VN, McCall IW. Longitudinal study of vertebral type-1 end-plate changes on MR of the lumbar spine. Eur Radiol 2004;14:1574–81.

96. Fayad F, Lefevre-Colau MM, Rannou F, et al. Relation of inflammatory Modic changes to intraal steroid injection outcome in chronic low back pain. Eur Spine J 2007;16:925–31.

97. Wybier M. Imaging of lumbar degenerative changes involving structures other than disk space. Radiol Clin North Am 2001;39:101–14.

98. Weishaupt D, Zanetti M, Boos N, et al. MR imaging and CT in osteoarthritis of the lumbar facet joints. Skeletal Radiol 1999;28:215–9.

99. Friedrich KM, Nemec S, Peloschek P, et al. The prevalence of lumbar facet joint edema in patients with low back pain. Skeletal Radiol 2007;36:755–60.

100. Pathria M, Sartoris DJ, Resnick D. Osteoarthritis of the facet joints: accuracy of oblique radiographic assessment. Radiology 1987;164:227–30.

101. Lakadamyali H, Tarhan NC, Ergun T, et al. STIR sequence for depiction of degenerative changes in posterior stabilizing elements in patients with lower back pain. AJR Am J Roentgenol 2008;191:973–9.

102. D'Aprile P, Tarantino A, Jinkins JR, et al. The value of fat saturation sequences and contrast medium administration in MRI of degenerative disease of the posterior/perispinal elements of the lumbosacral spine. Eur Radiol 2007;17: 523–31.

103. Weishaupt D, Zanetti M, Hodler J, et al. Painful lumbar disk derangement: relevance of endplate abnormalities at MR imaging. Radiology 2001; 218:420–7.

104. Van Rijn JC, Klemetsö N, Reitsma JB, et al. Observer variation in MRI evaluation of patients suspected of lumbar disk herniation. AJR Am J Roentgenol 2005;184:299–303.

105. Carrino JA, Lurie JD, Tosteson AN, et al. Lumbar spine: reliability of MR imaging findings. Radiology 2009;250:161–70.

106. Modic MT, Obuchowski NA, Ross JS, et al. Acute low back pain and radiculopathy: MR imaging findings and their prognostic role and effect on outcome. Radiology 2005;237: 597–604.

Imaging in Pre- and Post-operative Assessment in Joint Preserving and Replacing Surgery

Adnan Sheikh, MD*, Mark Schweitzer, MD

KEYWORDS

- Arthroplasty • Cartilage repair • High tibial osteotomy
- Computed tomography • Magnetic resonance imaging

The number of joint replacement surgeries performed throughout the world continues to rise annually. Joint replacements are among the most common surgical procedures in most developed countries. From 1% to 5% of these patients develop such complications as fracture, particle disease, and infection, which may require revision.[1] A basic understanding of these surgical procedures and devices is important for imaging evaluation.

The detection of complications can be challenging because these patients usually present with nonspecific and subtle clinical symptoms, such as pain and decreased range of motion. Conventional radiography, arthrography, scintigraphy, ultrasound, CT, and MRI can be used to assess the orthopedic prosthesis and, to some degree, the adjacent osseous and soft tissue structures. With the transition from salvage to reconstruction techniques, the role of imaging in the preoperative assessment increases. The knowledge of utility, limitations, and optimization of technique is essential to diagnose pathology in postoperative patients. This article reviews the radiographic, ultrasound, CT, and MRI appearance of knee and hip joint–preserving surgeries.

IMAGING TECHNIQUES
Conventional Radiography

Conventional radiography remains the cornerstone of postoperative musculoskeletal imaging. A minimum of two views of the affected joint should be obtained to assess the orthopedic hardware and adjacent bone. Serial radiographs play an important role in the evaluation of hardware complications. Fracture and osteolysis can be more easily diagnosed when baseline imaging is available. The radiographic findings of hardware loosening include lucency of greater than 2 mm at the bone-metal or cement-bone interface, fracture of the cement, and change of alignment or migration of the component.[2,3] Well-defined radiolucencies around a hardware component suggest particle disease. Most cases of loosening from modern arthroplasties are sequelae of particle disease. Careful attention should be paid to the relative position of the femoral head within the acetabulum component to assess for polyethylene wear.

Arthrography

Arthrography can be performed concurrently with aspiration to distinguish infection from loosening. The presence of contrast material between the bone-metal or cement-bone interface suggests loosening,[4–6] especially as it goes more distal. This is not diagnostic. The major role of arthrography is to guide and confirm joint aspiration. The more contrast fills sacculations around the joint, however, the more likely there is to be secondary loosening.

Department of Diagnostic Imaging, The Ottawa Hospital, General Campus, University of Ottawa, 501 Smyth Road, Ottawa, Canada KIH 8L6
* Corresponding author.
E-mail address: asheikh@ottawahospital.on.ca (A. Sheikh).

Radiol Clin N Am 47 (2009) 761–775
doi:10.1016/j.rcl.2009.05.001

Scintigraphy

Scintigraphy can be used in the assessment of painful arthroplasty. Although technetium Tc 99m methylene diphosphonate (Tc-MDP) can show increased uptake around the arthroplasty component in the early postoperative period, little imaging is done during that time. When the first two phases are normal, a three-phase bone scan is more useful to exclude infection than it is to diagnose infection. The more unilateral the uptake is, the closer it is to the joint line, and the more lateral the uptake is, the more likely the changes are related to particle disease. The presence of increased activity after an injection of gallium- or indium-labeled leukocytes suggests infection.[7,8] However, usually these studies should be combined with sulfur colloid scanning to distinguish this "inflammatory" uptake from displaced marrow. All scintigraphic examinations are more accurate in the hip than the knee, with knee arthroplasties especially prone to false-positive scintigraphies. Currently, gallium is infrequently used even for chronically infected arthroplasties.

Ultrasound

Ultrasound can also be used in the assessment of painful arthroplasty as it's an excellent modality to assess soft tissues. Ultrasound can be used in the assessment and therapeutic intervention of periprosthetic collection and bursitis.[9–11] The integrity of the adjacent tendons and ligaments can also be assessed. Ultrasound plays mainly a secondary role to see if joint fluid is present and to guide the aspiration of this fluid.

CT

In the past, CT was considered to be of limited utility in patients with metallic hardware. The present-generation multidetector CT, along with improved computer software, is able to overcome the attenuation of x-ray beam by the metal.[9,12] The type of metal also has an effect on these artifacts. The more recent titanium prosthesis has a lower x-ray coefficient compared with steel and cobalt-chrome devices.[10] Radiation dose is drastically increased when an arthroplasty is present. CT is helpful in the evaluation of fracture mapping and assessment of osteolytic lesions.[10] Metal artifact reduction techniques include:

- Positioning the patient in the gantry such that the x-ray beam courses through the smallest diameter of the hardware
- Using high kilovolts and milliamperes with thin overlap slices, thus minimizing noise,

which contributes to degradation of image quality
- Reformatting the images in multiple planes with slice thickness greater than originally acquired, which decreases streak artifact and thereby improves visualization of structures around the hardware
- Using soft tissue reconstruction kernels rather than bone algorithm and wide windows when viewing images to reduce metal artifact[9–11]

MRI

MRI once had a limited role in postoperative assessment due to severe susceptibility artifact. However, the modification of imaging parameters has led to less motion degradation of image quality and improved diagnostic images. MRI is currently widely used in postoperative patients because of its multiplanar imaging capability, better contrast resolution, and lack of ionizing radiation when compared with CT.[9,13] The metallic artifact can be reduced by:

- Using a higher bandwidth
- Using fast spin echo instead of spin echo sequences
- Avoiding gradient echo sequence
- Using short tau inversion recovery (STIR) instead of a T2 fat-saturated sequence
- Lowering echo time
- Using a large-frequency encoding matrix
- Orienting frequency encoding direction along the longitudinal axis of the implant[9–11,14,15]

ARTHROPLASTY

Arthroplasty is an orthopedic procedure to partially or completely resurface, remodel, rebuild, or replace an arthritic, dysfunctional, or necrotic joint. We focus on the hip and knee joints in this article. The components of arthroplasty are held in position using a cemented, noncemented, or hybrid procedure, depending on the clinical indication and age of the patient.

In a cemented procedure, the components are fixed with polymethyl-methacrylate, which allows the implant to fit to the irregularities of the bone. This type of replacement is stable and immediate full weight bearing is possible. However, should the component become loose, some bone will grind away, making revision more difficult.[15] In a noncemented procedure, the components have a roughened porous surface to allow bone to grow into it. These types of implants are press fit against the bone. In case of loosening, bone loss is minimal and bone stock is preserved.[15] Currently, few hip arthroplasties are fully cemented.

Knee Arthroplasty

Unicompartmental knee arthroplasty is one of several options in the treatment of unicompartment arthritis in young patients. The advantages of unicompartmental arthroplasty over total knee arthroplasty are smaller incision, more rapid recovery, and, more importantly, loss of less than 75% of bone and cartilage.[2] By retaining all the undamaged parts, the joint bends and functions more naturally. Unicompartmental knee arthroplasty is commonly used to treat medial compartment arthritis. However, it may also be used to treat lateral compartment osteoarthritis and, more recently, patella-femoral disease. Indications for medial unicompartmental knee arthroplasty include medial compartment arthritis, intact anterior and posterior cruciate ligaments, intact lateral compartment, correctable varus deformity, and less than 10° of fixed flexion.[16,17] Contraindications include inflammatory arthropathy, high tibial osteotomy, tibial and femoral shaft deformity, and sepsis.[16–18] Clinical trials by Savard and colleagues[19] and Berger and colleagues[20] have indicated a success rate of 95% and 98% respectively.

Medial compartment osteoarthritis affects the anteromedial aspect of the tibial plateau. In the lateral compartment, the femoral side is usually affected.[20] Preoperative radiographic assessment includes a weight-bearing anteroposterior and tunnel views to evaluate for cartilage narrowing. A lateral radiograph should be obtained to assess for posterior bone loss. Long leg radiographs to assess for malalignment may also be obtained.[2,18] White and colleagues described the features of anteromedial arthritis of the knee. An anteroposterior view should show a central erosion of the tibia. The lateral view should show an intact posterior tibial plateau. This finding is important because it suggests that the tibia cannot sublux anteriorly on the femur, and that the anterior cruciate ligament is intact.

Total knee arthroplasty is usually provided for patients with severe osteoarthritis. The aim is to resurface the damaged tibiofemoral surface with metal components and provide low-friction articulation with a polyethylene liner. Patellar resurfacing is also indicated if severe patellofemoral disease is present. Preoperative radiological evaluation with standing anteroposterior view, lateral view, and skyline radiographs to assess the patellofemoral joint is obtained. A long leg view to assess for malalignment, a Rosenberg view, and standing radiographs in 45° of flexion can also be obtained to assess for cartilage degeneration.[21] Indium In 111 scintigraphy can help to rule out infection, but is not usually necessary.[22–24] A CT is occasionally performed to assess bone stock.

Postoperatively, anteroposterior views are taken in supine and standing positions along with lateral and skyline views of the patella for follow-up of patients and to assess for fracture, loosening, component dislocation, liner wear, and infection in knee arthroplasty.

Complications of Knee Arthroplasty

Thromboembolism

Deep venous thrombosis, with potential to propagate a pulmonary embolism, is the most feared complication of knee arthroplasty. The incidence of deep venous thrombosis without prophylaxis ranges from 40% to 88%, with symptomatic pulmonary embolism ranging from 0.5% to 3%. Related mortality is 2%. Deep venous thrombosis can be easily diagnosed on ultrasound.[21]

Fracture

Periprosthetic fractures incurred either during surgery or in the postoperative period can be diagnosed with conventional radiography. Occasionally, a CT may be required for better delineation of the fracture. Most fractures are seen later through areas of particle disease.

Joint instability

An asymmetric widening of the prosthetic joint space suggests ligamentous imbalance and varus-valgus instability. This accounts for 1% to 2% of primary instability following total knee arthroplasty.[21]

Patellar complications

Stress fracture of the patella and loosening and dislocation of patellar components are the most common complications. Patellar stress fractures, commonly seen in older patients, are reported in 21% of cases.[3,25] These can be easily detected on radiographs. Fatigue fractures are not uncommonly seen with metal-backed prosthesis, usually at the peg-plate junction.[3,25] Patellar subluxation and tilt, recognized on tangential view of the patella, are caused by an imbalance of soft tissue (tight lateral retinaculum) and malpositioning and malalignment of components. The thin polyethylene liner may wear or get displaced from the metal backing into the Hoffa fat pad. The liner wear results in rubbing of the femoral metal component against the metal backing of the patellar component, resulting in metallosis. This is visible radiographically as a line of linear opacity outlining the distended joint effusion (metal line sign).[3] Patellar and quadriceps tendon rupture, resulting in abnormal positioning of the patella, has also been reported. This can be seen on radiographs and confirmed with ultrasound. Fibrosis and scarring of the Hoffa fat pad may result in a low-lying patella (patella baja).[21]

Prosthesis loosening

Prosthesis loosening can be seen along both the tibial and femoral components as a result of stress shielding, infection, and osteolysis.[26] This is more commonly seen with uncemented tibial components along the medial side, resulting in varus angulations. From 1 to 2 cm of lucency at the bone-cement interface is normal.[2,26] It is secondary to cement shrinkage and endotermal injury to the adjacent bone. Widening of greater than 2 cm at the bone-cement, metal-cement, and prosthesis-bone interfaces on serial weight-bearing radiographs is suggestive of loosening (Fig. 1).[26] A bone scan can also be used to diagnose loosening. The presence of contrast between the bone-cement and bone-metal interface on arthrography also indicates loosening.

Prosthesis wear

Increased weight and physical activity, irregularities of the surface condylar component articulating with the polyethylene liner, and abnormal alignment of the condylar component each contribute to liner wear. This wear involves shedding of metal or polyethylene, resulting in hypertrophic synovium, which incites histocytic response, leading to osteolysis.[2,21] Osteolysis can occasionally be appreciated on radiographs, although it is not visible until far along in the process. Various studies have shown CT to be more sensitive in detection and quantification of osteolysis. Polyethylene wear is evaluated by measuring from the femoral condyles to the tibial base plate on serial radiographs. Interval narrowing of the joint space suggests polyethylene wear. Ultrasound can also be used to assess the polyethylene liner and osteolysis, but this is difficult in practice.

Infection

Infection is the most common cause of failure of knee arthroplasty. The prevalence of infection ranges from 0.5% to 2%.[21] The radiographic appearance of infection can be variable. In most patients, radiographs are normal. Serial radiographs may show periosteal reaction, progressive periprosthetic widening, and osteolysis, but this is rare (Fig. 2). Joint aspiration is the most useful confirmatory test. However, false-negative results have been seen and are quite common, particularly if saline irrigation is required. The sensitivity and specificity of joint aspiration can vary. Sensitivity ranges from 67% to 82%. Specificity ranges from 91% to 95%.[21,27] Bone scan may be positive for years following arthroplasty.

However, increased activity following injection of gallium- and indium-labeled leucocytes is suggestive of infection. Combined sulfur colloid scanning with indium-labeled white blood cells (In-WBC) offer the best accuracy—up to 95%.[21,28] When the uptake on both studies is similar, it indicates no infection as the changes represent displaced marrow. Increased In-WBC activity in relation to sulfur colloid is sensitive of infection. Fluorodeoxyglucose positron emission

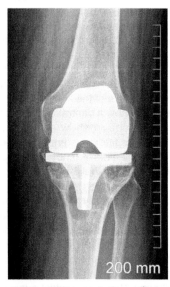

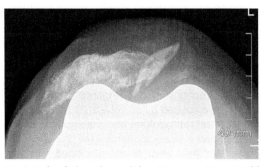

Fig. 1. Polyethylene liner dislocation in a 50-year-old man with knee pain. Sunrise patellofemoral joint view shows liner dislocation and lateral subluxation of the patella.

Fig. 2. Loosening. Anteroposterior radiograph of the knee shows increased lucency surrounding the tibial stem and under the tibial tray in keeping with loosening of the hardware.

tomography (FDG-PET) studies have shown sensitivity and specificity of 100% and 86% respectively in limited numbers.[28] Nearly all hip arthroplasties show uptake about the neck on PET images. Ultrasound can be used to assess for periprosthetic infection for limited indications. CT and MRI can also be used to assess the extent of soft tissue infection and collections and marrow outside of that in close proximity to the arthroplasty.

HIP ARTHROPLASTY

Hip arthroplasty is one of the most frequently performed reconstructive surgeries. It is estimated that 1.5 million procedures are performed worldwide.[11] Different types of prosthesis are used, depending on the pathophysiology and age of the patient. Unicompartment arthroplasty, which is used in the elderly to treat femoral neck fracture, involves replacement of femoral head and neck. A bipolar hemiarthroplasty is used to replace the femoral head and neck with an acetabular component that is not attached to the acetabulum. Normal motion can be seen between the acetabular cup and femoral head as well as between the acetabular cup and native acetabulum.[2,15] It is indicated in avascular necrosis of the hip and displaced femoral neck fracture in risk of developing avascular necrosis. A total hip arthroplasty is recommended when both the acetabular and the femoral head are affected, as in osteoarthritis. The prosthesis has an acetabular component, a ceramic cup, a polyethylene liner, and a femoral component. The present-day acetabular component is cementless and may accommodate a press fit or have a roughened surface for bone ingrowth. The femoral component may be fixed with cement or may be a press-fit type.

An anteroposterior view of the pelvis centered over the pubis and a true lateral view of the hip are used to assess the hip prosthesis postoperatively.[2]

Component Position

Acetabular inclination angle indicates the tilt of the acetabular component to a horizontal base line. An angle of 40° to 50° is considered neutral, an angle of greater than 40° suggests horizontal orientation, and an angle of less than 50° suggests vertical orientation.[2,29,30]

Mediolateral position of the hip is measured as a distance along the interteardrop line from the teardrop to the intersection with a perpendicular from the center of the femoral head. A change of more than 2 mm is considered significant.[2,30]

Anteversion angle, measured on the lateral view, is the angle between the axis of the acetabular marker wire and a perpendicular to the base line. There is normally 5° to 25° of anteversion.[31–33] The tip of the femoral component should be ventrally placed on an anteroposterior projection or be directed medially (valgus).[2] The anteversion angle can also be measured on CT while the patient is supine with the extremities in neutral position. A single CT is obtained that includes both hips and knees. Helical images of 5-mm thickness at 5-mm intervals are obtained from just above the femoral heads to the lesser trochanter and also from the level of the distal femoral physis to the tibial head. On a section through the femoral neck and upper portion of greater trochanter, a line is drawn through the femoral neck, using the femoral neck and greater trochanter as a guide. The angle that line forms with the horizontal line determines the relative angle of anteversion/retroversion of the femoral head. On CT sections through the femoral condyles, at the intercondylar notch, a line is drawn through the posterior margins of the condyles. The angle formed by this line and the horizontal line determines the degree of internal or external rotation of the extremity. True angle of version is calculated from these two angles. If the knee is in internal rotation, the sum of the angles yields the angle of anteversion. If the knee is externally rotated, then the angle obtained at the knee is subtracted from the angle obtained at the hip.

Complications of Hip Arthroplasty

Loosening

Loosening is the most common problem with cemented prosthesis. Lucency of less than 2 mm at the bone-cement interface outlined by a thin sclerotic demarcation line is normal and represents fibrous tissue. Lucency wider than 2 mm or progression of lucencies on serial radiographs suggests loosening. Acetabular loosening is identified by component migration. A 2-mm continuous lucency suggests impending loosening. Cement fracture and motion of the components on stress views or fluoroscopy also suggest loosening. On arthrography, extension of contrast material along the prosthesis-cement or bone-cement interface below the intertrochanteric line is suggestive of loosening (Fig. 3).[2,34]

Infection

Identification of lucency greater than 2 mm is suggestive of infection, loosening, or particle disease. It is usually difficult to distinguish between these three entities. Rapidly developing

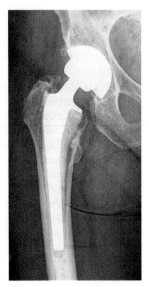

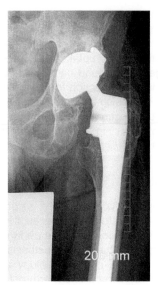

Fig. 3. Loosening. Anteroposterior radiograph of the right hip shows increased widening at the cement-bone interface in keeping with loosening.

Fig. 4. Aggressive granulomatous disease. Anteroposterior radiograph of the left hip demonstrates loosening of the femoral and acetabular components with well-defined focal areas of endosteal erosions in the proximal femur and ischium, indicating granuloma formation. Wear of the polyethylene acetabular cup is also present.

cement-bone lucency, endosteal scalloping, and periostitis may indicate infection. Joint aspiration and bone scan recommend for confirmation as described earlier. Ultrasound, CT, and MRI may also be used to assess for other soft tissue markers for infection, such as soft tissue collection, bursitis, and joint effusion.[35–39]

Osteolysis
Osteolysis, as described in the knee section, is related to polyethylene or metal debris phagocytized by macrophages, which accumulate to form foreign body granulomas. These granulomas stimulate osteoclastic activity and cause periprosthetic erosions (Fig. 4). CT, due to its multiplanar capabilities, has a detection rate of 82% when compared with radiograph, which has a detection rate of 52%.[2,11,38,40]

On CT, osteolysis manifests as well-defined lucencies devoid of trabaculae with associated soft tissue mass ranging from −40 to 100 Hounsfield units. Following contrast administration they show marked peripheral enhancement (Figs. 5 and 6).[11,40] On MRI they are typically low signal on T1-weighted sequences and intermediate-to-high signal on T2-weighted sequences[11,41] and enhance.

MRI plays a significant role in the assessment of the soft tissues adjacent to the prosthesis. Trochanteric bursitis (Fig. 7), avulsion of the gluteus tendons (Fig. 8), and short external rotators can easily be identified on MRI.[11] Psoas tendon impingement secondary to friction against the anterior acetabular spur or extruded cement

can easily be seen on CT. A pseudomass in the iliopsoas tendon sheath due to polyethylene wear has also been reported.[2,11,42] Lymphadenopathy secondary to dissemination of a large amount of polyethylene and metallic debris can easily be identified with cross-sectional imaging.

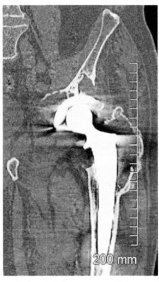

Fig. 5. Extensive granulomatous disease. Coronal CT reformat shows granuloma formation in the proximal femur and acetabulum.

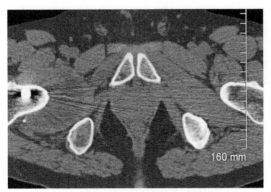

Fig. 6. Iliopsoas pseudomass. Axial CT scan shows complex cystic mass in the right iliopsoas tendon sheath in a patient with metal-on-metal surface replacement.

Other complications

Other complications of hip arthroplasty include periprosthesis fracture (Figs. 9, 10, 11), metallosis, acetabular liner wear (Fig. 12), prosthetic dislocation (Fig. 13), and heterotrophic bone (Fig. 14). Each can usually be identified on radiographs.

Resurfacing Hip Arthroplasty

A resurfacing hip arthroplasty is a metal-on-metal type of hip replacement that replaces the arthritic surface of the joint but removes far less bone than with traditional hip replacement. The ideal candidate is a young active adult with good bone quality and morphology.[42] Contraindications include proximal femoral osteoporosis, tumor, erosive and inflammatory arthritis, poor bone stock, short femoral neck, and acetabular dysplasia.

Postoperative Assessment

A review of literature suggests that there are six radiographic features of the component that should be monitored:[42–46]

- Peg femoral angle. The orientation of the peg should be parallel to the trabecular bone. Progressive change in the angle between the peg and femoral shaft, particularly varus, suggests loosening or fracture.
- Implant subsidence. Progressive reduction in the distance between the peg and the lateral femoral cortex over time suggests subsidence and instability.
- Femoral neck narrowing. This is commonly seen following hip arthroplasty and can be seen up to 3 years following the procedure. Progressive narrowing of the femoral neck beyond 3 years should be carefully monitored. This may be secondary to stress shielding, loosening, and femoroacetabular impingement or due to inflammatory response and metal hypersensitivity.
- Femoral neck scalloping. This can be superior or inferior and is related to bony remodeling. Superior scalloping is secondary to bony resorption or femoroacetabular impingement.
- Radiolucent lines. Similar to the femoral stem in total arthroplasty, the peg can be divided into three zones. Widening of more than 2 mm in any zone suggests loosening.
- Periprosthetic osteolysis. It can be located superior, inferiorly, or adjacent to the peg. This is secondary to liner wear–related or metal sensitivity–related tissue reactions.

Complications

Femoral neck fracture, the most common complication, is seen in 12% of resurfacing hip arthroplasties, and is more common in females (Fig. 15).[42–45] It may be related to osteoporosis and poor secondary operative technique, such as notching of the superior portion of the femoral neck and varus position of the femoral peg. Component loosening and femoral impingement are the other complications.[46]

IMAGING OF CARTILAGE REPAIR

Cartilage research has assumed increased importance because of better understanding of cartilage biology and function and because of improved

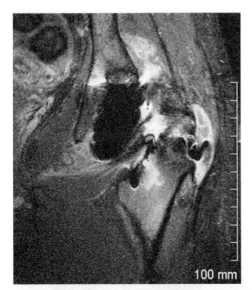

Fig. 7. Trochanteric bursitis. Coronal fat-suppressed T2-weighted MRI shows trochanteric bursitis following resurfacing arthroplasty.

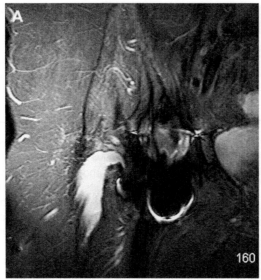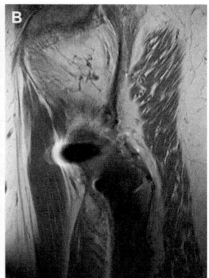

Fig. 8. (A) Coronal fat-suppressed T2-weighted MRI and (B) sagittal T1-weighted MRI show evidence of rupture of the gluteus medius tendon after total hip arthroplasty.

cartilage repair techniques and pharmacologic therapies. Advanced imaging techniques have improved recognition of treatable injuries, hence improving chances for full restoration of joint function.

The hyaline cartilage is an avascular and aneural connective tissue composed mainly of water, chondrocytes, collagen, and proteogylcans. The articular cartilage is divided into four zones: superficial, intermediate, deep, and calcified. The calcified zone attaches to the subchondral bone. The tidemark separates the deep zone from the calcified zone. The composition and organization of the collagen and cells in these zones also make the mechanical properties of the zones different. The superficial zone has the maximum water content and resistance to shear force. The intermediate zone is the thickest with maximum proteoglycans and resistance to compressive force. The deep zone resists compressive force. The calcified zone is the deepest layer and contains collagen X, which is associated with mineralization. Disruption of the normal articular property leads to cartilage degeneration.

Imaging of the cartilage has evolved significantly in recent years. The usefulness of conventional radiographs and CT in the assessment of cartilage is limited. MRI is the standard method for postoperative assessment of success of implantation and cartilage healing as it allows clinicians to assess the repair cartilage morphology, thickness, volume, and subchondral bone. MRI evaluation of cartilage can be performed by using the same accusation technique as used for native cartilage,

as recommended by the International Cartilage Repair Society.[47]

The most commonly used sequences are the intermediate-weighted fast spin echo (FSE) and three-dimensional (3D) fat-suppressed gradient echo sequences. In the FSE sequence, the articular cartilage shows lower signal than fluid, resulting in high contrast between joint fluid and cartilage, and between cartilage and bone marrow. The advantages of FSE are short acquisition time and relative insensitivity to magnetic

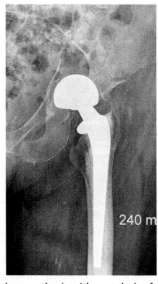

Fig. 9. Bipolar prosthesis with acetabular fracture. The bipolar prosthesis has migrated superomedially.

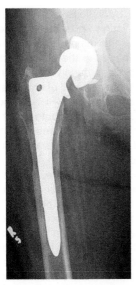

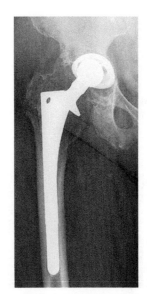

Fig. 10. Acetabular disruption. Anteroposterior radiograph of the right hip shows displacement of the bone ingrowth acetabular component from the bone.

Fig. 12. Liner wear. Anteroposterior radiograph of the right hip demonstrates eccentric position of the femoral head within the acetabular component in keeping with liner wear.

susceptibility artifact. The newer 3D FSE sequence, SPACE (sampling perfection with application-optimized contrast using different flip angle evolution), with isotropic voxels allows multiplanar reformatting in any plane without loss of resolution.[48–50] The 3D gradient-recalled echo (GRE) sequence using fat suppression (3D SPGR) or water excitation (3D fast low-angle shot water excitation [FLASH WE] or 3D dual echo in the steady state water excitation [DESS WE]) provides higher resolutions and contrast-to-noise ratios than two-dimensional acquisition.[50] New 3D isotropic GRE sequences, such as true fast imaging with steady state precision (FISP), volumeninterpolierter 3D-GRE (VIBE), and 2D multiple echo data image combination, seem to be promising in cartilage imaging.[49] Three-dimensional GRE offers the advantages of being easy to

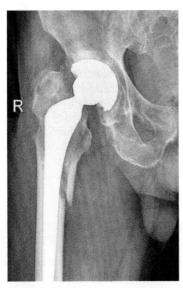

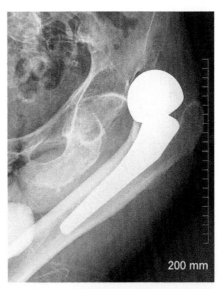

Fig. 11. Anteroposterior radiograph of the right hip shows periprosthetic fracture.

Fig. 13. Dislocation of bipolar prosthesis. Anteroposterior radiograph of the left hip shows superolateral dislocation of the bipolar prosthesis.

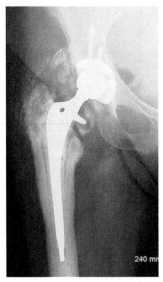

Fig. 14. Anteroposterior radiograph of the right hip shows extensive heterotopic bone formation after total hip arthroplasty.

perform, requiring no postprocessing, and allowing 3D visualization and volume measurements.[49,51–54] Indirect magnetic resonance–arthrography has been used postoperatively to differentiate between delamination of the base of the graft and normal high-signal repair tissue following autologous chondrocyte implants.[54] The biomechanical changes in the cartilage can

be assessed by various tissue parameters. The T1 and T2 relation times and apparent diffusion constants change during cultivation of cartilage, suggesting change in the biomechanical properties of the cartilage during maturation.[55] Delayed gadolinium-enhanced MRI of cartilage (dGEMRIC) techniques and sodium MRI have been used to assess the proteogylcan content within the cartilage. T2 mapping by assessing the collagen content and T1rho imaging have also seen used to evaluate cartilage repair.

In the dGEMRIC technique, double-dose gadolinium is injected. Then, after 10 minutes of exercise and 90 minutes of delay, a T1 map is obtained using specialized inversion recovery spin-echo sequence.[49,56] In T2 mapping, the loss of structural framework of the collagen and loss of tissue isotropy result in increased T2 value. Both sodium MRI and, to a lesser degree, T1rho image the proteoglycan content directly.

MRI of cartilage repair should be performed at a high resolution to detect early surface change.[49] To evaluate the cartilage, a 1.5-T magnet with a high-performance gradient and an extremity coil should be used. A 3-T magnet is more efficient as it can generate images with high resolution and high signal-to-noise ratio.[49] The follow-up MRI should be performed at 3 to 6 months postoperatively to assess the volume and integration of repair tissue and at 1 year to evaluate the maturation of graft and to identify any complication.[49]

The surgical options for cartilage injury used by orthopedic surgeons are microfracture surgery, chodral abrasionoplasty, autologous osteochondral allograft transplantation (mosaicoplasty), autologous chondrocyte implantation, autologous perichondral or periosteal transplantation, and transplantation of bioabsorbable screws.

MRI is a noninvasive technique to assess the cartilage repair by evaluating the surface integrity, contour, cartilage thickness, characteristics of graft substance, and underlying bone. Because of its excellent interobserver reproducibility, magnetic resonance observation of cartilage repair tissue (MOCART) is a widely accepted system for standardization of reports of the imaging features of cartilage repair.[57]

Bone Marrow Stimulation

Microfracture
Microfracture repair is the most commonly performed cartilage repair procedure.[47] The chondral defect is debrided to a stable articular margin. The base of the defect is debrided through the calcified

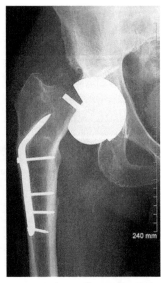

Fig. 15. Anteroposterior radiograph of the right hip shows femoral neck fracture related to resurfacing arthroplasty.

cartilage layer and three to four perforations are made per square centimeter.[58,59]

Chondral abrasion

In chondral abrasion, 1 to 3 mm of subchondral bone is removed beneath the cartilage defect, resulting in formation of a fibrin clot. The pluripotent stem cells migrate to the defect from the marrow, thereby promoting formation of fibrocartilaginous repair tissue.

On MRI, the signal changes can be variable. Early MRI may show bone marrow edema and hyperintense repaired cartilage compared with the native cartilage because the matrix of the repaired cartilage is less organized and water in the repaired cartilage has more mobility. The follow-up MRI shows a progressive decrease in subchondral edema and filling of the defect.[48,60–62] Persistent edema and incomplete filling of the defect with thin repair tissue are considered failure.[48,60–62]

Autologous osteochondral allograft transplantation

In autologous osteochondral allograft transplantation (mosaicoplasty), osteochondral cylinders are harvested from a non–weight-bearing surface and transplanted in an articular defect. This is recommended for chondral lesion between 1.5 to 4.0 cm.[2] It is predominantly used to treat osteochondral lesions in the ankle and knee.[63–65] MRI evaluation should include graft incorporation, cartilage contour, subchondral bone, and the donor site. A well-incorporated plug has uniform fatty signal intensity.[48,66] Bone marrow edema, synovitis, and joint effusion may be seen in the early postoperative period. This shows gradual reduction in the follow-up scan. Presence of persistent bony edema, fluid between the cartilage and bone, incongruity of the articular surface, subchondral cyst and subsidence of the graft suggest poor graft integration. Osteonecrosis of the graft can also be detected on magnetic resonance, but this is an uncommon complication.[48]

Autologous chondrocyte implantation

Autologous chondrocyte implantation was first described in 1990 in Sweden by Dr. Peterson for treatment of full-thickness chondral defect. It consists of two stages. First, the healthy chondrocytes are harvested from the non–weight-bearing surface and cultured for 4 to 5 weeks. In the second stage, the articular cartilage is debrided and implanted with the culture's chondrocytes. This is then covered by a periosteal graft. If successful, a hyalinelike cartilage similar to native cartilage forms. This procedure is used to treat defects of 2 to 12 cm.[2,67]

In the early postoperative period, bony edema and subchondral bone plate irregularity can be seen. The bone marrow edema progressively disappears but can last up to 1 year. In the late phase, the repair cartilage has signal intensity similar to that of native cartilage. Complete edge integration with native cartilage may take up to 2 years. The presence of fluid between the bone and repaired cartilage is suggestive of delamination. This usually occurs during the first 6 months. Subchondral bone cyst formation, worsening surface defects, loose fragments, and underfilling of the defect are signs of graft incongruity. Intra-articular adhesions and synovitis are the less common complications.[48,68–71]

HIGH TIBIAL OSTEOTOMY

High tibial osteotomy has been the accepted method of treatment for osteoarthritis of the knee since 1958 after studies by Jackson and Waugh.[72] It is a surgical procedure to realign a bone to change the biomechanics of a joint by changing the transmission force through the joint.

The surgical indications are relatively young (less than 60 years) active patients with osteoarthritis with varus or valgus deformity. Typical candidates for high tibial osteotomy are patients with medial compartment osteoarthritis (MCOA); patients with medial compartment osteoarthritis and deficiency in the anterior cruciate ligament, the posterior cruciate ligament, or both; patients with painful medial knee and with either meniscal pathology or cartilage defect; and patients with osteochondritis dissecans lesions.[73] Knee replacement is generally offered for patients over 65 years old.[74]

The general consensus is that osteotomy provides best results in mild to moderate unicompartmental osteoarthritis.[75] Patients with bone attrition (more than 1 cm), tibiofemoral subluxation, patellofemoral degenerative disease, patella baja, more than 15° of flexion contracture, and moderate to severe lateral compartment osteoarthritis have shown poor results.[75,76]

Surgical Technique

The goal of osteotomy is to reposition the weight-bearing line so that the load distribution is through the knee, thus minimizing stress to the affected compartment.

Medial open wedge tibial osteotomy

In medial open wedge tibial osteotomy, a wedge osteotomy is performed through the proximal tibia just proximal to the tibial tubercle. The space is filled with bone graft and plate and screws are applied.

Lateral closing wedge osteotomy

With lateral closing wedge osteotomy, the bony varus alignment is corrected by removing a lateral wedge of bone and closing the defect. The degree of correction and the amount of bone to be removed is assessed from the preoperative radiographs. As a result of leg shortening, a fibular shaft osteotomy or fibular head resection is also performed.

Distal femoral osteotomy

A distal femoral osteotomy is performed when there is valgus deformity associated with osteoarthritis. Pins are inserted through the femoral condyles and shaft to create an angle that is required for correction of deformity and 1° to 2° of overcorrection. After osteotomy, the proximal fragment is impacted to the distal one until the pins are parallel. A compression plate is then applied.

Correction with external fixator

A correction with external fixator involves an external ring fixator for high tibial osteotomy with the plane of the osteotomy being distal to the tibial tuberosity.

Preoperative Radiographic Assessment

Knee radiographs are essential for preoperative assessment. Bilateral weight-bearing anteroposterior views in extension, bilateral weight-bearing posteroanterior tunnel views in 30° of flexion, true lateral views with superimposition of the medial and lateral condyles, and skyline views must be obtained.

In addition. the presence of joint effusion, loose bodies, and tibiofemoral subluxation should be documented to assess the degree of osteoarthritis. The patellofemoral joint space and other joint spaces should be evaluated. The following axis and angles should be determined to assess the angle of deformity:

- Mechanical axis of lower extremity. This is the line from the center of the femoral head to the center of the talus. Normally it should pass through the tibial spine.
- Femorotibial angle. This is the angle between the anatomic axes of the femur and tibia. The medial angle subtended at the point at which these two lines meet in the center of the tibial spines is the anatomic angle. A normal femorotibial angle is 182° to 184°.

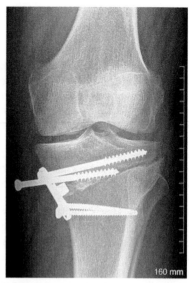

Fig. 16. Hardware failure. Anteroposterior radiograph of the left knee shows retraction of the screw transfixing the high tibial osteotomy.

- Posterior tibial slope angle. This is measured in the lateral view. It is the angle between the line drawn perpendicular to the tangential line of the posterior tibial cortex and the posterior slope of the tibial plateau.

After the preoperative mechanical and anatomic axes are measured, calculation should be made of the angular correction necessary for restoration of a normal mechanical axis with overcorrection of about 3° to 5°.

Various analyses have shown that by 5 years, nearly half of patients who underwent high tibial osteotomy require total knee replacement. Complications from this procedure are infrequent (Fig. 16). Fracture or ischemic necrosis of the proximal tibial fragment may occur, but infection and nonunion are rare. The average healing time for high tibial osteotomy is 9 weeks.[2]

SUMMARY

Various imaging modalities can be used in the assessment of orthopedic patients. Postoperatively, serial plain radiographs remain the modality of choice to evaluate patients with arthroplasty. With proper imaging modification techniques, CT and MRI with their superior resolution and increased sensitivity can evaluate the joint and surrounding osseous and soft tissue structures. CT can assess the subtle fractures and extent of osteolysis better than radiographs. The ability to demonstrate both intraosseous and soft tissue abnormalities has given MRI an edge over other imaging modalities. Ultrasound offers dynamic evaluation and can provide real-time guidance for percutaneous procedures. Injection and aspiration of the joint, along with scintigraphy, are important for the preoperative diagnosis of infection. In recent years, cartilage imaging has become one of the leading areas of research interest. With the development of newer surgical therapies and the improved cartilage imaging techniques, MRI is playing a pivotal role in the evaluation of cartilage abnormalities and postoperative assessment.

REFERENCES

1. Loone RJ, Boyd A, Totterman S, et al. Volumetric computerized tomography as a measurement of periprosthetic acetabular osteolysis and its correlation with wear. Arthritis Res 2002;4(1):59–63.
2. Weissman BN. Orthopedic imaging. In: Resnick D, editor. Diagnosis of bone and joint disorders. 4th edition. Philadelphia: Saunders; 2002. p. 595–644.
3. Tigges S, Stiles RG, Roberson JR. Complications of hip arthroplasty causing periprosthetic radiolucency on plain radiographs. AJR Am J Roentgenol 1994; 162:1387–91.
4. Miller TT. Imaging of hip arthroplasty. Semin Musculoskelel Radiol 2006;10:30–46.
5. Weissman BN. Imaging of total hip replacement. Radiology 1997;202:611–23.
6. Weissman BN, Sledge CB. The hip. Orthopedic radiology. Philadelphia: WB Saunders Co; 1991. p. 385–495.
7. Rosenthall L. Radionuclide investigation of osteomyelitis. Curr Opin Radiol 1992;4:62–9.
8. Kirchner PT, Simon MA. Radioisotopic evaluation of skeletal disease. J Bone Joint Surg Am 1981;63: 673–81.
9. Sofka CM. Optimizing techniques for musculoskeletal imaging of the postoperative patient. Radiol Clin North Am 2006;44:323–9.
10. White LM, Miller M, Schweitzer M. In: White LM, Miller M, Schweitzer M, editors. Imaging of joint replacement. Diagnostic musculoskeletal imaging. New York: McGraw Hill; 2004. p. 417–32.
11. Cahir JG, Toms AP, Marshall TJ, et al. Diagnostic musculoskeletal radiology. Clin Radiol 2007;62(12): 1163–71.
12. White LM, Kim JK, Mehta M, et al. Complications of total hip arthroplasty: MR imaging, initial experience. Radiology 2000;215:254–62.
13. Buckwalter KA, Parr JA, Choplin RH, et al. Multichannel CT imaging of orthopedic hardware and implants. Semin Musculoskelet Radiol 2006;10: 86–97.

14. Naraghi AM, White LM. Magnetic resonance imaging of joint replacements. Semin Musculoskelet Radiol 2006;10:98–106.
15. Jacobson JA. Hip replacement. Available at: e-medicine. Accessed May 1, 2008.
16. Ahlback S. Osteoarthrosis of the knee. A radiographic investigation. Acta Radiol Diagn 1968; 277(Suppl):7–72.
17. Amin AK, Patton JT, Cook RE, et al. Unicompartmental or total knee arthroplasty: results from a matched study. Clin Orthop Relat Res 2006;451:101–6.
18. White S, Ludkowski PF, Goodfellow J. J Bone Joint Surg.Br 1991;73:582–6.
19. Savard UC, Price AJ. Oxford medial unicompartmental knee arthroplasty. A survival analysis of an independent series. J Bone Joint Surg.Br 2001;83: 191–4.
20. Berger RA, Nedeff DD, Barden RM, et al. Unicompartmental knee arthroplasty. Clinical experience at 6- to 10-year follow-up. Clin Orthop 1999; 367:50–60.
21. Feiock DA, Newman JS, Newberg AH, et al. Radiological evaluation of total knee arthroplasty. In: Bono J, Scott RD, editors. Revision total knee arthroplasty. New York: Springer; 2005. p. 36–52.
22. Duus BR, Boeckstyns M, Kjaer L, et al. Radionuclide scanning after total knee replacement: correlation with pain and radiolucent lines, a prospective study. Invest Radiol 1987;22:891–904.
23. Kantor SG, Schneider R, Insall JN, et al. Radionuclide imaging of asymptomatic versus symptomatic total knee arthroplasties. Clin Orthop Relat Res 1990;260:118–23.
24. Schneider R, Soudry M. Radiographic and scintigraphic evaluation of total knee arthroplasty. Clin Orthop 1986;205:108–20.
25. Brick GW, Scott RD. The patellofemoral component of knee arthroplasty. Clin Orthop 1988;231: 163–78.
26. Schneider R, Hood RW, Ranawat CS. Radiological evaluation of knee arthroplasty. Orthop Clin North Am 1982;13:225–44.
27. Hanssen AD, Rand JA. Evaluation and treatment of infection at the site of a total hip or knee arthroplasty. J Bone Joint Surg Am 1998;80:1127–39.
28. Love C, Tomas MB, Marwin SE, et al. Role of nuclear medicine in diagnosis of the infected joint replacement. Radiographics 2001;21:1229–38.
29. Herrlin K. Space orientation of total hip prosthesis. Acta Radiol 1986;27:619–27.
30. McLaren RH. Prosthetic hip angulation. Radiology 1973;107:705–6.
31. Fackler CD, Poss R. Dislocation in total hip arthoplasties. Clin Orthop 1980;151:169–78.
32. Ghelman B. Radiographic localization of the acetabular component of a hip prosthesis. Radiology 1979; 130:540–2.

33. Mian SW, Truchly G, Pflum FA, et al. Computed tomography measurement of acetabular cup anteversion and retroversion in total hip arthroplasty. Clin Orthop 1992;276:206–9.

34. Kitamura N, Pappedemos PC, Duffy PR 3rd, et al. The value of anteroposterior pelvic radiographs for evaluating pelvic osteolysis. Clin Orthop Relat Res 2006;453:239–45.

35. Van Holsbeeck MT, Eyler WR, Sherman LS, et al. Detection of infection in loosened hip prostheses: efficacy of sonography. AJR Am J Roentgenol 1994;163:381–4.

36. Foldis K, Balint P, Gaal M, et al. Ultrasonography after hip atrhroplasty. Skeletal Radiol 1992; 21:297–9.

37. Graif M, Schwartz E, Strauss S. Occult infarction of hip prothesis: sonographic evaluation. J Am Geriatr Soc 1991;39:203–4.

38. Huo MH, Gilbert NF, Parvizi J. What's new in total hip arthroplasty. J Bone Joint Surg Am 2007;89: 1874–85.

39. Tigges S, Stiles RG, Roberson JR. Appearance of septic hip prostheses on plain radiographs. AJR Am J Roentgenol 1994;163:377–80.

40. Claus AM, Totterman SM, Synchterz CJ, et al. Computed tomography to assess pelvis lysis after total hip replacement. Clin Orthop 2004;422:167–74.

41. Mueller PR, Stark DD, Simeone JF, et al. MR-guided aspiration biopsy: needle design and clinical trials. Radiology 1986;161:605–9.

42. Shimmin A, Beaulé PE, Campbell P. Metal-on-metal hip resurfacing arthroplasty. J Bone Joint Surg Am 2008;90:637–54.

43. Wank R, Miller TT, Shapiro JF. Sonographically guided injection of anesthetic for iliopsoas tendinopathy after total hip arthroplasty. J Clin Ultrasound 2004;32:354–7.

44. Amstutz HC, Beaulé PE, Dorey FJ, et al. Metal-on-metal hybrid surface arthroplasty: two to six-year follow-up study. J Bone Joint Surg Am 2004;86: 28–39.

45. Pollard TC, Baker RP, Eastaugh-Waring SJ, et al. Treatment of the young active patient with osteoarthritis of the hip. A five- to seven-year comparison of hybrid total hip arthroplasty and metal-on-metal resurfacing. J Bone Joint Surg Br 2006;88: 592–600.

46. Hing CB, Young DA, Dalziel RE, et al. Narrowing of the neck in resurfacing arthroplasty of the hip: a radiological study. J Bone Joint Surg Br 2007;89: 1019–24.

47. Bobic V. ICRS articular cartilage imaging committee. ICRS MR imaging protocol for knee articular cartilage; 2000. p. 12.

48. Choi YS, Potter HG, Chun TJ. MR imaging of cartilage repair in the knee and ankle. Radiographics 2008;28:1043–59.

49. Potter HG, Chong le R. Magnetic resonance imaging assessment of chondral lesions and repair. J Bone Joint Surg Am 2009;91(Suppl 1):126–31.

50. Recht M, Bobic V, Burstein D, et al. Magnetic resonance imaging of articular cartilage. Clin Orthop Relat Res 2001;(Suppl 391):S379–96.

51. Peterfy CG, van Dijke CF, Lu Y, et al. Quantification of the volume of articular cartilage in the metacarpophalangeal joints of the hand: accuracy and precision of three-dimensional MR imaging. AJR Am J Roentgenol 1995;165:371–5.

52. Kawahara Y, Uetani M, Nakahara N, et al. Fast spin-echo MR of the articular cartilage in the osteoarthritic knee. Correlation of MR and arthroscopic findings. Acta Radiol 1998;39:120–5.

53. Peterfy CG, Majumdar S, Lang P, et al. MR imaging of the arthritic knee: improved discrimination of cartilage, synovium, and effusion with pulsed saturation transfer and fat-suppressed T1-weighted sequences. Radiology 1994;191:413–9.

54. Trattnig S, Huber M, Breitenseher MJ, et al. Imaging articular cartilage defects with 3D fat-suppressed echo planar imaging: comparison with conventional 3D fat-suppressed gradient echo sequence and correlation with histology. J Comput Assist Tomogr 1998;22:8–14.

55. Yao L, Gentili A, Thomas A. Incidental magnetization transfer contrast in fast spin-echo imaging of cartilage. J Magn Reson Imaging 1996;6:180–4.

56. Gillis A, Bashir A, McKeon B, et al. Magnetic resonance imaging of relative glycosaminoglycan distribution in patients with autologous chondrocyte transplants. Invest Radiol 2001;36:743–8.

57. Marlovits S, Singer P, Zeller P, et al. Magnetic resonance observation of cartilage repair tissue (MOCART) for the evaluation of autologous chondrocyte transplantation: determination of interobserver variability and correlation to clinical outcome after 2 years. Eur J Radiol 2006;57:16–23.

58. Bert JM. Abrasion arthroplasty. Op Tech Orthop 2001;11:90–5.

59. Mithoefer K, Williams RJ 3rd, Warren RF, et al. The microfracture technique for the treatment of articular cartilage lesions in the knee: a prospective cohort study. J Bone Joint Surg Am 2005;87: 1911–20.

60. Alparslan L, Winalski CS, Boutin RD, et al. Postoperative magnetic resonance imaging of articular cartilage repair. Semin Musculoskelet Radiol 2001;5: 345–63.

61. Fuchsjager MH, Mlynarik V, Marlovits S, et al. High field MR imaging in reconstituted articular cartilage: evaluation of cartilage maturation for determination of optimal transplantation time. Radiology 2004; 233:442–8.

62. Potter HG, Linklater JM, Allen AA, et al. Magnetic resonance imaging of articular cartilage in the

knee. An evaluation with use of fast-spin-echo imaging. J Bone Joint Surg Am 1998;80:1276–84.

63. Takahashi T, Tins B, McCall IW, et al. MR appearance of autologous chondrocyte implantation in the knee: correlation with the knee features and clinical outcome. Skeletal Radiol 2006;35:16–26.

64. Trattnig S, Millington SA, Szomolanyi P, et al. MR imaging of osteochondral grafts and autologous chondrocyte implantation. Eur Radiol 2007;17: 103–18.

65. Potter HG, Foo LF. Magnetic resonance imaging of articular cartilage: trauma, degeneration, and repair. Am J Sports Med 2006;34:661–77.

66. Link TM, Mishung J, Wortler K, et al. Normal and pathological MR findings in osteochondral autografts with longitudinal follow-up. Eur Radiol 2006; 16:88–96.

67. Brittberg M, Peterson L, Sjogren-Jansson E, et al. Articular cartilage engineering with autologous chondrocyte transplantation: a review of recent developments. J Bone Joint Surg Am 2003; 85(Suppl 3):109–15.

68. Peterson L, Minas T, Brittberg M, et al. Two- to 9-year outcome after autologous chondrocyte transplantation of the knee. Clin Orthop Relat Res 2000;374:212–34.

69. Peterson L, Minas T, Brittberg M, et al. Treatment of osteochondritis dissecans of the knee with autologous chondrocyte transplantation: results at two to ten years. J Bone Joint Surg Am 2003;85(Suppl 2):17–24.

70. Henderson I, Gui J, Lavigne P. Autologous chondrocyte implantation: natural history of postimplantation periosteal hypertrophy and effects of repair-site debridement on outcome. Arthroscopy 2006;22: 1318–24.

71. Alparslan L, Minas T, Winalski CS. Magnetic resonance imaging of autologous chondrocyte implantation. Semin Ultrasound CT MR 2001;22: 341–51.

72. Amendola A, Panarella L. High tibial osteotomy for the treatment of unicompartmental arthritis of the knee orthop. Clin N Am 2005;36:497–504.

73. Hernigou P, Medevielle D, Debeyre J, et al. Proxima tibial osteotomy for osteoarthritis with varus deformity: a ten to thirteen-year follow-up study. J Bone Joint Surg Am 1987;69:332–54.

74. Magyar G, Ahl TL, Vibe P, et al. Open-wedge osteotomy by hemicallotasis or the closed-wedge technique for osteoarthritis of the knee: a randomised study of 50 operations. J Bone Joint Surg Br 1999; 81:444–8.

75. Dugdale TW, Noyes FR, Styer D. Preoperative planning for high tibial osteotomy: the effect of lateral tibiofemoral separation and tibiofemoral length. Clin Orthop 1992;274:248–64.

76. Ogata K, Yoshii I, Kawamura H, et al. Standing radiographs cannot determine the correction in high tibial osteotomy. J Bone Joint Surg Br 1991; 73:927–31.

Index

Radiol Clin N Am 47 (2009) 777–782
doi:10.1016/S0033-8389(09)00108-0

Moving?

Make sure your subscription moves with you!

To notify us of your new address, find your **Clinics Account Number** (located on your mailing label above your name), and contact customer service at:

E-mail: elspcs@elsevier.com

800-654-2452 (subscribers in the U.S. & Canada)
314-453-7041 (subscribers outside of the U.S. & Canada)

Fax number: 314-523-5170

Elsevier Periodicals Customer Service
11830 Westline Industrial Drive
St. Louis, MO 63146

*To ensure uninterrupted delivery of your subscription, please notify us at least 4 weeks in advance of move.

ELSEVIER

Printed and bound by CPI Group (UK) Ltd, Croydon, CR0 4YY

03/10/2024

01040361-0005